INFANT AND CHILD NUTRITION WORLDWIDE:
Issues and Perspectives

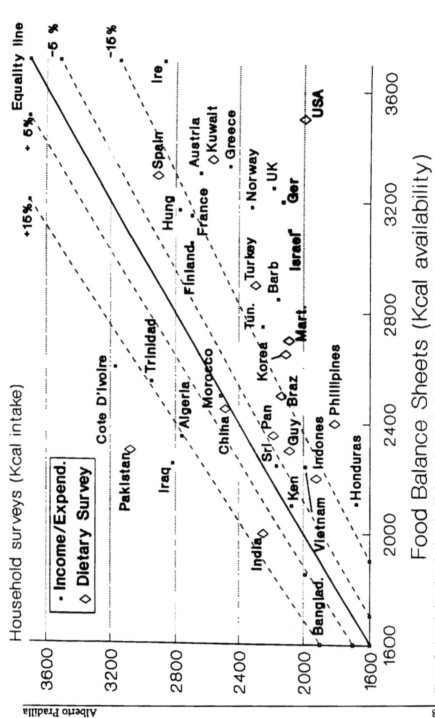

Figure 2. Association of results from food balance sheets indicating energy availability, with dietary and income expenditure surveys.

INFANT AND CHILD NUTRITION WORLDWIDE:
Issues and Perspectives

Edited By

Frank Falkner

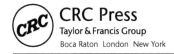

CRC Press
Taylor & Francis Group
Boca Raton London New York

CRC Press is an imprint of the
Taylor & Francis Group, an **informa** business

Published 1991 by CRC Press
Taylor & Francis Group
6000 Broken Sound Parkway NW, Suite 300
Boca Raton, FL 33487-2742

First issued in paperback 2019

No claim to original U.S. Government works

ISBN 13: 978-0-367-45048-9 (pbk)
ISBN 13: 978-0-8493-8814-9 (hbk)

Visit the Taylor & Francis Web site at
http://www.taylorandfrancis.com

and the CRC Press Web site at
http://www.crcpress.com

Library of Congress Cataloging-in-Publication Data

Infant and child nutrition / edited by Frank Falkner.
    p. cm.
    Includes bibliographical references.
    Includes index.
    ISBN 0-8493-8814-7
    1. Infants--Nutrition. 2. Breast feeding. 3. Infant formulas--
Health aspects. 4. Children--Nutrition. 5. Children--Nutrition--
Social aspects.   I. Falkner, Frank, 1918-
    [DNLM: 1. Breast Feeding. 2. Child Nutrition. 3. Infant Food.
4. Infant Nutrition.   WS 115 I43]
RJ216.I493   1991
649'.33--dc20
DNLM/DLC
for Library of Congress   90-11288
                              CIP

Library of Congress Card Number 90-11288

Contents

Preface   vii
Foreword   ix
Contributors   xiii

1   Breast Feeding Practices During
    Industrialisation 1800-1919
Valerie Fildes   1

2   The Geographic Distribution of Malnutrition
Alberto Pradilla   21

3   Maternal Undernutrition and Reproductive
    Performance
Barbara Abrams   31

4   Breast-feeding: An International and
    Historical Review
Joe D. Wray   61

5   Science and Lactation
Frank Hytten   117

6   Contemporary Feeding Practices in Infancy
    and Early Childhood in Developing
    Countries
Jean King and Ann Ashworth   141

7   Social and Psychological Factors in
    Breast-feeding
Manuel Carballo and Gretel H. Pelto   175

8 Weaning: Why, When and What?
Angel Ballabriga   191

9 Development in Infant Nutrition
L.J. Filer, Jr.   231

10 The Infant Food Industry as a Partner in
   Health
Fred T. Sai   245

11 Direct Intervention Programmes to Improve
   Infant and Child Nutrition
Mahshid Lotfi and John B. Mason   263

Preface

Few would disagree that infant and child nutrition throughout the world is a subject of great importance. Mild to severe malnutrition in this age group can lead not only to increased young morbidity and mortality, it has at last been realized that prevention in childhood of adult health problems is a key to improvement of a population's health.

The International Association of Infant Food Manufacturers (IFM), which includes in its objectives the dissemination of knowledge on infant and young child nutrition, proposed publication of a book containing current thinking on the subject. The Editor was to, and did, have sole choice of contributors, complete freedom in editorship and stood alone in the important relationship involved between contributors and editor. No contributor was to be from, nor associated with, any member of IFM.

It is commonplace that worldwide infant and child nutrition has a vast multifactorial background. At one end of the scale, government policy and agriculture; at the other end, maternal-fetal protein transport. It was therefore decided that this book's title would be appropriate for the subject at hand; particularly the secondary title of "Issues and Perspectives." The hoped-for goal has been to highlight some areas that need to be addressed. One example: Not only does child health precede and influence adult health, so too does fetal health precede infant and child health.

The incidence of the infant-of-low-birth-weight (ILB) in the developing world is twenty-fold higher than the developed world. As important, of the developing world's ILB, 75 to 80% are infants who have suffered from intra-uterine growth retardation (IGR), as opposed to being born too soon and hence small. This incidence is fourfold over the developed world. If it is accepted that the major causes of IGR are nutrition-infection, the condition is reversible.

This publication was conceived while I took sabbatical leave in the Family Health Division of WHO, Geneva. I am most grateful for the help and graciousness I received there, as well as to the University of California Berkeley for the granting of this leave. I owe untold thanks to the contributors, whose book this is, for the birth and for their labour(s). Our publisher was a model of patience and expertise.

Finally, my gratitude to James P. Grant, Executive Director of UNICEF, for agreeing to write the Foreword.

Frank Falkner
Berkeley, California

Foreword

There is no more important topic in development than the quality of life of children, because development is about the future, and children are the future - for every country and for the world. The first year of the last decade of the century is a good time to reflect on this theme. Near the start of the year the Governor of New York State recommitted himself to making this the Decade of the Child, proposing in his State of the State message an innovative community-based but state-supported programme. Towards the end of the year Heads of State or Government will gather at the United Nations in New York for an unprecedented World Summit - and the subject will be children. The purpose of the Summit - in the words of the Secretary General - is "to bring attention and promote commitment, at the highest political level, to goals and strategies for ensuring the survival, protection and development of children as key elements in the socio-economic development of human society."

This book could hardly be more timely. Its subject, infant and child nutrition, is central to the Summit's theme. Not only is good nutrition essential for the survival, protection and development of children, but the nutritional status of children, as reflected in their growth, is widely accepted as an "indicator with a human face" of socio-economic development. Thus nutrition can be seen as both a means and a measure.

If the foundation of good nutrition of the child is grounded in the nutrition of the mother, from the moment of birth it is ensured by the natural process of breast-feeding. Recent years have witnessed a much greater understanding of the intricacies and manifold benefits of this biological system, as well as attempts, which sometimes border on the brazen or bizarre, to provide alternatives. There is no doubt that this is a worldwide issue, with universal relevances, as my colleague Dr. Hiroshi Nakajima, Director-General of the World Health Organization, and I stressed in our Foreword to the 1989 joint statement by our two agencies on the special role of maternity services in protecting, promoting and supporting breast-feeding. We said that the principles affirmed in the statement "apply everywhere maternity services are offered, irrespective of such labels as 'developed' and 'developing', 'North' and 'South', 'modern' and 'traditional'"; and we spoke of the need "to sustain, or if necessary re-establish, a 'breast-feeding culture'."

The first two years of life are the most critical for the development of the child, for it is during this period that the pattern of its growth is established. Thus, the only way to reduce the prevalence of stunting is to take preventive action, ideally monitoring growth from birth, creating an environment of services and support such that mothers are enabled to breast-feed their children exclusively for the first four to six months of life, and ensuring that complementary foods in addition to breast milk are provided thereafter. Such foods need to be of appropriate quality and provided in appropriate quantity and at appropriate frequency. Growth and activity are dependent on the intake of nutrients from the diet (and perhaps from nutritional supplements), but are also influenced by exposure to infection, which affects intake and the utiliza-tion of nutrients by the body. Therefore each household or family must be able to enjoy food security, meaning insurance of foods to meet the needs of all its numbers throughout each season of the year, and also health security, meaning access to appropriate health services, in a healthy environment. But in addi-tion a third component is essential, which may be termed caring capacity, encompassing knowledge and understanding of the mother - and other mem-bers of the family - about the dietary, health, and social, psychological and cognitive needs of the infant or young child, coupled with the ability to provide child care. These characteristics are much influenced by attributes such as literacy, education, independent source of income, and - notably - sufficient time. And although these three components of Food, Health and Care are such necessary, in a sense the greatest of them is Care, for whatever foods and health services may be available they are unlikely to benefit the child below two years of age if care and developmentally sensitive interaction are lacking, while if care and commitment to the child are abundant then, even if food and health security are marginal, resources can more readily be mobilized in favor of the child. Moreover, developmentally sensitive interac-tion - interaction that includes early stimulation and satisfies a child's need to grow socially, psychologically and cognitively - has a direct and im-measurable impact on the health and nutritional status of the young child. Effective and sustainable programmes to improve the nutritional status of infants and young children must address simultaneously, therefore, all three needs: for food security, health security, and developmentally sensitive care.

This book makes an important, broadly balanced, contribution to under-standing and awareness of its subject. Not all will agree with all the judgments and points-of-view expressed. The subject is dynamic, and the present is a time of great activity, with new knowledge and fresh analyses deepening understanding - no collection of essays can claim to be fully comprehensive and completely up-to-date. Yet the material in this book provides much food for thought, and I hope it will be widely read.

James P. Grant
Executive Director, UNICEF
New York, March 1990

Contributors

Barbara Abrams
Public Health Nutrition Program
School of Public Health
University of California
Berkeley California 94720

Ann Ashworth
Centre for Human Nutrition
London School of Hygiene &
Tropical Medicine
London, England

Angel Ballabriga
Childrens Hospital
Vall d'Hebyon
Autonomous University
Barcelona, Spain

Manuel Carballo
Social & Behavioral Research
Global Programme on AIDS
W.H.O.
Geneva, Switzerland

Frank Falkner
Emeritus
Maternal and Child Health
Program
Department of Pediatrics
University of California
Berkeley. San Francisco
Berkeley, California 94720

Valerie Fildes
ESRC Cambridge Group for the
History of Population & Social
Structure
Cambridge, England

L.J. Filer, Jr.
Department Of Pediatrics
University of Iowa
College Of Medicine
Iowa City, Iowa 52242

Frank Hytten
Emeritus
Division of Perinatal Medicine
Clinical Research Centre
Harrow, England

Mahshid Lotfi
The United Nations
Administrative Committee on
Coordination
Sub-Committee on Nutrition
Geneva, Switzerland

Jean King
Agricultural and Food Research
160 Great Portland Street
London, England

John B. Mason
The United Nations
Administrative Committee on
Coordination
Sub-Committee on Nutrition
Geneva, Switzerland

Gretel H. Pelto
Department of Nutritional Science
University of Connecticut
3624 Horse Barn Road
Storrs, Connecticut 06269

Alberto Pradilla
Nutrition Programme
Family Health Division
W.H.O.
Geneva, Switzerland

Fred T. Sai
The World Bank
1818 H Street NW
Room S6065
Washington, DC 20433

Joe D. Wray
Center for Population and Family
Health
Columbia University
60 Hazen Avenue
New York, New York 10032

1

Breast-Feeding Practices During Industrialisation 1800-1919[1]

Valerie Fildes

ESRC Cambridge Group for the History of Population & Social Structure
Cambridge, England

1   Research for this chapter was supported by a grant from the Nestlé Nutrition Company
Ltd.

In pre-industrial European and colonial society, infant feeding practices remained relatively unchanged for many centuries. In most regions virtually all children were breast-fed, either by their mother or by a wet nurse (Fildes, 1986). Wealthy mothers who did not wish to breast-feed paid a married woman of lower social status to suckle their infants, either in the family home or, more usually, in the nurse's home. Abandoned children, bastards and orphans were also wet nursed, by the poor married women employed by foundling hospitals and municipal and parish authorities. A proportion of these disadvantaged infants, however, were artificially fed, either due to a shortage of wet nurses or because the authorities attempted to save money by employing dry nurses instead (Fildes, 1986; Fildes, 1988). Artificial feeding was universally accepted to be dangerous to life and, apart from these instances, was normally only employed in cases of necessity, such as where prematurity or congenital deformities made suckling impossible, or when a wet nurse could not be employed because the infant had syphilis (Fildes, 1986). There were also some clearly-defined regions in northern Europe where, by tradition, children were rarely or never breast-fed although the original reasons for this were lost in time. In addition, some infants were artificially fed when certain socially-privileged groups fleetingly experimented with feeding methods, but the vast majority of infants were not affected by these (Fildes, 1986). The duration of breast-feeding varied from 9-12 months in some areas to 2-3 years in others but most children were suckled, usually on demand, for at a year (Fildes, 1986; Fildes, 1988; Liestøl et al., 1988; Lithell, 1981; Rollet, 1981). This chapter will discuss how these breast-feeding practices were affected by industrialisation.

The industrial revolution began in England in the mid-18th century (Briggs, 1983). During the 19th century, although beginning at different times in different regions, many parts of Europe, North America and Australasia became increasingly mechanised and urbanised and, by the end of the first world war, a majority of the people in these continents were living in an industrialised society. The immense changes in lifestyle which occurred during this transition had a significant influence on infant feeding practices. Although some regions retained traditional habits until the mid-20th century, by the 1920s the feeding of most children was radically different from that of babies born a hundred years earlier (Apple, 1987; Cone, 1976; Fildes, 1988; Golden, 1984; Lewis, 1980; Kintner, 1985; Sussman, 1982; Van Eekelen, 1984).

Industrialisation involved large numbers of people moving away from their traditional communities to towns and cities and, in place of homebased work, both men and women working for long hours away from the home (Pinchbeck, 1981; Tilly & Scott, 1978). The explosion of the urban population resulted in public health problems, in particular those relating to overcrowding, poor sanitation, and the water and milk supply. Efforts to solve these led to the establishment of the specialty of public health, and the idea of preventing morbidity and mortality, including that of young children (Smith, 1979; Wohl, 1983).

Increasingly better demographic records were kept, particularly national registration of births and deaths and regular censuses (Wrigley & Schofield, 1981), which in some countries included details of infant feeding (Kintner, 1985). These, with the accompanying interest in epidemiology, meant that accurate figures relating to women's work, marital fertility and infant mortality became available for the first time. It was during industrialisation that the infant mortality rate became an index to the health and success of societies adapting to change (Garrison, 1965; Wohl, 1983).

Developments in education meant that more and more people, especially women, were able to read, and books, magazines and newspapers became universally available (Briggs, 1983), including those on infant care. Related to this was the mass-advertising of manufactured products, including infant feeding equipment and foods. In turn, consumer demand led to more experimentation by manufacturers, in conjunction with doctors and scientists, to produce new products and thus increase profits (Apple, 1987; Fildes, 1988; Van Eekelen, 1984).

Improvements in medicine led to many large hospitals being set up in towns and cities. In particular, the widespread provision of lying-in and children's hospitals made available populations of women and children for recording and experimenting with infant feeding methods (Budin, 1907; Fildes, 1988; Liestøl, 1988; Routh, 1860). Developments in science and medicine led to greater knowledge of nutrition and the causes of disease, and especially to solving the problem of supplying food and drink to large urban populations, particularly children, which was both nutritious and uncontaminated (Drummond & Wilbraham, 1957; Smith, 1979).

It is in the context of these great changes that the developments in infant feeding must be viewed. The most notable of these during the 19th century was the increasing difference between practices in rural and urban areas. While rural women largely continued to breast-feed as their mothers had done, and for a similar length of time, those who moved to the new manufacturing towns were more likely to supplement their breast milk with other foods early on, or to handfeed (Fildes, 1988; Rollet, 1981; Woodbury, 1962). However, it depended greatly upon the type of work in which the woman was employed; how close she lived to her place of work; whether a crèche was available; whether she had relatives nearby who could help with child care; and whether there was a tradition either of sending infants to be nursed in the country, or of employing caretakers during the day (Drake, 1908; Garrison, 1965; Fildes, 1988; Lithell, 1981; Tilly & Scott, 1978).

In the textile towns of Northern England women worked in the mills until shortly before childbirth and went back to work within a few days of delivery. The hours were long and in many places it was common to use very young girls or old women to care for infants during the day (Hewitt, 1958; Pinchbeck, 1981). Although some women breast-fed their babies in the morning and evening, they were fed with a variety of other foods during the day and frequently were also dosed with opiates which made suckling difficult in the evening (Fildes, 1988). In the 1890s and 1900s when vital statistics on feeding began to be compiled, the incidence of maternal breast-feeding (0-3 months) in some of these areas was as low as 50% (Jones, 1894; Newman, 1906). Although reliable figures for the earlier period are not available, observations by medical and lay writers suggest that these mothers often did not breast-feed at all, or supplemented with other foods from soon after birth, and that the duration of suckling was short. These towns had some of the highest infant mortality rates in the country and this was attributed principally to mothers not breast-feeding because they worked in the mills (Fildes, 1988; Garrison, 1965; Hewitt, 1958, Newman, 1906). Evidence which backed up these assertions was the dramatic fall in infant mortality during the Manchester Cotton Famine in the early 1860s. Because of the fall in raw cotton supplies due to the American Civil War, work in the mills was greatly reduced, women were forced to stay at home and were able to suckle their babies. When production resumed after the war, women went back to work, were no longer able to breast-feed and the infant mortality rate immediately rose again (Newman, 1906). This phenomenon was noted repeatedly by contemporaries. Where there was high infant mortality due to low breast-feeding rates, any social disruption which enabled urban mothers to remain at home and suckle their babies led to an immediate reduction in infant mortality even though child and adult mortality might increase (Garrison, 1965; Jones, 1894; Newman, 1906; Vincent, 1904).

There seems to have been considerable variation in the incidence of breast-feeding in different towns (see Table I) and also between different districts within towns (Drake, 1908; Newman, 1906; Thompson, 1984; Vincent, 1904; Woods et al., 1989). Figures from the later period show that these

Table I: Mode of feeding in the first three months of life: British towns 1894 - 1918 (data relating to all infants)					
Region	Town	Date	Breast milk only %	Other foods only %	Breast milk + other foods %
North	Liverpool	1894	50.0	30.0	20.0
	Salford	1907	85.2	9.7	5.4
		1908-10	85.1	7.4	7.4
	York	1911	77.5	14.6	7.8
	Middlesbrough	1909	97.9	1.2	0.9
		1914	92.9	4.2	2.9
		1915	98.0	-	-
Midlands	Derby	1900-03	63.3	19.5	17.2
	Birmingham	1916	87.0	-	-
S. Wales	Rhondda	1910	68.5	19.5	12.1
		1911	75.1	21.7	3.2
London	St. Pancras	1904	70.0	18.0	12.0
	Paddington	1904	77.0	12.0	11.0
	Finsbury	1905	82.5	7.8	9.7
	Hackney	1911-14	83.1	8.6	8.3
		1917-18	82.1	9.8	8.1
South	Brighton	1903-05	84.4	6.9	8.7
Median:			83.1	9.8	8.3
Range:			50.0-98.0	1.2-30.0	0.9-20.0

Sources: *Borough of Hackney*, 1911-18; Buchanan, 1985; Howarth, 1905; Jones, 1894; Local Government Board, 1913; Middlesbrough, 1903-18; Newman, 1906; Newsholme, 1906; Ross, 1986; Vincent, 1904.

were primarily related to the type of work in which women were employed. In some places it was feasible for mothers to at least partially breast-feed their children because they lived close to their place of work and were able to leave their infants sufficiently close by (often with a relative) to breast-feed in the middle of the day in addition to before and after work (Drake, 1908; Newman, 1906; Vincent, 1904). Provision of crèches by employers and municipal authorities was not common in Britain but in France, Austria, Italy and several other parts of Europe these were established from the 1840s onwards and enabled women to breast-feed if they wished to during breaks in their work (Garrison, 1965).

Table II: Mode of feeding in the first six months of life in the United States 1917 - 1919										
Type	Place	1 month or less			3 months			6 months		
		Breast milk only %	Other foods only %	Mixed %	Breast milk only %	Other foods only %	Mixed %	Breast milk only %	Other foods only %	Mixed %
	North-east									
Urban	Manchester, New Hampshire	82	15	3	61	33	6	36	47	17
Urban	New Bedford, Massachusetts	83	12	5	66	25	9	45	37	18
	Mid-west									
Urban	Saginaw, Michigan	88	9	3	75	16	9	54	24	22
Urban	Akron, Ohio	88	8	4	73	19	8	55	27	18
Rural	Kansas	92	2	6	83	6	11	61	13	26
Rural	S. Wisconsin	92	6	2	82	11	7	51	16	33
Rural	N. Wisconsin	89	6	5	76	9	15	49	16	35

Source: Apple, 1987.

Table III: Mode of infant feeding in Berlin 1885-1910						
Food received at time of the census	1885 %	1890 %	1895 %	1900 %	1905 %	1910 %
Breast milk	55.2	50.7	43.1	31.4	31.2	30.5
Wet nurses' milk	2.7	2.2	1.4	0.7	0.6	0.4
Mixed	6.7	4.8	9.9	14.4	4.2	3.7
Animal milk	33.9	42.3	45.3	49.7	63.7	62.6
Unknown	1.5	0.0	0.2	3.8	0.3	2.8
Percentage ever breastfed	78.9	79.5	72.3	67.3	65.6	71.8
Median duration (months)	8.6	7.4	4.6	2.2	1.9	2.1

Source: Kintner, 1985.

Although for most of this period there is little reliable data to support their view, the opinion of medical and lay observers was that the proportion of mothers who breast-fed declined steadily during the 19th century, particularly from the 1870s onwards when artificial feeding became a more viable alternative (Forsyth, 1911; Hope, 1899; Jones, 1894; Newman, 1906). From the 1890s infant feeding data, collected principally by medical officers of health, health visitors and infant welfare clinics, showed that in many urban areas over 80% of mothers did breast-feed, wholly or partially, especially during the first three months, although in certain towns, such as parts of Liverpool, Manchester and Birmingham, 40-50% of infants surveyed were completely weaned onto other foods by the age of six months (Jones, 1894; Newman, 1906; Vincent, 1904; Woods *et al.*, 1989). In less industrial towns, such as Brighton, only 30% of children aged 6-12 months were totally fed on foods other than breast milk (Newsholme, 1906). In rural areas almost all mothers were reported to breast-feed during the first three months and the majority of infants were still partly breast-fed at 9-12 months (Newman, 1906; Vincent, 1904).

Surveys in the United States showed a similar picture (See Table II). In Manchester, New Hampshire, where a high percentage of mothers worked in textile mills, 82% initiated breast-feeding but 47% had completely weaned their infants by 6 months (Apple, 1987; Garrison, 1965). In other urban areas 88% of mothers initiated breast-feeding and threequarters of their infants were still wholly or partially breast-fed at 6 months. In rural areas over 90% of mothers initiated breast-feeding and most were still suckling at 6 months (Apple, 1987; Woodbury, 1926).

In Germany, where details about infant feeding were included in the census, there was a decline in both the incidence and duration of breast-feeding in urban areas (Kintner, 1985). In Berlin between 1885 and 1910 there was a 27% decline in the infants receiving breast milk at the time of the census, and the median duration of suckling fell from 8.58 months to 2.11 months (See Table III).

In France, an increasing proportion of the thousands of children put out to country nurses was not breast-fed. In 1898, in 23 departments only 0-25% of nurslings were breast-fed (Sussman, 1982; see Figure 1). In some industrial areas of Northern France in 1907-10 less than 40% of infants were breast-fed at the time of death compared to over 60% throughout the rural south. The figure for the whole country was 55% (Rollet, 1981).

Apart from the urban-rural differences in suckling practices a consistent observation was the importance of traditional infant feeding customs in families who migrated to foreign cities. Where breast-feeding was the norm in their home country, immigrant mothers continued to suckle their babies and, often despite poorer living conditions, had a lower infant mortality rate than indigenous mothers in the same area who did not breast-feed. For example, Irish and Scottish mothers in Liverpool and London; Eastern and Southern European mothers in North American cities; and Jewish mothers in London, Manchester, Amsterdam and New York (Garrison, 1965; Newman, 1906).

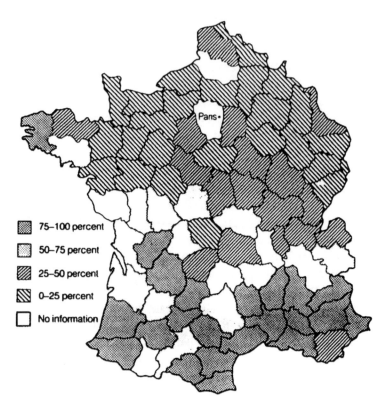

Figure 1. Proportion of French infants put out to nurse who were breast-fed, 1898 (Fildes, 1988).

Social class was also an important factor. In English-speaking countries, as artificial feeding became more popular, and apparently safer, middle class mothers who previously would have employed wet nurses increasingly chose to bottle feed their babies in order to avoid the domestic problems which often arose with these necessary servants (Apple, 1987; Fildes, 1988; Golden, 1984; see Figure 2). Physicians investigating infant feeding practices in Britain and North America between 1890 and 1919 repeatedly found that middle class mothers as a group were more likely to bottle feed their infants from birth than poorer mothers, and that this was frequently from choice rather than enforced by the mothers' poor health or need to work (Apple, 1987; Meyer, 1921; Newman, 1906; Vincent, 1904).

In many ways this was an unexpected finding. Infant feeding surveys were often instigated in response to high infant mortality rates in urban areas particularly those resulting from diarrhoeal disease. These always showed that

No More Wet Nurses!

Liebe's, Baron von Liebig's, *Soluble* Food—the most perfect substitute for *Mother's* milk. Prepared by T. Paul Liebe, Chemist, Dresden.

This food dissolves easily in warm milk, and is *at once ready* for the use of babies.

At all druggists. $1 per bottle.

Depot,   HEIL & HARTUNG,
                          390 PEARL STREET,
          Wholesale Druggists, New-York.

Figure 2. American advertisement for Liebig's food, promoting its use as an alternative to wet nurses, 1869 (*Hearth and Home*, 1, 207 (1869)).

most babies dying from diarrhoea were bottle fed, and that those dying from all causes were also more likely to have been bottle fed than infants in general (Hope, 1899; Howarth, 1905; Newman, 1906; Newsholme, 1906; Richards, 1903; Thomas, 1899; see Tables IV-VI). Investigators therefore expected to find that a high proportion of mothers, particularly among the poor, were not breast-feeding. The discovery that, even in many overcrowded industrial areas, the main group of women who did not breast-feed was the wealthy and middle class forced physicians to look in more detail at the substitute foods given, the method of administration, and especially the conditions in which infants were fed. Their conclusions were that, although a large proportion of well-to-do infants were not breast-fed, their parents were wealthy enough to provide them with adequate substitutes, such as clean milk and milk-based patent foods, a supply of suitably-constructed bottles, a clean sanitary environment and medical supervision. This largely protected them from illnesses arising from improper feeding and ensured prompt and appropriate treatment if they became ill (Apple, 1987; Howarth, 1905; Newman, 1906; Newsholme, 1906; Vincent, 1904). Thus they were less likely to appear in the mortality figures than poor infants who, in the absence of breast milk, received nutritionally inadequate substitutes, particularly farinaceous foods

Table IV: Mode of feeding of infants dying from diarrhoea in British towns 1894 - 1911					
Region	**Town**	**Date**	**Breast milk only %**	**Other foods only %**	**Breast milk + other foods %**
North	Liverpool	1894	4.2	54.5	41.4
		1899	6.9	-	-
	Wigan	1900-01	17.4	77.7	4.9
		1905	34.8	56.1	9.1
		1906	23.0	72.7	4.3
		1907	33.3	65.0	1.7
		1908	21.8	75.9	2.3
		1909	13.7	80.4	5.9
		1910	9.8	80.4	9.8
		1911	22.4	75.4	2.2
	Ince	1905	20.7	72.4	6.9
	Preston	1903	7.4	72.8	19.8
		1911	7.3	87.3	5.4
		1904	5.0	-	-
	Bootle	1903	19.6	80.4	-
	Middlesbrough	1903	22.0	78.0	-
Midlands	Chesterfield	1898	11.0	67.0	22.0
	Derby	1900-03	28.1	52.5	17.2
	Birmingham	1903	10.0	80.0	10.0
S. Wales	Rhondda	1899	15.0	-	-
	Aberdare	1907	12.5	79.2	8.3
London	Limehouse	1898	24.0	76.0	-
	Finsbury	1901-04	18.3	56.3	25.3
South	Croydon	1900-02	14.0	84.0	2.0
		1911	11.0	80.0	9.0
	Brighton	1903-05	6.5	88.5	5.0
Median:			14.5	76.0	7.6
Range:			4.2-34.8	52.5-88.5	1.7-41.4

Sources: Buchanan, 1985; Hope, 1899; Howarth, 1905; Jones, 1894; Local Government Board, 1913; Local Government Board, 1914; Middlesbrough, 1903-18; Newman, 1906; Newsholme, 1906; Richards, 1903; Roberts, 1984; Thomas, 1899; Vincent, 1904.

and skimmed condensed milk, administered in a dirty, unsuitably-constructed bottle in poor, overcrowded and insanitary conditions (Drake, 1908; Fildes, 1988; Newman, 1906; Thompson, 1984; Vincent, 1904; Woodbury, 1926).

Although the use of wet nurses declined in English-speaking countries in favour of artificial feeding this was not the case in much of continental Europe. Wealthy mothers, particularly in Catholic countries, who did not wish

Table V: Mode of feeding of infants dying from all causes in British towns 1891 - 1914					
Region	Town	Date	Breast milk only %	Other foods only %	Breast milk + other foods %
North	Salford	1903	54.2	31.9	13.9
	York	1905	11.0	84.0	5.0
	Wigan	1914	34.0	51.3	14.7
Midlands	Birmingham	1891	-	39.0	-
		1903	10.0	80.0	10.0
	Derby	1900-03	44.3	38.6	17.1
S. Wales	Rhondda	1910	37.2	43.8	19.0
		1911	30.5	58.8	10.7
London	Limehouse	1898	44.4	55.6	-
	Finsbury	1905	36.0	-	-
South	Croydon	1900-02	55.0	41.0	4.0
Median:			36.6	47.6	12.3
Range:			10.0-55.0	31.9-84.0	4.0-19.0

Sources: Buchanan, 1985; Howarth, 1905; Newman, 1906; Richards, 1903; Thomas, 1899; Vincent, 1904.

Table VI: Summary of mode of infant feeding in British towns 1891 -1918					
	Breast milk only %		Other foods only %		Breast milk + other foods %
	Median	Range	Median	Range	Median	Range
Infants 0-3 months	83.1	50.0-98.0	9.8	1.2-30.0	8.3	0.9-20.0
Infants in 5 towns	73.8	54.5-87.8	15.6	6.5-28.8	10.4	4.9-23.5
Infants dying from all causes	36.6	10.0-55.0	47.6	31.9-84.0	12.3	4.0-19.0
Infants dying from diarrhoea	14.5	4.2-34.8	76.0	52.5-88.5	7.6	1.7-41.4

Sources: Tables I, IV, V; Woods et al., 1989.

to breast-feed, paid other, poorer, mothers to suckle their children until the custom was irretrievably disrupted by the first world war. Although in France, where huge numbers of urban children of all classes were customarily placed out to country wet nurses, the incidence of breast-feeding by these nurses declined in favour of bottle feeding, the wealthy could afford to pay the higher rates of pay to employ a healthy wet nurse who did breast-feed. Poorer urban mothers who sent out their children could not afford these rates and their infants were usually bottle-fed by equally poor rural nurses. Similarly, the many European foundling hospitals which every year employed thousands of relatively poor wet nurses to feed their charges found that, with the increased availability and desirability of artificial feeding, their infants were less likely to be wholly or even partially breast-fed than in previous centuries (Fildes, 1988).

In most of continental Europe, therefore, the decline in breast-feeding was more likely to be confined to the infants of the poor since those of the wealthy continued to receive purchased breast milk. In English-speaking countries the decline in breast-feeding affected both the children of the wealthy and the urban poor, but the latter group suffered disproportionately because of their poverty and insanitary living conditions.

Although medical advice throughout this period was that maternal breast-feeding, preferably to the age of nine months, was the best and only safe method of feeding, the recommended alternative if this was not possible changed during this time. In the early-19th century most doctors thought that a wet nurse should be employed (Burns, 1811; Haden, 1827; Roberton, 1827) but as the century progressed more and more advised that artificial feeding was possible, and in many cases preferable, if mothers could not or would not suckle their own children (Apple, 1987; Fildes, 1988; Golden, 1984). By the early-20th century both medical and popular books on infant feeding and child care devoted substantial sections to the theory and practice of artificial feeding and minimal space to wet nursing (Holt, 1907; Pritchard, 1904; Vincent, 1904). In many instances the attention paid to the advantages and especially the practice of breast-feeding was also much less than had been usual in the earlier period. Although this partly reflected the increased prevalence of artificial feeding in society and the consequent need for accurate information, it also gave both medical readers and mothers the impression that bottle feeding was much safer than was actually the case in many domestic circumstances. It was principally left to the members of the emergent specialty of public health to investigate and underline the resulting dangers to infant life.

They identified three main reasons why the poor did not breast-feed:

1) Mothers had to work away from home
2) Artificial feeding was possible, was apparently easier to carry out than in the past, and seemed increasingly desirable
3) Mothers were ignorant and did not understand that if they did not breast-feed their infants they were more likely to die

An important factor associated with (1) was that, due to poverty, hard physical work and repeated childbearing, many mothers became debilitated. This was worsened by the widespread practice of their giving most of the family's food ration to their husband and children and led to emaciated women having a poor supply of breast milk, so that early supplementation and complete weaning became inevitable (Drake, 1908; Garrison, 1965; Howarth, 1905; Local Government Board, 1913; McCleary, 1905; McCleary, 1935; Newman, 1906; Vincent, 1904).

Worldwide concern about high infant mortality rates resulted in the international infant welfare campaign of 1900-1919 (Dwork, 1987; Garrison, 1965; McCleary, 1935). When, as an integral part of this movement, medical and lay workers wanted to stop the decline in the number of urban mothers who suckled their children, and attempt to increase the overall incidence of breast-feeding, they saw the main remedies to causes of the decline as

1) Education of mothers
2) Provision of crèches in or near factories together with nursing breaks for mothers (*English-speaking conference*, 1913; Newman, 1906; McCleary, 1935).

Education of mothers about breast-feeding was tackled on several fronts and was similar in most countries:

1) A system of nurses or voluntary women workers who visited women in their own homes
2) Information given by medical, nursing and lay personnel at infant consultations, infant welfare centres, schools for mothers and baby welcomes
3) Organisation of baby weeks, baby competitions, infant welfare exhibitions and poster displays accompanied by extensive advertising in newspapers and women's magazines
4) Regular pages in newspapers and women's magazines, written under medical supervision, which discussed and promoted breast-feeding and to which mothers could write for advice on feeding problems
5) Education of girls whilst they were still at school

Probably the most effective of these in raising the incidence, and ensuring the continuation, of maternal breast-feeding was the visiting of mothers in their own homes, especially in those countries which had passed a law enforcing notification of all births and where there were sufficient visitors to ensure visiting all or most of the children born in an area within a short time of birth. Most cities which had an effective visiting system showed a stable or

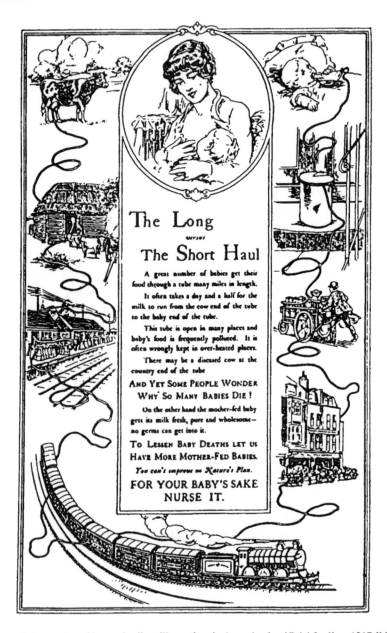

Figure 3. Promotion of breast-feeding, illustrating the hazards of artificial feeding, 1917 (*Maternity and Child Welfare*, 1 (1917)).

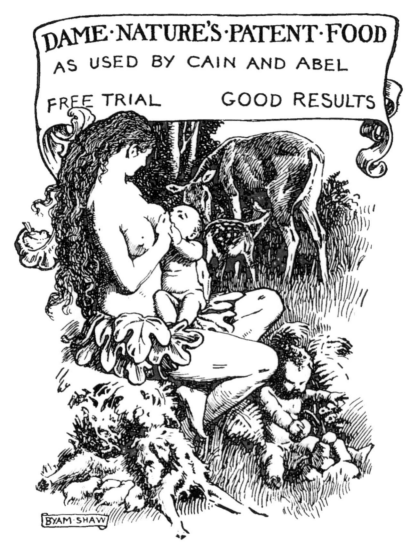

Figure 4. Promotion of maternal breast-feeding, 1918 (*Maternity and Child Welfare*, **2** (1918)).

increasing breast-feeding rate over the period 1900-1919 (Ashby, 1915; *Borough of Hackney*, 1911-18; Mackellar, 1917; Meyer, 1921; Middlesborough, 1903-18; Royal New Zealand, 1907-19).

Promotion of maternal suckling by infant welfare centres and similar institutions was less effective, because they were not universally available, there was no compulsion to attend and only a limited number of mothers in an area attended. Also, a major part of their work was to distribute milk which was safe for artificial feeding so that a large percentage of the mothers who attended were already bottle feeding their babies (Ashby, 1915; Budin, 1907; *English-speaking conference*, 1913; McCleary, 1905; Meyer, 1921). However, centres that provided free or low-cost dinners for nursing mothers were significant in helping physically-debilitated mothers to maintain their supply of breast milk (Dwork, 1987; *English-speaking conference*, 1913; McCleary, 1935; Reeves, 1979).

Provision of information in newspapers and women's magazines was probably more effective in reaching and influencing the middle classes than the poor (Apple, 1987). Although statutory education for girls was widespread by the early-20th century, oral and literary accounts of working class women rarely refer to the influence of written sources. Much more important was the experience and advice of mothers, women relatives and friends (Davies, 1978; Roberts, 1984). Promotion of breast-feeding in this medium also had to compete with commercial advertising of patent foods and feeding vessels printed alongside it, so that the message was inevitably diluted (Apple, 1987; *Maternity and Child Welfare*, 1917-19).

Certain countries, such as Germany and France, which instituted a system of nursing allowances and/or bonuses to be paid to mothers who successfully breast-fed their babies for a specified length of time, found these proved an effective incentive to mothers to breast-fed, especially those with illegitimate children (Garrison, 1965; Kintner, 1985), although this scheme was not adopted by a majority of countries.

Provision of crèches and nursing breaks was undertaken more energetically in some countries than others but the first world war proved an incentive to increase these in Britain and continental Europe because so many women were required to work in munitions and other factories that provision had to be made for nursing mothers (*Infant welfare in Germany*, 1918; *Maternity and Child Welfare*, 1917-19; *Welfare of the children*, 1919). The effectiveness of this measure is shown by the fact that the incidence of breast-feeding remained high in many areas where women worked in munitions and other industries during the war (Carnegie, 1917; Kintner, 1985; Middlesbrough, 1903-18).

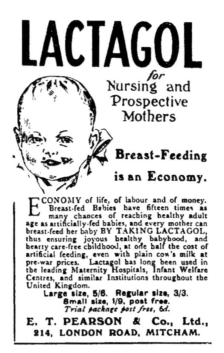

LACTAGOL

for
Nursing and
Prospective
Mothers

Breast-Feeding

is an Economy.

ECONOMY of life, of labour and of money. Breast-fed Babies have fifteen times as many chances of reaching healthy adult age as artificially-fed babies, and every mother can breast-feed her baby BY TAKING LACTAGOL, thus ensuring joyous healthy babyhood, and hearty care-free childhood, at one half the cost of artificial feeding, even with plain cow's milk at pre-war prices. Lactagol has long been used in the leading Maternity Hospitals, Infant Welfare Centres, and similar Institutions throughout the United Kingdom.
Large size, 5/6. Regular size, 3/3.
Small size, 1/9, post free.
Trial package post free, 6d.
**E. T. PEARSON & Co., Ltd.,
214, LONDON ROAD, MITCHAM.**

Figure 5. Food supplements for nursing mothers were an important feature of campaigns to increase breast-feeding among poor, physically-debilitated mothers (*Maternity and Child Welfare*, 2 (1918)).

By 1919, many countries which had perceived a decline in breast-feeding rates during the previous 20-30 years, and had made a concerted effort to increase the number of nursing mothers, particularly in poor urban areas, had been successful in their efforts to varying extents (Kintner, 1985; Mackellar, 1917; Royal New Zealand, 1907-19). However, although an increased proportion of women may have initiated breast-feeding, in most places they did so for a shorter period of time (Kintner, 1985; Liestøl *et al.*, 1988). Reasons for this included changes in the nature of women's work and lifestyle, the greatly increased safety of artificial feeding due to improved sanitation and sterilisation of milk and feeding vessels, and the influence of the medical profession who (largely because bottle feeding was now safer) often advised earlier supplementation and earlier weaning than before (Apple, 1987; Dwork, 1987; Fildes, 1988; King, 1918; McCleary, 1935; Newsholme, 1936).

The history of infant feeding in this period highlights some basic factors that form, and will always form, a background to further discussion on world wide infant nutrition in the 20th century.

REFERENCES

Apple, R. D. *Mothers and medicine. A social history of infant feeding, 1890-1950*, Madison, University of Wisconsin Press (1987).

Ashby, H. T. *Infant mortality*, Cambridge, Cambridge University Press (1915).

Baby-saving campaigns. A preliminary report on what American cities are doing to prevent infant mortality, Washington, Government Printing Office (1913).

Black, C. (Ed.), *Married women's work*, Reprinted. London, Virago (1983).

Borough of Hackney, Reports on the sanitary condition of, London (1911-18).

Briggs, A. *A social history of England*, London, Weidenfeld & Nicholson (1983).

Buchanan, I. Infant feeding, sanitation and diarrhoea in colliery communities, 1880-1911. In: D. J. Oddy and D. S. Miller (Eds.), *Diet and health in modern Britain*, London, Croom Helm, 148-177 (1985).

Budin, P. *The nursling. The feeding and hygiene of premature and full-term infants*, Trans. W. J. Maloney, London, Caxton (1907).

Burns, J. *Popular directions for the treatment of the diseases of women and children*, London (1811).

Carnegie United Kingdom Trust, *Report on the physical welfare of mothers and children*, Liverpool, C. Tinling (1917).

Cone, T. E. *200 years of feeding infants in America*, Columbus, Ohio, Ross Laboratories (1976).

Davies, M. L. (Ed.), *Maternity. Letters from working women*, Reprinted London, Virago (1978).

Drake, Mrs. A study of infant life in Westminster, *J. Roy. Stat. Soc.*, 71:678-686 (1908).

Drummond, J. C., and Wilbraham, A. *The Englishman's food. Five centuries of English diet*, London, Jonathan Cape (1957).

Dwork, D. *War is good for babies and other young children. A history of the infant and child welfare movement in England 1898-1918*, London, Tavistock (1987).

English-speaking conference on infant mortality held at Caxton Hall, Westminster, August 4 and 5 1913, Report of the proceedings of, London (1913).

Fildes, V. *Breasts, bottles and babies. A history of infant feeding*, Edinburgh, Edinburgh University Press (1986).

Fildes, V. *Wet Nursing. A history from antiquity to the present*, Oxford, Basil Blackwell (1988).

Forsyth, D. The history of infant feeding from Elizabethan times, *Proc. Soc. Med.*, 4:110-141 (1911).

Garrison, F. H. *History of pediatrics*, Philadelphia, W. B. Saunders Company, 84-170 (1965).

Golden, J. *From breast to bottle: the decline of wet nursing in Boston, 1867-1927*, PhD Dissertation, Boston University (1984).

Haden, C. T. *Practical observations on the management and diseases of children*, London (1827).

Hewitt, M. *Wives and mothers in Victorian industry*, Rockliff (1958).

Holt, L. E. *The care and feeding of children*, London, Sidney Appleton (1907).

Hope, E. W. Observations on autumnal diarrhoea in cities, *Pub. Hlth.*, 11:660-665 (1899).

Howarth, W. J. The influence of feeding on the mortality of infants, *Lancet*, 2:210-213 (1905).

Infant welfare in Germany during the war, London, HM Stationery Office (1918).

Jones, H. R. The perils and protection of infant life, *J. Roy. Stat. Soc.*, 57:1-103 (1894).

King, F. T. *Feeding and care of baby*, Auckland & London, Whitcombe & Tombs (1918).

Kintner, H. J. Trends and regional differences in breastfeeding in Germany from 1871 to 1937, *J. Fam. Hist.*, 10:163-182 (1985).

Lewis, M. The problem of infant feeding: the Australian experience from the mid-nineteenth century to the 1920s, *J. Hist. Med.*, 35: 174-187 (1980).

Lithell, U. -B. *Breast-feeding and reproduction. Studies in marital fertility and infant mortality in 19th century Finland and Sweden*, Doctoral Dissertation, University of Uppsala (1981).

Liestøl, K., Rosenberg, M., and Walløe, L. Breast-feeding practice in Norway 1860-1984, *J. Biosoc. Sci.*, 20:45-58 (1988).

Local Government Board, *Supplement to the forty-second Annual Report 1912-13, On infant and child mortality*, London, HM Stationery Office (1913).

Local Government Board, *Supplement to the forty-third Annual Report 1913-14, On infant mortality in Lancashire*, London, HM Stationery Office (1914).

Mackellar, C. K. *The mother, the baby and the state*, Sydney, Government Printer (1917).

McCleary, G. F. *Infantile mortality and infants' milk depots*, London, P. S. King & Son (1905).

McCleary, G. F. *The maternity and child welfare movement*, London, P. S. King & Son Ltd. (1935).

Maternity and Child Welfare, 1-3 (1917-19).

Meyer, E. C. *Infant mortality in New York City. A study of the results accomplished by infant-life saving agencies 1885-1920*, New York, Rockefeller Foundation (1921).

Middlesbrough Maternal and child welfare files, Public Record Office MH 48 262 (1903-18).

Newman, G. *Infant mortality: a social problem*, London, Methuen (1906).

Newsholme, A. Domestic infection in relation to epidemic diarrhoea, *J. Hyg.*, 6:139-148 (1906).

Newsholme, A. *Fifty years in public health*, London, George Allen & Unwin (1936).

Pinchbeck, I. *Women workers and the industrial revolution 1750-1850*, Reprinted London, Virago (1981).

Pritchard, E. *The physiological feeding of infants*, London, Henry Kimpton, 2nd edn. (1904).

Reeves, M. P. *Round about a pound a week*, Reprinted London, Virago (1979).

Richards, H. M. The factors which determine the local incidence of fatal infantile diarrhoea, *J. Hyg.*, 3:325-346 (1903).

Roberton, J. *Observations on the mortality and physical management of children*, London (1827).

Roberts, E. *A woman's place. An oral history of working-class women 1890-1940*, Oxford, Basil Blackwell (1984).

Rollet, C. Infant feeding, fosterage and infant mortality in France at the end of the 19th century, *Population. Selected Papers*, 7:1-14 (1981).

Ross, E. Labour and love: rediscovering London's working-class mothers, 1870-1918. In: J. Lewis (Ed.), *Labour and love. Women's experience of home and family, 1850-1940*, Oxford, Basil Blackwell, 73-96 (1986).

Routh, C. H. F. *Infant feeding and its influence on life: or, the causes and prevention of infant mortality*, London, John Churchill (1860).

Royal New Zealand Society for the Health of Women and Children, *Annual Reports*, Dunedin (1907-19).

Smith, F. B. *The people's health 1830-1910*, London, Croom Helm (1979).

Sussman, G. D. *Selling mother's milk. The wet-nursing business in France 1715-1914*, Urbana, University of Illinois Press (1982).

Thomas, D. L. On infantile mortality, *Pub. Hlth.*, 11:810-816 (1899).

Thompson, B. Infant mortality in nineteenth-century Bradford. In: R. Woods and J. Woodward (Eds.), *Urban disease and mortality in nineteenth-century England*, London, Batsford, 120-147 (1984).

Tilly, L. A., and Scott, J. W. *Women, work and family*, New York, Holt, Rinehart & Winston (1978).

Van Eekelen, A. De Knecht -, *Naar een rationale zuigelingenvoeding.* *Voedingsleer en kindergeneeskunde in Nederland 1840-1914*, Doctoral Thesis, Catholic University of Nijmegen, G. H. Thieme, 375-382 (1984).

Vincent, R. *The nutrition of the infant*, London, Bailliere, Tindall & Cox (1904).

Welfare of the children of the women employed in factories in France and Germany, London, HM Stationery Office (1919).

Wohl, A. S. *Endangered lives. Public health in Victorian Britain*, London, Methuen (1983).

Woodbury, R. M. *Infant mortality and its causes*, Baltimore, Williams & Wilkins Company, 1-22, 75-101 (1926).

Woods, R. I., Watterson, P. A., and Woodward, J. H. The causes of rapid infant mortality decline
   in England and Wales, 1861-1921. Part II, *Popul. Stud.*, 43:113-132 (1989).
Wrigley, E. A., and Schofield, R. S. *The population history of England*, London, Edward Arnold
   (1981).

2

The Geographic Distribution of Malnutrition

Alberto Pradilla

Nutrition Programme
Family Health Division
W.H.O.
Geneva, Switzerland

INTRODUCTION

The term malnutrition is, and has been, utilized to describe the prevalence of a number of indicators that, either directly or indirectly, are associated with physiological reality. In medical terms, malnutrition is used to refer to a number of conditions, each with a specific cause related to one or more nutrients and each characterized by a cellular imbalance between the supply of nutrients and energy, and the demand for them to ensure growth, maintenance, activity and specific functions. Malnutrition has clearly defined anthropometric, clinical and biochemical signs and symptoms, and can be treated by an increase or decrease in the nutrient and energy supply.

The first physiological response to an imbalance is adaptation (Waterlow, 1985). Short periods of stress are handled without negative effects on basic functions. Severe or prolonged stress requires adaptation mechanisms for survival that could produce alterations in critical functions that are basic for individual welfare. Indicators of malnutrition are derived from the measurement of some of the clinical, biochemical or functional expressions of these adaptive mechanisms. The most commonly used indicators of malnutrition are those of body mass and physical growth, and in the case of vitamins and minerals, by clinical and biochemical measurements. For excesses or deficits of short duration, the basic mechanism is the utilization of storage capacity leading to small increases or decreases of weight or stores. Severe or prolonged stress in children leads to the slowing down of linear growth (Beaton, 1987). A block at any stage in the flow of nutrients and energy, from production to the final metabolic fate, or a change in the demand, increase or decrease, can disturb the balance. Food has to be produced, marketed and transported. Food has to be purchased, processed and distributed at the household level. Food has to be eaten, digested and the energy and nutrients absorbed and metabolized.

The number of factors that influence this process is such, and the possible number of combinations so large, that the interpretation of the causes is possible only in very homogenous conditions. Models of causality have been developed based on discrete studies and observations, and they actually reflect all possible interaction of factors (Beghin *et al.*). For individuals, or for special population groups, many of these factors may not apply. Group or national aggregates are basically the means of normal or skewed distributions of different variables. This results in a national indicator determined by a part of the population that is different from the one determining the average of another indicator.

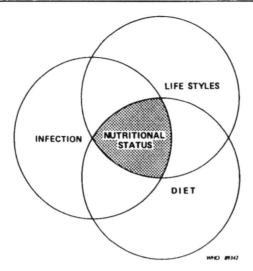

Figure 1. Interrelated factors influencing body mass.

In summary there are three interrelated factors influencing the manner in which body mass is built - diet, life-style, infection - and the determination of the balance as shown in Figure 1.

MAGNITUDE OF THE PROBLEM

There is general agreement that malnutrition is a world wide problem and that the causes lie in the social, economic, political and physical environment in which people live. Income, food availability, health care, the environment, food production, life-styles, etc., are obvious causal factors for nutritional status. Indices or indicators for such factors are frequently used at various levels of aggregation to estimate the number of malnourished. Recognizing the fact that the growth of children and the body mass of adults are outcomes reflecting the overall health of individuals, they have been included as indicators for Health for All 2000: Weight at birth, weight in relation to height, weight in relation to age, and height in relation to age.

The nutrition programme of WHO has been collecting and collating results of national or subnational studies to monitor the process of health development. Data has been collected at national levels by means of special studies, regular food and nutrition surveillance systems and school and health services records. The data has been processed in some cases to facilitate comparisons between countries or time periods (WHO weekly Epidemiological Record, 1987).

Anthropometric data is available now from more than 120 countries. In a number of cases these are also sufficient to permit an assessment of related trends in time. Data in obesity is presently being analyzed as well as breast-feeding prevalences and trends and dietary components associated with other health problems.

It was decided to prepare a series of cartograms to obtain a visual description of a combination of prevalences of each of the anthropometric indices. One of the variables is used to determine the relative size of the country, the other variable is expressed by a code. Thus, cartograms were developed to express the associations of factors with growth failure. In this case, diarrhoea, morbidity or energy availability determining the relative size of the country while anthropometric indicators are given a code (World Health Magazine, 1988).

Note: The cartograms presented throughout only describe the final out-come but indicate very little of the specific factor responsible for specific problems.

Birth Weight

Birth weight is probably the most critical factor determining infant mortality and morbidity. Recent studies suggest that prenatal factors and birth weight could be the most important determinant in the growth of a child to the age of 2 years (Calloway et al., 1988). Low birth weight has been defined as being below 2,500 gms. As birth weight is the result of the duration of gestation and growth rate the proportion of the two could be different. The lower the prevalence of children born weighing less than 2,500 gms the more likelihood there is of a high proportion of prematurity and/or intra-uterine growth failure. Prematurity, and stunted and wasted intrauterine growth retar-dation reflect the condition of the mother and her own environment (Kramer, 1987). For the purpose of monitoring progress it would be ideal to have data discriminating these conditions. This is not yet possible, however, and the Cartogram I presentation has codes only for prevalence of births with less than 2,500 gms.

The size of each country has been set according to the total number of live births. The code has been distributed in relation to the prevalence as percent of births. For comparison purposes a map on standard projection has been coded identically with the prevalence of low birth weight. When the world is seen in the cartogram a clear distortion is observed. India alone appears the size of the African continent, Mongolia the same size as Jamaica. The addition of the prevalence to the same cartogram depicts the fact that the highest number of low birth weight infants are born in a few large countries which have a very high prevalence, both WHO African and South East Asian Regions having the largest prevalences with a large number of births.

As in older ages, the causes of growth failure and malnutrition are many. Some factors are interdependent, others have a direct effect either on the length of gestation or on intrauterine growth. A recent review has suggested that the relative risk of each factor is similar in different locations and that the critical issue becomes the prevalence of that same factor in the location.

Wasting and Stunting

The association between weight and height and wasting, reflects acute changes in body mass. The relation is calculated in children by:

current weight   Current height or weight = W/A or H/A
ref. weight/height   ref. weight or height
                           for same age

For older children and adults the body mass index is utilized to describe this association (kg/m^2). Fasting, acute infections, intense exercise and any other situation producing either a decrease or an increase in stores of fluids or nutrients will modify this relation. The balance could be re-established very rapidly. This association essentially describes thinness or fatness and for that reason has been called an indicator of acute malnutrition or wasting, obesity, etc. As mentioned before, prolonged or severe stress initiates other functional changes that have repercussions on the health of the individual. Frequent or prolonged episodes of weight loss induce longitudinal growth arrest. The fact that arrest lines in long bones appear during periods of active nephrotic syndrome has been well documented. Stunted growth has been called chronic malnutrition although some evidence suggests specific nutrient deficits could also be used for this expression (Waterlow, 1988).

Because of the rapid growth of children and because of the likelihood that their health status indicates the overall conditions of their environment, the pre-school age group has been generally utilized as an indicator of the overall nutritional status of population groups. Cartograms II and III have been designed so that the area for each country corresponds to the total number of children under the age of six. (They could also be presented to reflect the total population). The codes express the proportion of children whose weight/height relation, or their height, is below 2 standard deviations from the mean of a reference population. With the assumption that these measurements have a normal distribution, it is expected that no more than 2.28% of the population is below this point or above +2 standard deviations.

It is clear that wasting, on national average, has essentially disappeared from most countries in the Americas, Europe, Western Pacific and large parts of the Eastern Mediterranean and African WHO Regions. South East Asia presents the largest prevalences as well as the area where most of the children are wasted. High prevalences in relatively less populated areas in the northern part of the African Region and Eastern Mediterranean are also present. This situation is quite different from the one observed 20 years ago where significant numbers of children had weights well below -3 standard deviations (equivalent approximately to Gomez III and II). National averages, on the other hand, may be misleading as they hide the presence of population pockets where prevalences are still high (Gorstein & Akre, 1988). Linear growth retardation and stunting, reflect the association of height and age. This indicator, though in decline, remains high throughout the world, the largest numbers living in South East Asia and in Africa. From the experience of some countries if appears that once wasting disappears, a downward trend of stunting begins.

GROWTH FAILURE AND INFECTION

Bacterial, viral and parasitic infections, through their effect on appetite, resultant of vomiting and/or diarrhoea, impairment of absorption, increased requirements and changes in metabolic processes, have significant impact on the nutrient balance (Food & Nutrition Bulletin, 1979). Weight loss during illness is a regular clinical feature. When the frequency of infection is low and they are of short duration, a balance could be reached in a short period during convalescence. In conditions when nutrient dense foods are not available, a high frequency of even mild diseases could have marked effects on the growth of children. Similar effects have been documented in relation to the stores of certain vitamins and minerals (Tomkins & Watkins, 1988).

Growth failure, on the other hand, is associated with the development and course of infection. Duration and severity of infections are related to impairments of the immune system brought about in particular by prolonged growth failure.

Because diarrhoea is one of the infections with higher prevalence throughout the world, it has been utilized as a proxy for general infections in Cartogram IV. The size of each country has been given by the number of estimated episodes of diarrhoea in children under five. For contrast, the colour code indicates the percentage of children below minus 2 standard deviations of weight for height (wasting). It is evident that communities who are more affected by the diet infection cycle, are usually more deprived in terms of distribution of resources, opportunities for earning and access to a good

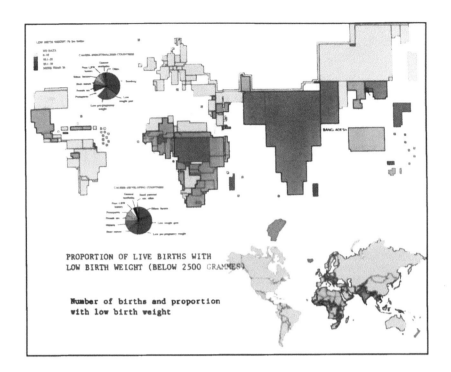

Cartogram I.

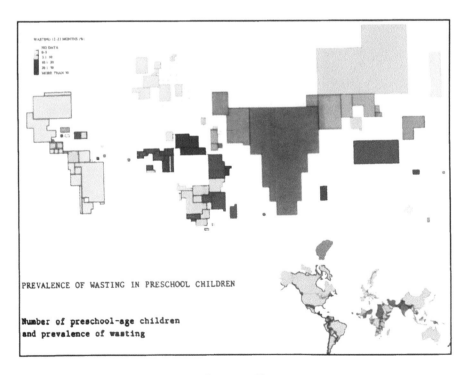

Cartogram II.

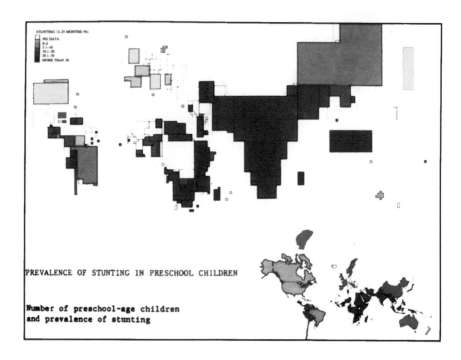

Cartogram III.

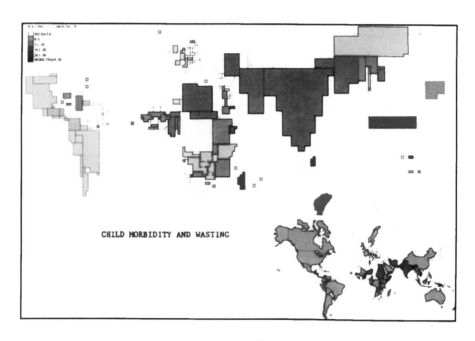

Cartogram IV.

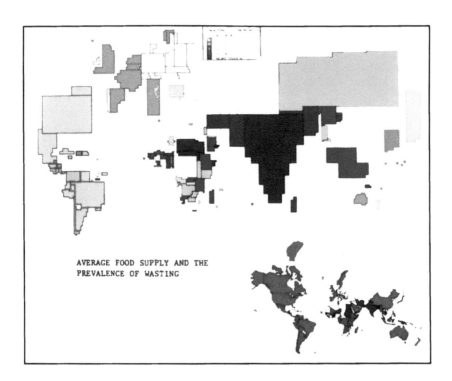

Cartogram V.

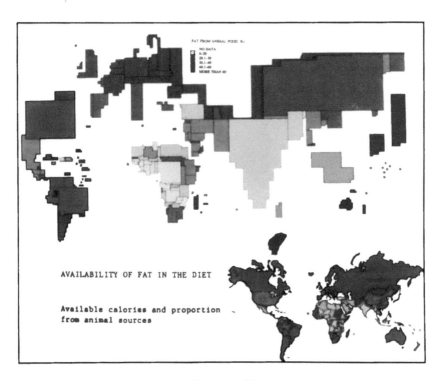

Cartogram VI.

environment and health services and to an appropriate diet. Improvements in growth performance have been obtained through a combination of policies aimed at reducing poverty, improving the availability of services, education and primary health care and food supply.

Cartogram IV, through the distortion of size of countries, emphasizes this point. Often, if not always, a relative decrease in country size in the Cartogram is associated with a low percentage of wasting. The WHO South East Asia and African Regions exhibit a combination of increased relative size and more than 20% prevalence. In contrast, most countries in America and in the Western Pacific depict a smaller size and prevalences below 10% wasting.

DIET AND GROWTH PERFORMANCE

The composition of a diet as well as its quantity is and has been one of the major determinants of individual health, and also of the interaction of population groups and countries. A number of limitations appear when assessing the appropriateness of diet. It is only during strict diet control that it is possible to document individual consumption. A number of flaws have been revealed in the different techniques of dietary surveys. Other flaws have been detected in household food-purchase surveys. There are problems not only in the way in which data are obtained or estimated for availability of different foods at the macro level, but also the fact that these data say little in relation to distribution. Food composition tables used to calculate nutrients, do not in general, specify the variety analyzed or the method of analysis used. Figure 2 demonstrates the extreme differences observed when the two different methods of dietary survey and food balance sheets are used.

As in the case of anthropometry, the problem lies not in techniques but in the manner in which results are utilized. Food balance sheets were developed with specific purposes with known characteristics. If these are utilized to determine the proportion of the population malnourished, the results are clearly different from actual measurements of growth failure as well as from data derived from dietary surveys.

Substantial progress has been made during the last 25 years in increasing food production and improving health status. Whereas in the 1950s there were more than 30 countries that produced less than 2000 calories per capita per day, in the last Food and Agriculture Organisation Food Survey. The only 16 are in that range. The populations (Ref) of China, India, Nigeria and Brazil have more than 2000 calories available per capita. More needs to be done towards increasing the access to adequate diets for all, for in many countries in fact, a large sufficient availability of nutrients is still not reflected in individual consumptions.

Scientific evidence continues to accumulate that support the important role of diet in the prevention of the most common causes of premature and disability and death in those areas where infectious diseases have been mostly controlled: cardiovascular diseases and cancer (WHO Study Group). The dynamic relationship between changes in a population's diet and changes in its health has been well reflected in the rapidly changing profiles of migrant populations and in many countries of Asia, Africa and the Americas (Waterlow, 1985).

Cartograms V & VI have been designed so that the size of each country represents the total number of calories available per day. The colour code in cartogram V expresses the calories available per person per day. Most of the industrialized and a number of developing countries have more than 2400 KCals available per person/day. Highly populated countries have sometimes limited per capita availability although there is high total country availability.

Cartogram VI indicates by its colour coding the proportion of fat of animal origin in the total energy available per person/day. An almost reverse colour, as can be expected, is portrayed. The Americas, Western Pacific, Europe and the Eastern Mediterranean Regions have more than half of their fat from animal sources. In most of these countries, some of the noncommunicable diseases are among those with the highest mortality. Although this is clearly not the only major factor, there are recent population based indications that there is a link between fat consumption, salt intake and hypertension, between high energy dense foods and diabetes; and on the intake of total calories, dietary fats and alcohol in certain types of cancers. These problems, which were of particular concern in industrialized countries, are rapidly increasing in most parts of the world, and since prevention must start in fetal, infant and child health, this picture includes those individuals, groups and population components.

CONCLUSION

The methodology of depicting world wide nutritional issues with the cartograms used in this chapter, puts into perspective figuratively how these issues and problems are spread across countries and populations allowing comparisons between them.

REFERENCES

Beaton, G. *Small but Healthy. Are we asking the right question?* American Anthropological Association Symposium, (November 1987).

Beghin *et al.*, *Nutritional Assessment.* WHO publication. (Date)

Calloway, D. H., *et al.*: *Food Intake and Human Function: A Cross Country Perspective.* University of California, Berkeley, (1988).

Food and Nutrition Bulletin: Protein energy requirements under conditions prevailing in developing countries: *Current Knowledge and Research needs*. Supplement 1, (1979).

Gorstein, J., and Akre, J. *WHO Statistics Quarterly*, vol. 41 No. 2, pp. 48-88 (1988).

Kramer, M. S.: Determinants of low birth weight. Methodological assessment and meta-analysis. *WHO Bulletin* 65(5):663-737 (1987).

Tomkins, A., and Watson, F. Interaction of Nutrition and Infection. In: *Report of ACC Subcommittee on Nutrition*. (in press) (1988).

Waterlow, J. C. *What do we mean by adaptation in nutritional adaptation man*. In: Blaxter, K., Waterlow, J. C. (Eds.), pp. 1-11. John Libbey London, Paris (1985).

Waterlow, J. (eds.): *Linear Growth Retardation in Less Developed Countries*. Nestle Nutrition Workshop Series, vol. 14. Raven Press, New York (1988).

WHO Study Group, *Diet, Nutrition, and the Prevention of Chronic Diseases*, (in press) (1990).

WHO Weekly Epidemiological Record. Part I, No. 7, pp. 37-38 (1987); Part II, no. 8, pp. 45-50 (1987); Part III, no. 9, pp. 57-59 (1987); Part IV, no. 10, pp. 64-66 (1987); Part V, No. 11, pp. 71-73 (1987); Part VI, no. 12, pp. 78-80 (1987).

World Health Magazine, (May 1988).

3

Maternal Undernutrition and Reproductive Performance

Barbara Abrams

Public Health Nutrition Program
School of Public Health
University of California
Berkeley, California 94720

Table I: Energy and protein requirements during pregnancy						
	FAO/WHO/UNU, 1985			NRC RDA, 1989		
	Refer-ence weight	Average energy range (kcal/day)[1]	Safe level of protein intake (g/day)	Refer-ence weight	Energy (kcal/day)	Protein (g/day)
Nonpregnant	55 kg	1850-2850	41	55 kg	2200	44
Pregnancy						
full activity		+285	+6		+300[2]	+10
reduced activity		+200	+6			
Lactation						
first 6 months		+500	+17.5		+500	+15
after 6 months		+500	13		+500/+600[3]	+12

[1] range is based on activity level
[2] during the 2nd and 3rd trimesters unless pregancy is begun with depleted energy stores
[3] 650 kcal suggested for women with suboptimal prenatal weight gain or with body weight below standard for height

Recommended dietary allowances for adult women (NRC, 1989)						
	Thiamin (mg)	Riboflavin (mg)	Niacin (mg)	VitA (mcg)	VitC (mg)	Calcium (g)	Iron (mg)
Nonpregnant	1.1	1.3	15.0	800	60	0.8	18
Pregnant	1.5	1.6	17.0	800	70	1.2	30
Lactation	1.6	1.8	20.0	1300	95	1.2	15

World Health Organization, Energy and Protein Requirements. Report of a Joint FAO/WHO/UNU Expert Consultation. Technical Report Series 724. WHO, Geneva (1985).
National Research Council, Recommended Dietary Allowances 10th ed. National Academy Press, Washington, D.C. (1989).

INTRODUCTION

Pregnancy and lactation increase nutritional requirements. At the same time, maternal physiological adjustments in nutrient absorption, excretion and metabolism may conserve nutrients. Current evidence suggests that when women begin pregnancy adequately nourished, modest but important increases in maternal dietary requirements are associated with successful pregnancy and lactation. (Table I) However, millions of pregnant and lactating women around the world are undernourished. The majority of these women live in developing countries, but women within developed nations are also at risk. The etiology, prevalence and severity of undernutrition differs from place to place, and within population subgroups.

Undernutrition occurs when dietary intake cannot meet nutritional requirements. The synthesis of maternal and fetal tissue or breast milk, and the associated costs of maternal maintenance increase nutrient requirements during pregnancy and lactation. Nutrient requirements are also increased by high levels of physical activity, such as the heavy physical labor regularly performed by pregnant or lactating women in many agricultural societies. In developing countries, poor sanitation and limited health care increase the risk of illness, especially infections and parasitic infestations which tend to increase nutrient requirements but decrease nutrient absorption. In developed countries, poor maternal health or nutritional status may often accompany, and exacerbate, the effects of cigarette smoking, abuse of alcohol or illicit drugs.

Acute or seasonal food shortages and inadequate resources to purchase food can produce insufficient dietary intake. Even if adequate amounts of food are available, cultural taboos, poor individual food selection or unequal food distribution favoring males over females within the household, may restrict maternal food intake during pregnancy or lactation. Urbanization, industrialization and migration also have important impacts on livelihood, lifestyle, and dietary intake, leading to negative changes in maternal health and nutritional status (Williams *et al.*, 1985).

This chapter examines the influence of maternal undernutrition on pregnancy outcome, especially low birth weight (<2500 grams), which is the most important determinant of infant mortality and morbidity(Committee to Study the Prevention of Low Birth Weight, 1985; McCormick, 1985). In the United States, two thirds of all neonatal deaths, and 20% of all postneonatal deaths can be attributed to low birth weight (LBW) (Committee to Study the Prevention of Low Birth Weight 1985), and a study of infant mortality in eight Latin American countries estimated that 60% of neonatal deaths were linked to low birthweight (Puffer and Serrano, 1973). Less conclusive information is available regarding the effect of maternal nutritional deficiencies on fetal congenital anomalies, pregnancy complications or the health of the newborn infant, but where available, data on these outcomes have also been reviewed.

Maternal undernutrition and lactational performance is also discussed. Human milk is considered the optimal food for young human infants because of its unique nutritional and immunological characteristics. Breast milk plays a vital role in infant survival in communities where families cannot afford infant formula, especially where environmental conditions increase the risk of contamination of breast milk substitutes. Since millions of infants around the world depend on the milk of mothers who themselves are undernourished, it is important to understand the relationship between maternal nutritional status and lactation performance, which is defined by both the quantity of breast milk produced and its quality. A brief review of the literature relating maternal undernutrition to lactational amenorrhea is also provided.

COMPLEXITIES IN THE LITERATURE

Although many attempts have been made to understand the relationship between maternal nutritional status, and human reproduction, the literature is replete with conflicting, and sometimes confusing, results. To really understand this topic, it is important to read some of the excellent critical reviews that have been written about research on low birthweight (Kramer, 1987a; Kramer, 1987b), nutrient utilization during pregnancy (King *et al.* 1987), nutritional supplementation (Rush, 1982), breast milk production and quality (Jelliffe and Jellifffe, 1978; Lonnerdal, 1986; Whitehead, 1983; WHO Collaborative Study on Breastfeeding, 1985), and women and nutrition in developing countries (Hamilton *et al.*, 1984). Some of the most important limitations in the literature are described below.

Well Controlled Experiments Cannot Be Conducted to Directly Determine the Influence of Undernutrition on Fertility, Human Pregnancy or Lactational Performance

It is obvious that women cannot be experimentally starved in order to study the effect of poor nutrition on pregnancy or lactational performance. Nutrient deficiencies can be induced experimentally in other animals, but the applicability of these studies is limited due to differences in reproductive and nutritional physiology. Furthermore, the magnitude of deficiency provoked in animal studies is often more severe than might be encountered by humans under most conditions, and interactions with the myriad other confounding variables that human women experience cannot be well studied in animals. Findings in animals, however, that a vitamin or mineral deficiency produces a poor outcome, such as congenital malformation, stillbirth, or impaired growth and development, suggests that the potential exists for a similar effect in humans. Descriptions of possible links between maternal nutrition and reproductive performance in humans consist primarily of case reports describing the possible effect of nutrient deficiency or excess, observational studies linking a specific nutrient to certain outcomes, or experimental trials of nutritional supplementation. Observational studies attempt to understand how maternal characteristics (such as socio-economic class, nutritional status, or age) influence birth weight, other fetal outcomes, or estimates of the output and/or composition of breast milk. But, when malnutrition is the result of multiple deficiencies of many nutrients, or when poor reproductive performance is associated with many problems, it is hard to assign responsibility to one factor alone. Experimental studies can test the effect of specific maternal dietary supplements on outcomes such as pregnancy performance, the quality and quantity of breast milk, return of ovulation or occurrence of pregnancy. A well-designed trial attempts to control for other, potentially confounding variables by using experimental techniques and a randomized study design. However, many problems can interfere with the experiment. Maternal diet supplementation studies are difficult to interpret because the food supplement may replace part of the diet rather than complement it, the length of treatment, timing, or quantity or composition of the supplement may be inappropriate, or the diet supplement may not be correctly related to the degree of malnutrition(WHO Collaborative Study on Breastfeeding, 1985). In addition, no matter how carefully a study is designed, humans cannot be controlled, and many trials suffer from problems with subject compliance, loss to follow-up, and other sources of inconsistency and bias.

It is Difficult to Obtain Accurate and Reliable Measurement of Nutritional Status

There is no perfect way to measure maternal nutritional status. Assessment can be based on physical examinations for clinical indicators of nutritional disease, anthropometry, laboratory analyses of blood, urine or other tissues to estimate nutrient levels, and estimates of dietary intake. Each technique has its own strengths and weaknesses, and detailed discussions on nutrition assessment methodology have been written (Christakis, 1973; Jelliffe, 1964; Rush, 1975). Assessment of food intake data is limited by difficulties in obtaining accurate measures of intake and lack of accurate food composition data. Assessment of laboratory measures of nutritional status is limited by methodological problems in the biochemical assay of certain nutrients. Of additional concern are the changes in nutrient serum levels and urinary excretion, which occur as normal physiological adaptations to pregnancy, but which resemble signs of deficiency in nonpregnant individuals (Hytten and Chamberlain, 1980; Hytten and Leitch, 1971; Winick, 1986). For example, even when maternal iron status is adequate, hemoglobin and hematocrit levels decrease as a result of hemodilution, and decreased levels of vitamins during pregnancy do not necessarily reflect dietary intake, and may represent a "normal" response to pregnancy. Finally, studies of energy balance and requirements are difficult to conduct and interpret. Even when similar methods have been used, estimates of maternal body composition, metabolism, physical activity and dietary intake vary between pregnant populations, as demonstrated by the recently published Five-Country Study

(Durnin, 1987). Some studies in developing countries report that despite high levels of physical activity, energy balance can be maintained on dietary intakes that are much lower than recommended, suggesting that some populations may have the ability to adapt to low energy intake by increasing metabolic efficiency, and that people in developing countries could be more efficient than those in developed countries (Prentice, 1984). Evidence refuting this relationship also exists (Collaborative Research Support Program, 1988).

It is Difficult to Obtain Accurate and Reliable Definition of Pregnancy Outcomes, Lactational Performance and Related Confounding Variables

Both the definition and ascertainment of specific pregnancy outcomes vary around the world. Even under the best circumstances, reliable estimates of variables such as gestational age are difficult to obtain. For rare events, such as congenital anomalies, very large numbers of observations are required. Many factors in addition to nutrition influence birth weight and other pregnancy outcomes. A recent review identified 43 different factors, many interrelated with each other, that were linked, in the literature, to low birth weight (Kramer, 1987).

The difficulties in accurately measuring breast milk output have been well described (Jelliffe and Jelliffe, 1978; Whitehead 1983; WHO Collaborative Study on Breastfeeding 1985). Common techniques for collection of human milk include test-weighing the mother or infant before and after each feeding, measuring samples of milk obtained through manual or machine expression, and estimating breast milk adequacy by measuring the rate of growth of an exclusively breast-fed infant. Each of these methods has limitations. Because both test- weighing and expression interfere with the normal mode of feeding, their use can unintentionally influence milk production. In a solely breast-fed infant, adequate maternal milk output is required for optimal infant growth, but other factors beside food, especially the health status of the infant, also have important influences. Estimating the nutrient composition of the milk is also difficult for several reasons: in addition to differences attributable to normal variation between healthy women, nutrient content also varies over the course of lactation, through- out the day, between breasts, and within a feed. Thus, an ideal sample would contain all milk produced within a 24 hour period. Since it is invasive and logistically difficult to obtain 24 hour milk samples, many studies of breast milk quality are based on more limited collections, and this may explain the substantial variability in reported nutrient values. Currently, infant test-weighing has been the most commonly used method for estimating human milk production. However, the deuterium dilution technique, which estimates infant fluid consumption by administering a stable isotope and measuring its content in infant saliva, is most promising for large field studies because it does not interfere with the feeding process, demands little maternal cooperation, and provides accurate estimates of intake(Vio *et al.*, 1986).

Even when the measurement of milk samples is reasonably accurate, determining the actual influence of maternal nutrition is difficult, because the production of breast milk is extremely sensitive to other factors. The infant's size, health status and activity determines the frequency and length of feeding, strength of sucking and appetite, which are vital stimulants to milk production. The timing of introduction, type and amount of supplementary foods consumed by the infant are also important, as are maternal emotional state and physical health, which can influence both milk production and let-down, (Delgado, 1983). These variables are so inter- related that attempts to determine the individual effect of one factor are almost impossible.

The Effect of a Nutritional Insult May be Based on Its Timing

Studies that attempt to relate undernutrition to reproductive performance must consider the timing and intensity of the nutritional insult on fertility, pregnancy outcome or breast milk production. For example, since organogenesis occurs during the first trimester of pregnancy, any dietary effect on fetal congenital anomalies would be related to maternal dietary intake or nutrient stores prior to pregnancy or soon after conception. It has been suggested that adequate increases in blood volume, protein tissue and maternal fat stores are required during the first half of pregnancy to ensure fetal growth later in pregnancy, and these parameters have been shown to be limited by undernutrition in human pregnancy (Winick, 1986). Most observational studies have been based on simply one measurement of nutritional status, and many intervention studies have provided supplements only during a specific period of pregnancy. Yet, the importance of the timing of a nutritional insult on pregnancy outcome is illustrated by data from the Dutch famine, which occurred for six months during the Second World War (Stein *et al.*, 1975). Although the Dutch population was considered well-nourished prior to the famine, shortly after its onset the number of births decreased. An increase in the incidence of preterm birth, still-birth, early neonatal death and congenital anomalies was associated with exposure to the famine at conception or early in pregnancy, while fetal growth retardation was increased in pregnancies which were conceived prior to the famine but exposed to under-nutrition later in gestation. The possible importance of timing is also illustrated by the results of a study which showed that birth weight was significantly increased in a group of women who were provided with nutritional supplements before and during pregnancy, compared to those who were supplemented only during pregnancy (Caan, 1987).

The Effect of a Nutritional Insult may be Based on Its Severity

Mild or chronic undernutrition is often characterized by low but stable body weight and relatively normal biochemical measures of most nutrients, despite dietary intake below that recommended to meet theoretical nutritional requirements. Severe or acute malnutrition, resulting from extreme nutritional deprivation, is usually accompanied by extremely low weight-for-height, muscle wasting, and abnormal biochemical values for iron, protein and other nutrients. Mild undernutrition is common in many developing countries and among disadvantaged subgroups of developed societies, while severe or acute undernutrition occurs less frequently, often in association with famine or with anorexia nervosa. The influence of acute undernutrition on reproductive outcome is much more dramatic and easier to detect in research studies than the influence of chronic malnutrition.

It Is Difficult to Interpret the Independent Role of Nutrition

Because numerous genetic, social, cultural, and economic factors inter-relate and influence human reproductive performance, it is difficult to isolate the independent effect of maternal nutrition. For example, women who are poor tend to be shorter, weigh less, eat less, work harder and suffer from more infections than those who are economically advantaged. Even if nutrition plays an important role in fetal growth or lactation, simply improving the diet may not compensate for the other factors. The same thing could be said about intervention on other factors, but not diet. Interpreting studies is also challenging because of the many methodological issues previously described.

It is also essential to remember that demonstrating an independent association does not prove that the factor of interest actually caused the observed outcome. For example, a low breast milk output may be associated with infant growth retardation, but one must question whether the low volume is causing slow growth in a small infant, or the infant's low demand is causing the smaller output?

MATERNAL UNDERNUTRITION AND BIRTH WEIGHT (LBW)

In 1982, 16% (20 million) of the 122 million live births world-wide were LBW, and 90% occurred in developing countries, with the highest incidence in Asia and Africa, and the lowest in North America and Europe (World Health Organization, 1982). LBW can result from shortened gestation,

Table II. Incidence of LBW (≤2500 gm) in developing and developed areas			
	Developing countries	Developed countries	Risk ratio
No. populations studied	25	11	
Total LBW (average)	23.63%	5.90%	4.0
IUGR-LBW (average)	16.97%	2.57%	6.6
Preterm LBW (average)	6.66%	3.32%	2.0
Source: Villar and Belizan, 1982.			

retarded intrauterine growth, or both. Preterm birth is usually defined as less than 37 completed weeks gestation. Intrauterine growth retardation (IUGR) is commonly defined as a birth weight of less than 2500 grams with a gestational age of 37 weeks or birthweight less than the 10th percentile for gestational age. Discrimination of the type of LBW is important if clues to its etiology are to be identified.

A recent study estimated the proportion of LBW attributable to preterm birth or IUGR by examining available data on both birthweight and gestational age in 11 developed countries and 25 developing countries (Villar and Belizan, 1982) (Table II). Overall, although LBW was four times more likely to occur in developing than developed countries, the incidence of preterm birth (5-7%) tended to be stable across all the populations. The authors concluded that when the overall incidence of LBW was higher than 10%, the increase could be attributed to IUGR low birth weight. The incidence of IUGR was 6.6 times higher in developing than in developed countries.

Maternal nutritional factors that have been linked with low birth weight are stature, prepregnancy weight or weight-for-height, weight gain during pregnancy, other anthropometric values, and dietary deficiencies of energy, protein, and vitamin and minerals. Each of these factors are briefly reviewed below.

Maternal Stature

There is general agreement that a positive relationship exists between maternal height and mean birth weight; most of the evidence suggests that maternal short stature is associated with an increased risk of IUGR rather than preterm birth (Anderson et al., 1984; Kramer, 1987a; Kramer, 1987b; Villar, 1986). It has also been demonstrated that among marginally nourished mothers, a low maternal head circumference predicted IUGR but not preterm low birthweight (Villar et al., 1986). Although factors such as genetics and health history also influence skeletal size, low maternal height and head circumference may reflect maternal stunting secondary to undernutrition during childhood.

Maternal Prepregnancy Weight and Body Mass

A positive and significant relationship between maternal prepregnancy weight or prepregnancy weight-for-height (body mass index) and fetal size has been repeatedly observed in both well-nourished and poorly-nourished populations (Abrams and Laros, 1986; Brown *et al.*, 1981; Committee to Study the Prevention of Low Birth Weight, 1985; Eastman and Jackson, 1968; Edwards *et al.*, 1979; Kleinman and Madans, 1985; Kramer, 1987a; Kramer, 1987b; Niswander *et al.*, 1969; Taffel, 1986; Villar and Belizan, 1982). The highest risk of delivering a low birth weight infant has been observed among women who begin pregnancy with a low weight-for-height, or simply a low prepregnancy weight. This risk appears to relate to both IUGR low birth weight, and to preterm low birth weight, although the data for IUGR are more consistent.

Weight Gain During Pregnancy

Although an average pregnancy weight gain of 12.5 kg has been proposed as optimal, women in developing countries have been reported to gain an average of between 3 and 7 kg. (Subcommittee on Maternal and Infant Nutrition in Developing Countries, 1983; Collaborative Research Support Program, 1988). A recent series of studies in five countries (Scotland, the Netherlands, Thailand,the Philippines and the Gambia) estimated that although the absolute mean maternal weight gain during pregnancy was lower in the less developed compared to more developed countries, (7-9 kg compared to 10-12 kg), when weight gain was expressed as a proportion of mean maternal prepregnancy weight, women in Scotland, the Netherlands, Thailand and the Philippines gained a similar proportion of their pregravid weight, while women from the Gambia gained somewhat less (Durnin 1987).

A strong association between maternal weight gain and birth weight has been consistently reported, with low mean birth weights and a higher incidence of low birth weight associated with low gestational weight gains (Abrams and Laros, 1986; Anderson *et al.*, 1984; Committee to Study the Prevention of Low Birth Weight, 1985; Eastman and Jackson, 1968; Hytten and Chamberlain, 1980; Kramer, 1987a; Kramer, 1987b; Niswander *et al.*, 1969; Rosso, 1985; Taffel, 1986). Most of the evidence relates pregnancy weight gain to term births; weight gain (adjusted for gestational age) may also be associated with preterm birth, but only limited data address this issue (Hediger, *et al.*, 1989, Abrams, *et al.*, 1989, Berkowitz, 1981; Papiernik *et al.*,

1974; Van den Berg and Oechsli, 1984). Some factors seem to modify the influence of weight gain on birthweight. Underweight women with a low gestational weight gain are at highest risk of delivering a low birth weight infant, and this risk decreases with increasing weight gain (Brown *et al.*, 1981; Edwards *et al.*, 1979). Although a linear relationship between maternal weight gain and birth weight has been observed for all categories of maternal body mass, as prepregnancy body mass increases, the influence of gestational weight gain appears to become less important (Abrams and Laros, 1986; Anderson *et al.*, 1984; Eastman and Jackson, 1968; Hytten and Chamberlain, 1980; Kramer, 1987a; Kramer, 1987b; Niswander *et al.*, 1969; Rosso, 1985; Taffel, 1986). Rosso (Rosso 1985) has proposed that optimal fetal growth can be expected when women reach at least 120% of their ideal pregravid weight for height at term. The practical application of this theory would imply that as weight-for-height decreases, proportionately more weight gain during pregnancy would be required to support fetal growth.

There is some evidence that adolescents may also need more weight gain during pregnancy. If an adolescent mother is not yet fully grown, her own nutrient requirements may compete with those of her fetus (Frisancho *et al.*, 1983; Frisancho *et al.*, 1985; Naeye, 1981). Thus it has been proposed that adolescents may require more nutrients than mature women to produce similar size infants. In a recent study of 696 adolescents, as gestational weight gain increased from less than 9 kg to more than 20 kg, the risk of low birth weight at term decreased 86% (Scholl *et al.*, 1988). Both the total amount and pattern of gestational weight gain may differ in adolescents when compared to mature women (Meserole *et al.*, 1984).

Other Maternal Anthropometric Values

Compared to the large amount of data on prepregnancy weight and gestational weight change, relatively few studies have assessed the relationship between other aspects of maternal body composition and pregnancy outcome. Potentially relevant measures of body composition include maternal arm circumference and skinfolds. Arm circumference can be used to estimate muscle mass or protein reserves, and allow assessment of mild versus severe malnutrition. Skin folds estimate subcutaneous fat. A combination of the arm circumference and triceps skinfold measurements is required to assess fat and lean tissue reserves. Both methods have methodological and practical limitations, especially during pregnancy.

Longitudinal studies suggest that skinfold measurements increase during the first three quarters of pregnancy, and then tend to stabilize or diminish (Pipe *et al.*, 1979; Taggart *et al.*, 1969). Changes in skinfolds appear to depend on prepregnancy fatness, parity, and the specific site of measurement. Data from Guatemala suggest that a maternal arm circumference of less than 21.4 cm was significantly associated with a doubled risk of preterm low birth weight, and a 1.8 times increased risk of intrauterine growth retardation (Villar *et al.*, 1986). Another study of poorly nourished pregnant Guatemalan women indicated that a maternal arm circumference measurement of less than 23.5 cm at any point in pregnancy was associated with increased risk of delivering a LBW infant (Lechtig, 1988). However, other maternal parameters, including fundal growth (uterine height for gestational age), and maternal weight gain adjusted for weight-for-height, were better predictors of LBW. A recent comparison of skin folds and arm circumference data in 100 U.S. adolescents suggested that normal birth weight was associated with increased skin folds and arm circumference, suggesting fat deposition during pregnancy, while those who delivered low birth weight infants either deposited no fat during pregnancy, or showed evidence of mobilizing body fat, presumably to meet the needs of the growing fetus (Maso *et al.* 1988).

Other data suggest that the relationship between maternal fat stores and fetal growth may not be a simple one. A study conducted in Senegal, West Africa, found that after controlling for a variety of factors, maternal triceps skinfolds measured shortly after birth were negatively correlated with birth weight, suggesting that the fattest women gave birth to the smallest infants (Briend, 1985). Based on these findings, the author hypothesized that maternal lean body mass, rather than maternal fat stores, was associated with fetal growth. Several other studies have reached similar conclusions (Frisancho *et al.*, 1977; Langhoff-Roos *et al.*, 1987).

Dietary Energy Deficiency

Energy requirements increase during pregnancy, and when the diet does not provide adequate calories, the metabolism and utilization of other nutrients is affected. For example, if energy needs are not met, dietary protein will be utilized for energy, rather than for tissue synthesis. A variety of factors, including maternal size, pregravid maternal energy stores, and maternal physical activity make energy requirements particularly difficult to study. The cumulative extra cost of pregnancy has been estimated to be about 85,000 kcal (Hytten and Chamberlain, 1980). However, results of the recent Five Country Study, which used standard methods to study energy balance in pregnant women in Scotland, the Netherlands, Thailand, the Philippines and the Gambia, suggest that the energy cost of pregnancy was lower (Durnin 1987).

Despite various methodological problems, the best data on the relationship between dietary intake and birth weight come from experimental supplemental feeding trials. In a study in Guatemala, for example, women who consumed more than 20,000 supplemental kcal delivered infants more than 100 grams heavier than those who consumed less than 20,000 kcal; this was accompanied by a decrease in the incidence of low birth weight (Lechtig *et al.*, 1975). An effect on gestational age with supplementation was also reported (Delgado *et al.*, 1982). In a randomized controlled trial in undernourished Colombian women, supplementation during the third trimester produced a significant (95g) increase in birth weight associated with increased energy intake for male children only (Mora, 1979). When the most underweight women were analyzed separately, birth weight increased 181 g. Women in the Gambia who were given an high-energy supplement during pregnancy showed a highly significant (225g) increase in birth weight, but only when the supplement was provided during the wet season when they experienced negative energy balance resulting from a combination of heavy work and limited food intake (Prentice, 1987). Maternal energy supplementation has also been associated with increased mean birth weight among marginally nourished women in India (Bhatnagar, 1983; Iyenger, 1967), Thailand (Tontisirin, 1987) and Chile (Mardones-Santander *et al.*, 1988). Supplementation has not been significantly related to birth weight in trials among women living in developed countries (Adams *et al.*, 1978; Rush *et al.*, 1980; Veigas, 1982), and the influence on mean birth weight, when significant, averages about 50 grams (Rush, 1981; Rush, 1982). Studies on the Women Infants and Children Special Supplemental Feeding Program (WIC) suggest that the program consistently increases mean birth weight by 30-60 grams and decreases low birth weight 1-2% (Rush, 1988). Taken as a whole, the data suggest that maternal energy supplementation is associated with increased mean birth weight, presumably though enhanced fetal growth rather than through an effect on gestational age. The greatest benefits of supplementation appear to occur among the most undernourished women. Based on published data, Kramer estimated that the influence of maternal dietary energy on birth weight for undernourished women was 99.7g/100 kcal supplement per day compared to only 34.6 g/100 kcal supplement per day for women who were considered adequately nourished, and every 100 kcal of supplement per day could decrease the risk of IUGR by almost half in undernourished women, but by only about 20% in well nourished women (Kramer 1987a).

Dietary Protein Deficiency

Dietary protein provides increased nitrogen and amino acids required for maternal and fetal tissue synthesis. There is little evidence that protein supplementation improves either gestational age or fetal growth (Lechtig *et al.*, 1975; Zlatnik, 1983). There is, however, some evidence that an excessive concentration of protein in the diet may decrease intrauterine growth (Kramer, 1987a; Rush, 1982).

Vitamin and Mineral Deficiencies

Iron

In 1979, WHO estimated that more than 60% of pregnant women in developing countries had hemoglobin concentrations indicative of iron deficiency anemia (World Health Organization, 1979). Another study estimated that the incidence of anemia ranged from 5% to 15% in the United States and 20 to 80% in other countries (Bothwell, 1981). Additional iron is required during pregnancy to allow expansion of maternal red blood cell mass, for the development of the placenta, and other supportive tissues, and for transfer to the fetus. Some of this increased requirement can be met by iron conserved due to the cessation of menstrual losses, and improved dietary iron absorption. When women begin pregnancy with poor iron stores, however, it is difficult to meet these increased requirements, especially if the major dietary sources of iron are vegetable foods which are poorly absorbed. Anemia is even more probable if the mother suffers from parasitic infections. Two large epidemiologic studies in developed countries have examined the relationship between hemoglobin/hematocrit levels before 24 weeks gestation, and both have reported that an increased incidence of low birth weight, preterm birth and perinatal death was associated with both low (< 10 g/dl) and high (> 13 g/dl) hematocrit levels (Garn *et al.*, 1981; Murphy, 1986), with low values probably representing iron deficiency, and with high values probably reflecting abnormalities in maternal blood volume expansion. Since the process of hemodilution is associated with a decrease in hemoglobin/hematocrit values during the first two trimesters, and then a gradual increase as women approach term, studies that use hematocrits recorded at delivery may be confounded by the relationship between hematocrit and gestational age. Kramer concluded that the available data were unsatisfactory to determine whether supplementation with iron could benefit birth weight in countries with a high prevalence of iron deficiency anemia (Kramer, 1987a).

Aside from iron, little is known about the relationship between specific vitamin or mineral deficiencies and birth weight in human pregnancy.

Zinc

Some studies suggest an association between maternal zinc status and fetal growth; others, including clinical trials of zinc supplementation, do not (Kramer, 1987a; Solomons et al., 1986; Winick, 1986).

Folate

Fetal growth retardation can result from maternal megaloblastic anemia (Lillie, 1962). The incidence of low birth weight decreased by 50% with daily supplementation of 500 μg of folate in studies conducted in India (Iyengar and Rajalakshmi, 1975) and among South African Bantus (Baumslag et al., 1970). In the South African study, supplementation had no effect on a population with better nutrition.

Vitamin A

Although it has been reported that maternal vitamin A status might relate to both fetal growth and gestational age (Shah, 1984) there is little evidence for effects on fetal birth weight despite relatively widespread deficiency of vitamin A in the developing world.

Vitamin C

Low serum levels of vitamin C or low intake (<20 mg/day) have been associated with increased risk of preterm birth (Wideman et al., 1964).

Other Vitamins and Minerals

Kramer found little evidence that other nutrients, including calcium, phosphorus, vitamin D, vitamin B-12, Copper, vitamin B-6 or other vitamins and minerals were associated with fetal growth or gestational age (Kramer, 1987a). Routine supplementation of the diet of women in developed countries with vitamin-mineral supplements have not been shown to improve dramatically either fetal growth or gestational age (Hemminki, 1982).

MATERNAL UNDERNUTRITION AND CONGENITAL ANOMALIES

Evidence from animal studies suggests a link between both undernutrition and over-nutrition of specific nutrients with various congenital anomalies (Hurley, 1980; Worthington-Roberts et al., 1985; Sellar, 1987), but because studies in humans are difficult to conduct, only limited and conflicting data are available. The theory that maternal folate deficiency is associated with neural tube defects (Smithells, 1985) has been more intensively studied recently; two reports suggest that use of multivitamin supplements prior to conception was associated with a significant decrease in the risk of these birth defects (Milunsky et al., 1989; Mulinare et al., 1988), while a third found no association (Mills and Jelliffe, 1989). Studies of pregnancies complicated by acrodermatitis enteropathica, an inborn error of zinc metabolism, provide evidence that zinc deficiency increases fetal wastage and congenital anomalies (Hambidge, 1985). Goiter results from either an iodine deficient diet or presence of excessive quantities of goitrogens in certain types of cassava or cabbages which form the basis of local diets in some parts of the world (Williams et al., 1985). As many as 800 million people in the developing world are at risk (Editorial, 1986). Iodine deficiency can produce endemic cretinism, which is associated with mental retardation, deafness and stunted growth. Supplementation with iodine prenatally through fortification of salt or other foods can decrease the risk of this disorder. The recent popularity in the US and Europe of vitamin A analogues to treat acne has increased understanding that excessive doses of vitamin A can act as a teratogen, producing spontaneous abortion, facial abnormalities and other problems (Lammer et al., 1985).

MATERNAL UNDERNUTRITION AND PREGNANCY COMPLICATIONS

It is generally believed that in areas where acute or chronic undernutrition is prevalent, improved nutrition in women would reduce the morbidity and mortality associated with infectious disease and pregnancy complications (Hamilton et al., 1984). However, very little is actually known about the relationship between maternal undernutrition and maternal morbidity and mortality. Some of the studies linking poor maternal nutrition and other complications in the human mother or infant are summarized below.

In a large study of 144,000 Missouri births delivered between 1978 and 1979, underweight (< 90% ideal weight for height prior to pregnancy) women were at significantly higher risk of antepartum hemorrhage, premature rupture of the membranes, and preterm delivery (Schramm, 1981). Compared to women of average weight, the neonatal death rate was significantly elevated in underweight white, but not nonwhite women. The incidence of anemia and infection was also elevated, though not significantly, in the underweight women. In this study, overweight women were also at higher risk of complications. In a smaller US study, underweight pregnant women had significantly higher rates of cardiac-respiratory problems, anemia, premature rupture of the membranes and endometritis (Edwards *et al.*, 1979).

Several hypotheses exist linking maternal nutrient deficiencies with complications of pregnancy, but too few studies have been conducted to provide a clear view of these relationships. Some, but not all, studies have linked low maternal zinc levels with pregnancy-induced hypertension, amniotic fluid infections, and labor abnormalities (Lazebnik *et al.*, 1988; Solomons *et al.*, 1986, Hunt *et al.*, 1985). It has also been theorized, but not directly proved, that low maternal calcium intake may increase the risk of pregnancy-induced hypertension, and that prenatal calcium supplementation might reduce its incidence (Belizan *et al.*, 1988). Lower serum levels of vitamins A, B-6, and thiamin have been reported in women with pregnancy-induced hypertension, but results are not consistent (van den Berg, 1988). There is little evidence in humans that protein intake is associated with pregnancy-induced hypertension (Zlatnik and Burmeister, 1983). Folate deficiency has been firmly associated with increased risk of megaloblastic anemia, and there are also data suggesting links with toxemia, spontaneous abortions and antepartum hemorrhage (Hibbard, 1975; Iyengar and Rajalakshmi, 1975), although other studies have not confirmed this (Giles, 1966; Scott and Usher, 1966, Prichard, 1970). It has been estimated that megaloblastic anemia develops during pregnancy in 1-5% of women in developed countries, and rates as high as 50% have been reported in developing countries (van den Berg, 1988). Various maternal vitamin deficiencies have also been associated with abrupto placenta (vitamin A, E, C, folacin), hyperemesis (vitamin B-6, thiamin), impaired glucose tolerance (vitamin B-6), maternal depression (vitamin B-6) and low infant Apgar scores (vitamin B-6) (van den Berg, 1988), but the data are extremely limited.

MATERNAL UNDERNUTRITION DURING PREGNANCY AND INFANT HEALTH

Data on the impact of maternal deficiency during pregnancy on infant health are also limited. Winick has described the impact of severe maternal deficiencies of individual nutrients on human infant health (Winick, 1986). Thiamine deficiency, which still occurs in some developing countries where rice is the main staple food, can result in an increased incidence of infantile beri-beri, even when there are no clinical signs of deficiency in the mother. Although pernicious anemia is rare, low biochemical measures of vitamin B_{12} have been seen early in life among infants of women who had followed vegan (no animal protein) diets for an extended period. Reduced fetal bone density, neonatal hypocalcemia and even fetal rickets have been associated with maternal deficiencies of vitamin D and calcium, usually the result of a deficient diet combined with lack of exposure to sunlight. The fetus can be affected even if the mother shows no clinical signs of deficiency, but this can be prevented or treated through supplementation. Infants of iron deficient mothers may require supplementation with iron after birth to reduce the chance of developing iron deficiency.

MATERNAL UNDERNUTRITION AND LONGTERM MATERNAL HEALTH

By emphasizing fetal well being through studies of birth weight, and infant well-being through studies on breast-feeding performance, most research studies of maternal nutritional status have failed to describe the long term impact of maternal undernutrition on the mother. Maternal depletion syndrome can result from the combination of repeated pregnancies and lactation, infection, and hard work unrelated necessarily with inadequate nutrition (Williams *et al.*, 1985). Although maternal depletion has been said to increase the risk of goiter, osteomalacia, anemia, fatigue, infection and, potentially, long term morbidity and early mortality, few studies have described its epidemiology.

MATERNAL UNDERNUTRITION AND BREAST MILK VOLUME

Women can still produce breast milk even under extremely difficult circumstances. Lactation continued during the Dutch famine, and although the volume of milk was slightly decreased, its chemical composition was reported to be normal (Smith, 1941). Studies suggest that exclusively breast-fed infants of adequate birth weight grow in a similar manner in developed and developing countries (Seward and Serdula, 1984). Growth was actually slightly more rapid in infants from developing compared to developed countries during the first three months, but somewhat slower from months four through six. It has been pointed out that breast milk output in both developed and developing countries does not meet theoretical energy requirements of 3 month old infants, yet in many studies infants have grown adequately beyond that time (World Health Organization, 1985). The quantity of breast milk produced in the Gambia during the dry season is similar to that of well-nourished mothers in England, even Gambian maternal energy intakes are much lower than currently recommended (Prentice, 1984).

There is also evidence that poor maternal nutrition negatively affects the quantity of milk produced. Although growth of breast-fed infants during the first three months tends to be excellent in developing countries, the slower rate from four to six months is considered to be growth faltering by some researchers. Studies of breast milk output during the first six months suggest an average output of 600-900 ml per day in developed countries compared to 400 to 700 ml/day in developed countries (Jelliffe and Jelliffe, 1978; Whitehead, 1983). This difference of 100-200 ml may be due to better maternal nutrition, but other possible explanations include measurement variation, infant birth weight (presumably better nourished women deliver larger infants who in turn demand more milk), or the possibility that women who exclusively breast-feed in developed countries are a relatively select group that may be more motivated and better milk "producers" than average.

Several studies have compared milk volume by nutritional status among women within the same developing country. It has been reported that the breastmilk output of well nourished Egyptian women was 922 ml/day, compared to only 733 ml/day among women who were considered clinically malnourished (Hanafy et al., 1972). A similar difference of approximately 200 ml/day was observed between well-nourished and poorly nourished women in New Guinea (Bailey, 1965). A survey of well-nourished British women indicated that "successful" breast-feeders increased their energy intakes during lactation while "unsuccessful" mothers did not, and an immediate reduction in milk supply was noted by women who attempted weight-reduction diets (Whichelow, 1975; Whichelow, 1976).

In a study of 130 pregnant and lactating Gambian mothers, Prentice found that during the dry season, dietary intake among lactating women averaged 1650-1700 kcal per day, and this was associated with maternal weight gain, some repletion of fat stores, and an average breast milk output of 850 ml/24 hours (Prentice et al., 1980). During the wet season, when agricultural work was heavy and food intake decreased to 1200-1300 kcal/day, maternal weight loss and depletion of fat stores was observed, and average milk output was 550 ml/day. This 40% decrease in milk output supports the concept that when maternal energy is very low, lactational performance is compromised. A similar seasonal influence was observed among very poorly nourished women in Zaire (World Health Organization, 1985).

There is also some evidence that maternal fat stores resulting from adequate nutrition during pregnancy influence lactational performance. A study of 30 nursing Gambian women during the last trimester of pregnancy and during the first 3 months of lactation, suggested a complex relationship between maternal energy intake and milk output (Paul et al., 1979). In this report, although the women worked harder, ate less and lost weight during the wet season, breast milk output was higher (320-600 ml/12 hours) than during the more abundant dry season (200-410 ml/12 hours) when the women consumed more energy and gained weight. Milk production was negatively and significantly correlated with maternal skinfold thickness. It was hypothesized that if during pregnancy women were unable to store fat required later for milk production, ingested energy during the lactational period might be used to replenish maternal fat stores rather than to produce breast milk.

Additional data from the Gambia also suggest that parity influences milk production (Whitehead, 1978). Among primiparous mothers, breast milk production increased for 9 months postpartum, but among the highest parity mothers, maximum breast milk production was observed at about 3 months. The investigators suggested that repeated pregnancies may have induced nutritional depletion in these women who were already malnourished, and this may in turn have reduced their capacity to produce adequate supplies of milk. The WHO Collaborative Study of Breast-feeding used a cross-sectional study design and standard methods of data collection to assess breast-feeding performance in mother-infant pairs of different ages and levels of income in Guatamala, Hungary, the Philippines, Sweden and Zaire (WHO Collaborative Study on Breastfeeding, 1985). Although attempts were made to include women of higher and lower socioeconomic status in the various countries, influences of maternal nutritional status were only observed in the poorest group in Zaire, where malnutrition was the most severe. In that group of nursing mothers, both low maternal weight-for height (body mass <18) and very low (<30 g/l) serum albumin values were associated with significantly lower breast milk outputs. Such low albumin levels were not observed in the other study groups. Unlike the observations in other countries, maternal weight-for-height did not decrease with longer lactation, suggesting that the Zaire sample did not mobilize fat stores to subsidize lactation.

Earlier studies in Zaire have suggested that exceptionally low intake of protein in the diet, producing primary protein deficiency, was associated with very low outputs of breast milk (Coward, 1984).

Intervention trials have been conducted to attempt to increase breast milk output by feeding the mother. As described in the earlier section on Research Complexities, such experiments are difficult to perform. Major problems in comparing studies include differences in maternal nutritional status (in some cases women were already producing adequate quantities of milk without supplementation), in the composition, amount and timing of the supplementation, and in provision of supplements to the infant, either intentionally or nonintentionally. The results of several of these trials are described below.

Increased protein intake in a small number of hospitalized, Nigerian women was associated with an increase in both measured milk output and infant growth (Edozian et al., 1976). Both milk output and infant growth increased (although the milk appeared to become more dilute) in a study of poorly nourished Mexican women who were given 300 supplementary kcal per day during pregnancy and lactation (Chavez *et al.*, 1975). However, other studies have not demonstrated important effects of supplementation on breast milk output (Whitehead, 1983; WHO Collaborative Study on Breastfeeding, 1985). In a recent study in the Gambia supplements of about 700 kcal per day were provided to lactating women, and although increased maternal weight gain was observed, no consistent improvement in breast milk output was observed (Prentice *et al.*, 1981). There was, however, some qualitative evidence that supplementation may have affected maternal health and work capacity (Coward, 1984). Additional research is needed to assess adequately the influence of maternal supplementation on breast milk output.

MATERNAL UNDERNUTRITION AND THE COMPOSITION OF BREAST MILK

Detailed reviews describing the influence of maternal nutrition on the nutrient content of breast milk are available (American Academy of Pediatrics Committee on Nutrition, 1981; Jelliffe and Jelliffe, 1978; Lonnerdal, 1986; Whitehead, 1983; WHO Collaborative Study on Breastfeeding, 1985). Although interpretation of the data and conclusions regarding individual nutrients vary somewhat from review to review, the following generalizations about the relationship between maternal diet and breast milk composition can be made:

The energy, protein, fat and lactose concentration of breast milk is relatively insensitive to diet and maternal nutritional status, but lower levels of protein in the milk of severely undernourished women have been reported, and there is some evidence that protein supplementation of maternal diet can increase the protein content of breast milk. The lipid content of milk is of interest because fat provides a concentrated source of calories, as well as fat-soluble vitamins and essential fatty acids. The data linking maternal undernutrition with the concentration of fat in breast milk is conflicting, with some studies suggesting that poorly nourished women produce milk with less fat, and some finding no difference between underprivileged and well nourished mothers. Differences in results may reflect diurnal variations, differences in timing of collection or differences in analytic methods. Maternal diet does appear to influence the fatty acid composition of breast milk. When the mother is well nourished, the fatty acid composition of her milk reflects her diet, but when she is not in energy balance, the lipid content reflects her subcutaneous fat stores. Cholesterol content in human milk is not influenced by maternal dietary intake. The water soluble vitamin content of breast milk is quite sensitive to maternal intake, and low levels of all water soluble vitamins have been observed in poorly nourished women. Recent data from the Gambia indicated that levels of most of the B vitamins in milk were reduced during the wet season, when dietary intake decreased. Likewise, supplementation with thiamin, riboflavin, niacin and vitamin C improved breast milk content of these nutrients among the poorly nourished women (Prentice *et al.*, 1982). Studies from other undernourished populations also suggest low levels of water soluble vitamins in the milk of poorly nourished women, and an improvement in milk concentration when vitamin supplements were provided.

Fewer studies have addressed the relationship between maternal diet and fat soluble vitamins, and results are not always consistent, but there is evidence that seasonal availability of food sources of retinol or beta carotene are related to vitamin A levels in breast milk, and some, but not all of the published evidence suggests that the vitamin A content of milk was significantly higher in better nourished women compared to those who were less privileged. Data on the relationship between vitamins E and D in maternal diet and breast milk content are less available.

There is little evidence that maternal intake or body stores of calcium, phosphorus, iron or zinc influence levels in breast milk. Taken as a whole, the data suggest that, even when maternal nutrition is not optimal, breast milk output tends to be reasonably good in promoting growth in infants during the first 4-6 months after birth. On the other hand, extreme maternal undernutrition decreases breast milk output. Diet supplementation of nursing mothers has sometimes, but not always, improved milk output. Maternal diet influences the levels of fatty acids, and some vitamins; very marginal diets may influence levels of protein, and fat.

MATERNAL UNDERNUTRITION AND LACTATIONAL AMENORRHEA

Results of Studies during World War II indicate that the acute malnutrition resulting from famines in Holland (Smith, 1947) and Leningrad (Antonov, 1947) was accompanied by a dramatic decrease in the number of women who became pregnant, and it is generally accepted that acute malnutrition significantly influences fertility. The influence of chronic malnutrition on fertility is less well understood, although comparisons across and within populations suggest that well-nourished women tend to reach menarche earlier than poorly nourished women (Chowdhury *et al.*, 1977; Tanner, 1968). The onset of menarche has been related to dietary intake (Frisch, 1972), height and/or weight (Chowdhury *et al.*, 1977; Frisch and McArthur, 1974; Hillman *et al.*, 1970; Zacharias *et al.*, 1976). Malnutrition and weight loss of more than 10 to 15% below ideal weight have also been associated with irregular menstrual cycles and more frequent anovulatory cycles. Frisch and McArthur have proposed that a minimal amount of body fat is necessary for the onset and maintenance of fertility, suggesting that the reduction of body fat accompanying periods of food shortages would decrease reproductive capacity, sparing the mother and fetus from severe malnutrition (Frisch and McArthur, 1974). Other studies have failed to confirm this "critical fat" hypothesis (Billewicz et al., 1976; Garn and LaVelle, 1983). Overall, birth rates in areas where chronic malnutrition is prevalent remain high, and a recent review concluded that although moderate malnutrition had a small effect on fecundity, fertility among well-nourished women is only slightly higher than among chronically malnourished women (Bongaarts and Delgado, 1980).

Breast-feeding has an important influence on birth spacing in societies where other means of contraception are inaccessible or unacceptable. It is thought that the contraceptive effect of breast-feeding is mediated at least in part through the hormone prolactin, which, secreted in response to suckling, both stimulates the production of breast milk and inhibits ovulation. Compared to women who do not nurse, those who breast-feed experience a longer period of amenorrhea, more anovulatory cycles and longer intervals between births. The frequency, timing and duration of lactation, as well as the use of supplementary feedings also influence the relationship between breast-feeding and postpartum fertility (Bongaarts and Delgado, 1980; Whitehead, 1983). These factors have not always been controlled for in analyses attempting to study the independent effect of maternal malnutrition on lactational amenorrhea.

Undernutrition, assessed by anthropometric measures of maternal nutritional status, has been associated with a small, but significant increase in the duration of postpartum amenorrhea in some, but not all, studies (Huffman, 1987). Poor maternal dietary intake of energy and protein was associated with decreased fertility in Zaire (Carael, 1980), and data from Mexico suggested that maternal dietary supplementation decreased the length of postpartum amenorrhea (Chavez and Martinez, 1973). These studies, though, are difficult to interpret because of methodological problems related to comparison groups in the Zaire research, and the fact that infants in the Mexico study probably reduced the frequency of nursing secondary to receiving supplementary foods. Maternal dietary supplementation in Guatemala reduced the average length of amenorrhea by less than 2 months (Delgado et al., 1979). A more recent, carefully controlled study conducted in the Gambia found that although dietary supplementation did not improve the yield of breast milk, it was related to both the length of lactational amenorrhea and plasma levels of prolactin (Lunn et al., 1980; Prentice et al., 1980). In this study, 33% of the

supplemented mothers became pregnant again within 18 months, compared to
18% of unsupplemented mothers, suggesting that improved maternal nutrition
in undernourished women may have contributed to a decrease in the duration
of lactational amenorrhea.

CONCLUSION

Research relating maternal undernutrition to pregnancy outcome, lactational performance and fertility is difficult to conduct and interpret. There is
good evidence that maternal nutritional status, reflected by short maternal
stature, low prepregnancy weight, low maternal weight gain during pregnancy, low maternal body stores and deficient energy intake, is associated with
low birth weight. There is also evidence that supplementing the maternal diet
with energy can increase fetal growth; while the effect is small in women who
are not significantly undernourished, results have been dramatic among
women with evidence of poor nutritional status. Although some studies show
effects, the influence of maternal undernutrition and congenital malforma-
tions, pregnancy complications and long-term maternal or fetal health is not
clear. Some studies show that maternal undernutrition during pregnancy or
lactation is associated with decreased milk production and poorer quality
breast milk, but others do not show effects except when maternal nutritional
deficiency is extreme. Improvements in maternal diet through supplementation during lactation have been inconsistent. Poorly nourished women have
been observed to experience longer periods of amenorrhea during lactation,
and there are hints in the literature that in some populations, dietary supplementation at this time might decrease this duration, possibly leading to
shorter inter-pregnancy intervals. However, the data are by no means consistent or well understood, and although undernutrition may influence fertility to
some extent, the effect is not dramatic.

Humans have evolved in ways that allow reproduction against many odds.
Overall, the literature suggests that even when women are undernourished,
their ability to reproduce is, on the whole, maintained. But, women who live
with chronic or acute malnutrition experience poorer health, pregnancy outcome, and lactational performance than women who are well nourished. It has
been proposed that women of reproductive age should begin pregnancy with
good health and dietary intake that allows them to achieve adequate muscle
mass, a minimum of 16-18% body fat, 300-500 mg of iron stores and adequate
stores of other nutrients (Subcommittee on Maternal and Infant Nutrition in
Developing Countries, 1983). Unfortunately, millions of women fall short of
this goal. Although the specific effects of particular nutrient deficiencies on
reproductive performance are still unclear, there is no question that adequate

maternal nutrition before, during and after pregnancy would improve health status and the quality of life for mothers and babies around the world.

ACKNOWLEDGEMENT

The author wishes to thank Gail Woodward for her assistance in preparing this manuscript.

REFERENCES

Abrams, B. and, Laros, R. K.: Prepregnancy Weight, Weight Gain and Birth Weight. *Am. J. Obstet. Gynecol.*, 154:504-509 (1986).

Abrams, B., Newman V., Key, T., and Parker, J.: Maternal Weight Gain and Preterm Delivery. *Obstet. Gynecol.*, 74:577-83 (1989).

Adams, S. O., Barr, G. D., and Huenemann, R.: Effect of nutritional supplementation in pregnancy. *J. Am. Diet Assoc.*, 72:144-147 (1978).

American Academy of Pediatrics Committee on Nutrition: Nutrition and Lactation. *Pediatrics*, 68:435-443 (1981).

Anderson, G. D., Blidner, I. N., McClemont, S., and Sinclair, J. C.: Determinants of Size at Birth in a Canadian Population. *Am. J. Obstet. Gynecol.*, 150:236-244 (1984).

Antonov, A. N.: Children Born during the Siege of Leningrad in 1942. *J. Pediatr.*, 30:250 (1947).

Bailey, K. V.: Quantity and Composition of breast milk in Some New Guinea Populations. *J. Trop. Ped.*, 11:135-149 (1965).

Baumslag N., and Mertz, J.: Reduction of Incidence of Prematurity by Folic Acid Supplementation in Pregnancy. *Br. Med. J.*, 1:16-17 (1970).

Belizan, J. M., Villar, J., and Repke, J.: The Relationship between Calcium Intake and Pregnancy-induced Hypertension: Up-to-date Evidence. *Am. J. Obstet. Gynecol.*, 158:898-902. (1988).

Berkowitz, G. S.: An Epidemiologic Study of Preterm Delivery. *Am. J. Epidemiol.*, 113:81-92 (1981).

Bhatnagar, S., Dharamshaktu, N. S., Sundaram, K. R., and Seth, V.: Effect of Food Supplementation in the Last Trimester of Pregnancy and early Post-natal Period on Maternal Weight and Infant Growth. *Indian J. Med. Res.*, 77:366-372 (1983).

Billewicz, W. Z., Fellowes, H. M., and Hytten, F. A.: Comments on the Critical Metabolic Mass and the Age of Menarche. *Ann. Human Biol.*, 3:51-59 (1976).

Bongaarts, J., and Delgado, H.: Does Malnutrition affect Fecundity? *Science*, 208:564 (1980).

Bothwell, T. H., Charlton, R. W., (Eds.), *International Anemia Consultive Group.Iron Deficiency in Women*. The Nutrition Foundation, Washington, D.C. (1981).

Briend, A.: Do Maternal Energy Reserves Limit Fetal Growth? *Lancet.*, January 5:38-40 (1985).

Brown, J. E., Jacobson, H. N., Askue, L. H., and Peck, M. G.: Influence of Prepregnancy Weight Gain on the Size of Infants Born to Underweight Women. *Obstet. Gynecol.*, 57:13 (1981).

Caan, B., Horgen, D. M., Margen, S., King, J. C., and Jewell, N. P.: Benefits Associated with WIC Supplementation feeding during the Interpregnancy Interval. *Am. J. Clin. Nutr.*, 45:29-41 (1987).

Carael, M. (1980). *Relations Between Birth Intervals and Nutrition in Three Central African Populations (Zaire). Nutrition and Human Reproduction.* New York, Plenum.

Chavez, A. and Martinez, C.: Nutrition and Development of Infants from Poor Rural Areas. III. Maternal Nutrition and its Consequences on Fertility. *Nutr. Rep. Internat.*, 7:1-8 (1973).

Chavez, M., Martinez, C., and Bourges, H.: Role of Lactation in the Nutrition of Low Socioeconomic Groups. *Ecol. Food Nutr.*, 4:159-169 (1975).

Chowdhury, A. K., Huffman, S. L., and Curlin, G. T.: Malnutrition, Menarche and Marriage in Rural Bangladesh. *Soc. Biol.*, 24:316-25 (1977).

Christakis, G.: Nutritional Assessment in Health Programs. *Am. J. Pub. Health.*, 63 (Supplement) (1973).

Collaborative Research Support Program in Egypt, Kenya and Mexico. *Food Intake and Human Function: A Cross Project Perspective.* University of California, Berkeley (1988).

Committee to Study the Prevention of Low Birth Weight, Institute of Medicine: *Preventing Low Birthweight.* Washington, D.C., National Academy Press (1985).

Coward, W. A., Paul, A. A., and Prentice, M.: The Impact of Malnutrition on Human Lactation: Observations from Community Studies. *Fed. Proc.*, 43:2432-2437 (1984).

Delgado, H., Martorell, R., Brtineman, E., and Klein, R. E.: Nutrition and the Length of Gestation. *Nutr. Res.*, 2:117-126 (1982).

Delgado, H., McNeilly, A. S., Hartmann, P. E.: *Non-nutritional Factors Affecting Milk Production. Maternal Diet, Breast-feeding Capacity, and Lactational Infertility.* United Nations, University Tokyo (1983).

Delgado, H., Lechtig, A., Brineman, E., Martorell, R., Yarbrough, C., and Klein, R.: *Nutrition and Birth Interval Components: The Guatemalan Experiences.* Nutrition and Human Reproduction. Plenum, New York (1979).

Durnin, J. V. G. A.: Energy Requirements of Pregnancy: An Integration of the Longitudinal Data from the Five-Country Study. *Lancet*, ii:1131-1133 (1987).

Eastman, N. J., and Jackson, E.: Weight Relationships in Pregnancy. *Obstet. Gynecol. Surv.*, 23:1003-24 (1968).

Editorial: Prevention and Control of Iodine Deficiency Disorders. *Lancet*, ii:433-434 (1986).

Edozian, J. C., Khan, M. A. R., and Waslien, C. L: Human Protein Deficiency: Results of a Nigerian Village Study. *J. Nutr.*, 106:312-328 (1976).

Edwards, L., Alton, I., Bariada, I. M., and Kakanson, Y. E.: Pregnancy in the Underweight Woman. Course, Outcome, and Growth Patterns of the Infants. *Am. J. Obstet. Gynecol.*, 135:297-302 (1979).

Frisancho, A. R., Klayman, J., and Matos, J.: Influence of maternal nutritional status on prenatal growth in a Peruvian urban population. *Am. J. Phys. Anthro.*, 46:265-274 (1977).

Frisancho, A. R., Matos, J., and Flegal, P.: Maternal Nutritional Status and Adolescent Pregnancy Outcome. *Am. J. Clin. Nutr.*, 38:739-746 (1983).

Frisancho, A. R., Matos, J., Leonard, W. R., and Yaroch, L. A.: Developmental and Nutritional Determinants of Pregnancy Outcome Among Teenagers. *Am. J. Phys. Anthro.*, 66:247-261 (1985).

Frisch, R. E.: Weight at Menarche: Similarity for Well-Nourished and Undernourished Girls at Different Ages. *Pediatr.*, 50:445-50 (1972).

Frisch, R. E., and McArthur, J. W.: Menstrual Cycles: Fatness as a Determinant of Minimum Weight for Health Necessary for Their Maintenance and Onset. *Science*, 184:949-51 (1974).

Garn, S. M., Ridella, S.A., Petzold, A. S., Falkner, F.: Maternal Hematological Levels and Pregnancy Outcomes. *Semin. Perinatol.*, 5:155-162 (1981).

Garn, S. M., and LaVelle, M.: Reproductive Histories of Low Weight Girls and Women. *Am. J. Clin. Nutr.*, 37:862-866 (1983).

Giles, C.: An account of 335 Cases of Megaloblastic Anemia of Pregnancy and the Puerperium. *J. Clin. Pathol.*, 19:1 (1966).

Hambridge, K. M: *Trace Minerals and Fetal Development. Feeding the Mother and Infant.* John Wiley and Sons, New York, Inc. (1985).

Hamilton, S., Popkin B.: *Women and Nutrition in Third World Countries.* Praeger Publishers division of Greenwood Press, Inc. Westport, Conn. (1984).

Hanafy, M. M., Morsey, M. R. A., Seddick, Y., Habib, Y. A., and el Lozy, M.: Maternal Nutrition and Lactational Performance. *J. Trop. Ped. and Envir. Health*, 18:187-191 (1972).

Hediger, M. L., Scholl, T. O., Belsky, D. H., Ances I. G., Salmon R. W.: Patterns of weight gain in adolescent pregnancy: Effects on birth weight and preterm delivery. *Obstet. Gynecol.*, 74:6-12 (1989).

Hemminki, E.: *Effects of Routine Haemantinic and Vitamin Administration in Pregnancy. Effectiveness and Satisfaction in Antenatal Care.* Spastics International Medical Publications: William Heinemann Medical Books Ltd. London, (1982).

Hibbard, B. M.: Folates and the Fetus. *S. Afr. Med. J.*, 49:1223-1226 (1975).

Hillman, R. W., and Nelson, M.: Season of Birth, Parental Age, Menarcheal Age and Body Form: Some Interrelationships on Young Women. *Hum. Biol.*, 42:570-80 (1970).

Huffman, S. J.: Risk of Pregnancy Associated with Maternal and Child Nutritional Status. *Int. J. Gynecol. Obstet.*, 25 (supp):57-75 (1987).

Hunt, L, Murphy, N., Cleaver, A., Faraji, M. Swendseid *et al.*: Zinc supplementation during pregnancy in low-income teenagers of Mexican descent: effects on selected blood constituents and on progress and outcome of pregnancy. *Am. J. Clin. Nutr.*, 42:815-828 (1985).

Hurley, L.: *Developmental Nutrition.* Prentice-Hall, Inc. Englewood Cliffs, New Jersey (1980).

Hytten, F. and Chamberlain, G.: *Clinical Physiology in Obstetrics.* Blackwell Scientific Publications. Oxford (1980).

Hytten, F. E. and Leitch, I. *The Physiology of Human Pregnancy.* Blackwell Scientific. Oxford (1971).

Iyengar, L. and Rajalakshmi, K.: Effect of folic acid supplement of birth weights of infants. *Am. J. Obstet. Gynecol.*, 122:322-336 (1975).

Iyenger, L.: Effects of Dietary Supplements Late in Pregnancy on the Expectant Mother and her Newborn. *Indian J. Med. Res.*, 55:85-89 (1967).

Jelliffe, D. B. *The Assessment of Nutritional Status of the Community.* WHO. Geneva (1964).

Jelliffe, D. B., and Jelliffe, E. R. P.: The Volume and Composition of Human Milk in poorly Nourished Communities: A Review. *Am. J. Clin. Nutr.*, 31:492-497 (1978).

King, J. C., Bronstein, M. N., Fitch, W. L., and Weininger, J.: Nutrient Utilization during Pregnancy. *Wld Rev. Nutr. Diet.*, 52:71-142 (1987).

Kleinman, J. and Madans, J. H.: The Effects of Maternal Smoking, Physical Stature, and Educational Attainment on the Incidence of Low Birth Weight. *Am J. Epidemiol.*, 121:843-855 (1985).

Kramer, M. S.: Determinants of Low Birth Weight: Methodological Assessment and Meta-Analysis. *Bull of the WHO*, 65:663-737 (1987a).

Kramer, M. S.: Intrauterine Growth and Gestational Duration Determinants. *Pediatrics*, 80:502-511 (1987b).

Lammer, E., Chen D. T., Hoar R. M.,: Retinoic acid embryopathy. *N Engl. J. Med.*, 313:837-41 (1985).

Langhoff-Roos, J., Lindmark, G., and Gebre-Medhin, M.: Maternal Fat Stores and Fat Accretion during Pregnancy in Relation to Infant Birthweight. *Br. J. Obstet. Gynecol.*, 94:1170-1177 (1987).

Lazebnik, N., Kuhnert, B. R., Kuhert, P. M., Thompson, K. L.: Zinc Status, Pregnancy Complications, and Labor Abnormalities. *Am. J. Obstet. Gynecol.*, 158:161-166 (1988).

Lechtig, A.: Predicting Risk of Delivering Low Birthweight Babies: Which Indicator is Better? *J. Trop. Ped.*, 34:34-41 (1988).

Lechtig A., Delgado, H., Klein, R. E.: Effect of Food Supplementation during Pregnancy on Birthweight. *Pediatr.*, 56:508-20 (1975).

Lillie, E. W.: Obstetrical Aspects of Megaloblastic Anemia. *J. Obstet. Gynecol. Br. Commonw.*, 69:736-40 (1962).

Lonnerdal, B.: Effects of Maternal Dietary Intake on Human Milk Composition. *J. Nutr.*, 116:499-513 (1986).

Lunn, P. G., Prentice, A. M., Austin, S., and Whitehead, R.: Influence of Maternal Diet on Plasma Prolactin Levels during Lactation. *Lancet.*, I:623-625 (1980).

Mardones-Santander, F., Rosso, A., Stekel, E., Ahumada, Llaguno, S., Pizassrro, F., Salina, J., Vial, I., and Walter, T.: The Effect of a Milk-Based Food Supplement on Maternal Nutritional Status and Fetal Growth in Underweight Chilean Women. *Am. J. Clin. Nutr.*, 47:413-419 (1988).

Maso, M. J., Gong, E. J., Jacobson, M. S., Bross, D. S., and Heald, F. P.: Anthropometric Predictors of Low Birth Weight Outcome in Teenage Pregnancy. *J. Adoles. Health. Care,* 9:188-193 (1988).

McCormick, M. C.: The Contribution of Low Birth Weight to Infant Mortality and Childhood Morbidity. *N. Eng. J. Med.*, 312:82-90 (1985).

Meserole, L. P., Worthington-Roberts, B. S., Rees, J. M., and Wright, L. S.: Prenatal Weight Gain and Postpartum Weight Loss Patterns in Adolescents. *J. Adoles. Health Care*, 5:21-27 (1984).

Mills, J. L., Rhoads, G. G., Simpson, J. L., et al. The Absence Of A Relation Between The Periconceptual Use Of Vitamins And Neural Tube Defects. *N. Engl. J. Med.*, 321:430-435 (1989).

Milunsky, A., Jick, H., Jick, S., Bruell, C. L., MacLaughlin D. S., Rothman K., Willett, W.: Multivitamin/Folic Acid Supplementation in Early Pregnancy Reduces the Prevalence of Neural Tube Defects. *JAMA*, 262:2847-52 (1989).

Mora, J. O., de Paredes, B., Wagner, M., de Navarro, L., Suescun, J., Christiansen, N., Herrera, M. G.: Nutritional Supplementation and the Outcome of Pregnancy. 1. Birth Weight. *Am. J. Clin. Nutr.*, 32:455-462 (1979).

Mulinare, J., Cordero J. F., Erickson J. D., Berry, R. J.,: Periconceptual use of multivitamins and the occurrence of neural tube defects. *JAMA*, 260:3141-3145 (1988).

Murphy, J. F., Newcombe, R. G., O'Riordan, J., Coles, E. C.: Relations of Hemoglobin Levels in First and Second Trimesters to the Outcome of Pregnancy. *Lancet*, 992-995 (1986).

Naeye, R. L.: Teenaged and Pre-Teenaged Pregnancies: Consequences of the Fetal-Maternal Competition for Nutrients. *Pediatrics*, 67:146-150 (1981).

Niswander, K. R., Singer, J., Westphal, M., and Weiss, W.: Weight Gain during Pregnancy and Prepregnant Weight. *Obstet. Gynecol.*, 33:492-91 (1969).

Papiernik, E., Kaminiski, M.: Multifactorial Study of the Risk of Prematurity at 32 Weeks Gestation. 1. A study of the Frequency of 30 Predictive Characteristics. *J. Perinat. Med.*, 2:30-36 (1974).

Paul, A. A., Muller, E. M., and Whitehead, R. G.: The Quantitative Effects of Maternal Dietary energy intake on Pregnancy and Lactation in Rural Gambian Women. *Trans. Roy. Soc. Trop. Med. Hyg.*, 73:686 (1979).

Pipe, N. G., Smith, T., Halliday, D., Edmonds, C. J., Williams, C., and Coltart, T. M.: Changes in Fat, Fat-Free Mass and Body Water in Human Normal Pregnancy. *Br. J. Obstet. Gynecol.*, 86:929-40 (1979).

Prentice, A. M. *Adaptations to Long-Term Energy Intake. Energy Intake and Activity.* Alan R. Liss. New York (1984).

Prentice, A. M., Cole, T. J., Foord, F. A., Lamb, W. H., Whitehead, R. G.: Increased Birthweight after Prenatal Dietary Supplementation of Rural African Women. *Am. J. Clin. Nutr.*, 46:912-925 (1987).

Prentice, A. M., Roberts, S. B., Prentice, A., Paul, A. A., Watkinson, M., Watkinson, A. A., and Whitehead, R. G.: Dietary supplementation of lactating gambian women. 1. effect on breast milk volume and quality. *.Hum. Nutr. Clin Nutr.*, 37C:53-64 (1982).

Prentice, A. M., Whitehead, R. G., Roberts, S. B., and Paul, A. A.: Dietary Supplementation of Lactating Gambian Women. *Am. J. Clin. Nutr.*, 34:2790-2799 (1981).

Prentice, A. M., Whitehead, R. G., Roberts, S. B., Paul, A. A., Watkinson, M., Prentice, A., Watkinson, A. A.: Dietary Supplementation of Gambian Nursing Mothers and Lactational Performance. *Lancet.* ii:886-888 (1980a).

Prichard, J. *Anemias Complicating Pregnancy and the Pureperium. Maternal Nutrition and the Course of Pregnancy.* National Academy of Sciences. Washington, D.C. (1970).

Puffer, R. P. and Serrano, C. B. *Patterns of Mortality in Childhood*. PAHO, Washington, D.C. (1973).

Rosso, P.: A New Chart to Monitor Weight Gain during Pregnancy. *Am. J. Clin. Nutr.*, 41:644-52 (1985).

Rush, D.: Maternal Nutrition during Pregnancy in Industrialized Societies. *Am. J. Dis. Child.*, 129:430-433 (1975).

Rush, D.: Nutritional Services during Pregnancy and Birthweight: a Retrospective Matched Pair Analysis. *Can. Med. Assoc. J.*, 125:567-574 (1981).

Rush, D.: Effects of Changes in Protein and Calorie Intake during Pregnancy on the Growth of the Human Fetus. Effectiveness and Satisfaction in Antenatal Care. Spastics International Medical Publications: William Heinemann Medical Books Ltd.London (1982).

Rush, D., Leighton, J., Sloan, N. L., Alvir, J. M., Garbowski, G. C.: Review of Past Studies of WIC. *Am. J. Clin. Nutr.*, 48:394-411 (1988).

Rush, D., Stein, Z., and Susser, M.: A randomized controlled trial of prenatal nutritional supplementation in New York City. *Pediatr.*, 65:683-697 (1980).

Scholl, T. O., Salmon, R. W., Miller, L. K., Vasilenko, P., Furey, C. H., and Christine, M.: Weight Gain during Adolescent Pregnancy: Associated Maternal Characteristics and Effects on Birth Weight. *J. Adolesc. Health Care.*, 9:286-290 (1988).

Schramm, W. J.: *Obesity. Leanness and Pregnancy Outcome*. Missouri Center for Health Statistics, Jefferson City (1981).

Scott, K. E., Usher, R.,: Fetal Malnutrition: Its incidence, causes and effects. *Am. J. Obstet. Gynecol.*, 94:951-63 (1966).

Seller, M. J.: Nutrition Induced Congenital Anomalies. *Proc. Nutr. Soc.* 46:227-235 (1987).

Seward, J., and Serdula, M. K.: Infant feeding and infant growth. *Pediatrics* (supplement) 74:728-762 (1984).

Shah, R. S. and Rajalakshmi, R.: Vitamin A Status of the Newborn in Relation to Gestational Age, Body Weight and Maternal Nutritional Status. *Am. J. Clin. Nutr.*, 40:794-800 (1984).

Smith, C. A.: Effects of Maternal Undernutrition upon Newborn Infants in Holland. *J. Pediatr.*, 30:229-33 (1941).

Smith, C. A.: Effect of Wartime Starvation in Holland on Pregnancy and its Product. *Am. J. Obstet. Gynecol.*, 53:599 (1947).

Smithells, R. W. *Vitamins and Neural Tube Defects. Feeding the Mother and Infant*. John Wiley and Sons. New York (1985).

Solomons, N. W., Helitzer-Allen, D. L., Villar, J.: Zinc Needs during Pregnancy. *Clin. Nutr.*, 5:63-71 (1986).

Stein, A., Susser, M., Saenger, G., and Marolla, F. *Famine and Human Development. The Dutch Hunger Winter of 1944-45*. Oxford University Press New York (1975).

Subcommittee on Maternal and Infant Nutrition in Developing Countries of the Committee on International Nutrition Programs. Maternal and Infant Nutrition in Developing Countries, with Special Reference to Possible Intervention Programmes in the Context of Health. Food and Nutrition Board, Commission on Life Sciences, National Research Council, National Academy of Sciences, Washington, DC (1983).

Taffel, S. *Maternal Weight Gain and the Outcome of Pregnancy*, United States, 1980. Vital and Health Statistics. Public Health Service, U.S. Government Printing Office Washington, D.C. (1986).

Taggart, N. R., Holliday, R. M., Bilewicz, W. Z., Hytten, F. E., and Thomsen, A. M.: Changes in Skinfolds during Pregnancy. *Br. J. Nutr.*, 21:439-451 (1969).

Tanner, J. M.: Early Maturation in Man. *Scientific American*, 218:21-27 (1968).

Tontisirin, K., Booranasubkajorn, U., Hongsumarn, A., Thewtong, D.: Formulation and Evaluation of Supplementary Foods for Thai Pregnant Women. *Am. J. Clin. Nutr.*, 43:931-939 (1987).

Van den Berg, B. J., Oechsli, F. W. *Prematurity. Perinatal Epidemiology*. Oxford University Press New York (1984).

Van den berg, H., Bruinse, H. W.: Vitamin Requirements in Normal Human Pregnancy. *Wld. Rev. Nutr. Diet*, 57:95-125 (1988).

Veigas, O. A. C., Scott, P. H., Cole, T. J., Mansfield, H. N., Wharton, P., Wharton, B. A.: Dietary Protein Energy Supplementation of Pregnant Asian Mothers at Sorrento, Birmingham. I. Unselective during the Second and Third Trimesters. *Br. Med. J.*, 285:589-92 (1982).

Villar, J. M.: Nutritional Factors Associated with Low Birth Weight and Short Gestational Age. *Clin Nutr.*, 5:78-85 (1986).

Villar, J. and Belizan, J. M.: The Relative Contribution of Prematurity and Fetal Growth Retardation to Low Birth Weight in Developing and Developed Societies. *Am. J. Obstet. Gynecol.*, 143:793-798 (1982).

Villar, J., Khoury, M. J., Finucane, F. F., and Delgado, H. L.: Differences in the Epidemiology of Prematurity and Intrauterine Growth Retardation. *Early Hum. Dev.*, 14:307-320 (1986).

Vio, F. R., Infante, C. B., Lara, W. C., Mardones-Santander, F., and Rosso, P. R. Validation of the Deuterium Dilution Technique for the Measurement of Fluid Intake in Infants. *Human Nutr. Clin. Nutr.*, 40C:327-332 (1986).

Whichelow, M. J.: Calorie Requriements for Successful Breast Feeding. *Arch. Dis. Child.*, 50:669-71 (1975).

Whichelow, M. J.: Success and Failure of Breast-feeding in Relation to Energy Intake. *Proc. Nutr. Soc.*, 35:62-63 (A) (1976).

Whitehead, R. J: *Maternal Diet, Breast-feeding Capacity, and Lactational Infertility*. Report to a Joint UNU/WHO Workshop. Tokyo (1983).

Whitehead R.: Factors Influencing Lactation Performance in Rural Gambian Mothers. *Lancet*, 2:178-81 (1978).

WHO Collaborative Study on Breastfeeding. *The Quantity and Quality of Breast Milk*. World Health Organization. Geneva (1985).

Wideman, C. L., Baird, G. H., Bolding O. T.: Ascorbic Acid Deficiency and Premature Rupture of Fetal Membranes. *Am. J. Obstet. Gynecol.*, 88:592 (1964).

Williams, C. D., Baumslag, N., and Jelliffe, D. B.: *Mother and Child Health: Delivering the Services*. Oxford University Press London (1985).

Winick, M.: *Nutrition in Pregnancy*. March of Dimes Defects Foundation. White Plains, New York, (1986).

World Health Organization. *The Prevalence of Nutritional Anemia in Developing Countries*. WHO, Geneva (1979).

World Health Organization: *The incidence of low birth weight:a critical review of available information*. World Health Statistics Quart., 33:197-224 (1980).

World Health Organization: The Incidence of Low Birth Weight: An Update. *Weekly Epidemiol. Record*, 59:201-211 (1984).

World Health Organization. (1985). *The Quantity and Quality of Breast Milk: Report of the WHO Collaborative Study on Breast-feeding*. Geneva, World Health Organization.

Worthington-Roberts, B. and Vermeersch, J. *Physiological Basis of Nutritional Needs. Nutrition in Pregnancy and Lactation*. Times Mirror/Mosby College Publishing. St. Louis, (1985).

Zacharias, L. W., Rand, W. M.: A Study of Sexual Development and Growth in American Girls: The Statistics of Menarche. *Obstet. Gynecol. Surv.*, 31:325-27 (1976).

Zlatnik, F. J., Burmeister, L. F.,: Dietary Protein in Pregnancy: Effect on Anthropometric Indices of the Newborn Infant. *Am. J. Obstet. Gynecol.*, 146:199-203 (1983).

4

Breast-feeding: An International and Historical Review

Joe D. Wray

Center for Population and Family Health
Columbia University
60 Hazen Avenue
New York, New York 10032

BACKGROUND: THE CONTEXT OF BREAST-FEEDING

Introduction

This chapter was prepared in response to an invitation to review "state of the art knowledge of the superiority of breast milk/breast-feeding." It is intended to serve as a link between others in this book that deal in detail with specific aspects of infant and child feeding. The focus in this chapter is on clinical or epidemiological studies that have compared the effects of different types of feeding methods on infants and very young children. These studies need to be considered carefully, in the light of what we know about human lactation and about nutrition in human infants. The chapter therefore begins with some caveats about how we perceive breast-feeding and its effects -- in the context of our biologic evolution; in the context of what we know about the nutrient requirements of the growing infant or young child; in the context of what we know about the immunology of breast milk, as well as the interactions of nutrition and infection; and finally, in the context of the environmental circumstances of the infant and how these interact with the type of feeding.

The caveats are followed by a review of some examples both of historical and of current clinical studies that have examined differences in morbidity and mortality among infants that were breast-fed, partially breast-fed or artificially fed. The purpose is not to scrutinize the methodologic minutiae of those studies, but rather to seek to understand the broader implications of the differences that have been observed in many parts of the world ever since the mid-19th century. There follows a review of current knowledge of the interactions between breast-feeding and fertility and the implications of this interaction for mothers and for children. Finally a brief note on the changing trends in the prevalence and duration of breast-feeding, and on recent studies of the factors that influence or modify those trends, a look at what we have learned about how to influence breast-feeding practices and our knowledge of effective measures to encourage and support breast-feeding, and a note on the policy implications of this knowledge.

The Evolutionary Context

The proposition that breast-feeding is superior can be considered first in the context of evolutionary biology. In evolutionary terms, human beings are viviparous mammals. The live birth of a human infant is the end result of a series of complex and marvelously intricate biological processes; breast-feeding, the biologic process for nourishing the newborn with which we were endowed by our mammalian evolution, is made possible by physiologic processes no less marvelous and intricate than those involved in reproduction. Fortunately for mankind, reproductive processes seldom fail; when there is a failure, we label it infertility and we take desperate measures to find ways to replace this, ranging from adoption, to artificial insemination, to *in vitro* fertilization and implantation, even to surrogate pregnancies. Meanwhile, however, there is never a question or doubt as to whether or not the basic biologic processes of reproduction are satisfactory.

Down through the millennia, lactation, too, has seldom failed, and to this day 97 or 98 percent of all newborns are successfully breast-fed, at least initially, in many human communities (Grant *et al.*, 1989; Baumslag and Putney, 1989; Millman, 1986). When lactation does fail, many alternatives are available. There is, however, a curious difference between our attitudes toward reproductive physiology and toward the physiology of lactation: Though questions are never raised about the adequacy of the biologic processes of reproduction, there are those who raise serious questions as to whether or not the physiologic processes of lactation and the quality of human milk are satisfactory. In spite of the fact that ever since mankind evolved, human milk has been the source of essential nutrients for the overwhelming majority of human beings who were born alive, it is deemed necessary in some quarters even to prove somehow that breast-feeding provides adequate nutrition for the human newborn, much less that it is optimum. The Jelliffes noted some years ago (1978) that,

> "... in the bottle-culture of the present-day Western
> world, differences between the two methods [breast-
> and bottle-feeding], which seem completely self-evi-
> dent and obvious, may not be considered sufficiently
> scientifically exact or mathematically proven. Stran-
> gely, the burden of having to produce proof that dif-
> ferences exist and are significant falls paradoxically
> on those advocating the natural method tested over
> millennia -- that is, breast-feeding." (Jelliffe and Jel-
> liffe, 1978).

The persistence of that mentality was suggested by Thapa *et al.* (1988), when they discussed the conservative recommendations concerning breast-feeding among HIV-positive women and suggested that "Such advice reflects the Western prejudice that *artificial milks are innocent until proven guilty, whereas breast milk is guilty until proven innocent."* (Emphasis added.) That doubt about the "innocence" of breast-feeding remains is apparent from the titles of a number of recent articles: "Birth weight and duration of breast-feeding: Are the beneficial effects of human milk being overestimated?" (Barros *et al.*, 1986); "Studies of breast-feeding and infections. How good is the evidence?" (Bauchner *et al.*, 1986); "Does breastfeeding really save lives, or are apparent benefits due to biases?" (Habicht *et al.*, 1986); "Does breast-feeding protect against infections in infants less than 3 months of age?" (Leventhal *et al.*, 1986). The issues were considered important enough to warrant the appointment of a Task Force on the Assessment of the Scientific Evidence of Problems of Infant Feeding. Its *Report* was published in 1984 as a Supplement to Vol. 74 of *Pediatrics*, and included extensive reviews of the studies of the relation between infant-feeding and infectious illness in industrialized countries (Kovar *et al.*, 1984) and less-developed countries (Jason *et al.*, 1984). The first of these concluded that a protective effect of breast-feeding in industrialized countries "if present, is apparently modest," while the latter review "found the evidence for an important protective effect of breast-feeding against infectious illness to be much stronger. This conclusion was reached despite serious problems in the design of many of the studies reviewed."

The Nutritional Context

In spite of the crucial role of lactation in infant nutrition, a role shaped by human evolution, it is important to recognize explicitly that lactation has physiologic limitations and that expectations must be realistic. The average, reasonably well nourished mother can produce a finite quantity of milk, which contains a variety of nutrients that meet the needs of the growing baby and provides around 70 to 75 calories per 100 ml. If a healthy infant needs a certain amount of nutrients and calories per kilogram of body weight to sustain normal growth, then there will come a point in time when the infant needs more nutrients and calories than the mother can produce. In the Third World, milk output from marginally nourished mothers may be significantly less; there are also exceptions at the other extreme, especially among well nourished mothers -- *i.e.*, there are mothers who are able to produce enough milk to sustain good growth almost through the first year of life.

It is interesting to contemplate how little we know about the actual quantities involved:

• There is unequivocal empirical evidence, based simply on observation of growth, that human milk output is sufficient to sustain normal growth -- and thus to meet the nutrient and caloric needs of infants at least up to six months of age, and often beyond that (Whitehead and Paul, 1984, provide what is probably the best current review of these issues). There is also strong, but non-quantitative empiric evidence that milk output varies with nursing frequency and vigor of suckling. In addition, we also know that milk production decreases when other foods, including bottle-feeds, are introduced, and reduce the infant's demand for the mother's milk, resulting in a decrease in frequency and vigor of sucking, as well as the completeness of breast emptying.

• We know that the measurement of milk output is extremely difficult. Breasts can be pumped, the milk measured, and estimates of daily output calculated, but this mechanical process quite probably affects output adversely, and there is uncertainty about how frequently to carry out the procedure or how long to continue it in order to obtain accurate estimates. Babies can also be weighed carefully immediately before and after each feeding, around the clock, and output estimates made. We know that studies, using these approaches, have shown that the volume of milk that a woman can produce varies widely, from as little as 400 to 600 ml per day (Gopalan, 1958; Bailey, 1964; Chavez and Martinez, 1973) to around 1200 ml per day (Edozian, 1976). The output varies, up to a limit, with the age of the baby, there are seasonal variations, and output has been observed to double during the week after admission to a hospital (Senecal, 1959).

• The measurement of the nutrient content of breast milk is much more straight-forward, depending on standard biochemical analyses, and has been done many times. What has been found, however, is that the nutrient content of breast milk is also quite variable -- differing in the specimens obtained early in a feeding from those late in the same feeding, differing with the age of the baby, and differing with the nutritional state of the mother (Jelliffe and Jelliffe, 1978).

• We know, too, that the human infant digests and absorbs human milk differently from cow's (and other) milks -- the stools of breast-fed babies differ in color, odor, acidity and volume, among other things, from those receiving formulas. Thus, estimates of the nutrient or caloric requirements for normal growth, based on meticulous metabolic studies of infants fed cow's milk-based formulas, do not necessarily apply to breast-fed infants. It is altogether possible that utilization of human milk is significantly more efficient, and there is evidence that an infant can grow normally on fewer calories if those calories and other nutrients come from human milk. The observations of Whitehead and Paul and other studies cited by them (1981 and 1984) show, for example, that breast-fed babies growing reasonably well may be receiving fewer than 80 calories per kilogram.

These issues are important because our estimates of infants' requirements, as these relate to mothers' production capacities, strongly affect our ideas about the nutritional adequacy of breast-feeding and how long exclusive breast-feeding can, or should be continued. Thus, if we start with the commonly accepted estimates of an average output volume of seven to eight hundred milliliters (ml) per day, with a caloric content of 70 to 75 calories per 100 ml, and if we assume that a normally growing infant needs around 100 to 120 calories per kilogram of body weight per day, we may then conclude that an average mother can produce five to six hundred calories per day and that this can sustain normal growth only until the infant weighs five or six kilograms at most. This is manifestly not the case: millions of exclusively breast-fed babies have gained weight according to Western reference values for at least six months, by which time they weigh 7.5 or 8 kilograms. Either our estimates of requirements are too high, or our estimates of the mothers' output are too low. Babies seem to grow better *in fact* than we think they should *in theory*.

Whitehead and Paul spoke to this paradox in 1981, when they took a "fresh approach" to the questions of infant growth and human milk requirements; they wrote,

> "... Using, for example, the W.H.O./F.A.O. recommendations for dietary energy, the theoretical milk need for a 50th centile male child at 3 months is 900ml/day and at 6 months 1250ml/day. Mean volumes of this magnitude from representative populations are not ... encountered even in well-nourished mothers, yet it is known that the great majority of women are quite capable of successfully breast-feeding ..." (Whitehead and Paul, 1981).

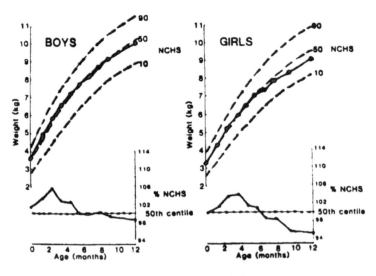

A. Cambridge (Whitehead & Paul, 1981)

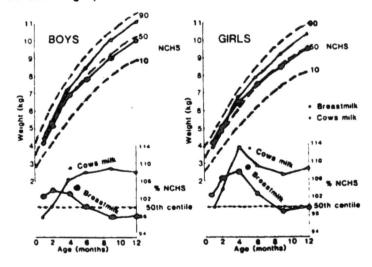

B. Finland (Saarinen & Siimes, 1979)

Figure 1. A. Mean weights, by month, and mean weights expressed as a percentage of expected weights for age, in boys and girls in Cambridge, England (Data from Whitehead and Paul, 1981). B. Mean weights, by month in breast-fed and cow's milk-fed boys and girls, and mean weights expressed as a percentage of expected weights for age, in boys and girls in Finland. Data from Saarinen and Siimes, 1979. Graphs re-drawn from Whitehead and Paul, 1984.

They recently presented a comprehensive review of these issues, based on their own work in Cambridge, England, and several other studies in Western as well as Third World countries (1984). It is not possible to do full justice to their study here, but at least three of their figures deserve consideration. Figure 1 shows the mean weight gain of a group of Cambridge boys and girls that were exclusively breast-fed for the first several months (Whitehead and Paul, 1981) and two groups of Finnish boys and girls, one fed breast milk and the other cow's milk, through the first year of life (Saarinen and Siimes, 1979). Both in Cambridge and Finland supplementary feedings were started at 3 to 4 months of age. The figure also shows the weight for both boys and girls expressed as a per cent of the National Centre for Health Statistics (NCHS) 50th centile values for the different feeding groups. Growth of the breast-fed babies in the two countries and the bottle-fed babies in Finland was similar for the first four months, and easily conformed to the NCHS norms, but it is clear that the bottle-fed babies grew more rapidly afterwards.

Figure 2 is a similar presentation of the growth pattern of exclusively breast-fed babies in Newfoundland (Chandra, 1982) and in Baltimore (Ahn and MacLean, 1980), that were followed prospectively from birth. As might be expected the number still exclusively breast-fed decreased each month, especially after six months and those still exclusively breast-fed toward the end of the first year were not a random sample. The Baltimore babies gained weight at a rate somewhat above the NCHS 50th centile levels until beyond the sixth month; the Newfoundland babies grew at a somewhat lower rate. In neither group did mean weights, expressed as a per cent of the NCHS 50th centile, fall below 95 per cent in the second six months. Considering that the NCHS standards were based on a population that included as many as ten per cent of babies that were obese it is clear that the breast-fed babies were growing quite well.

Observations from the Third World are shown in Figure 3 which combines the Whitehead and Paul presentation of the growth data from Bakau, a peri-urban area in The Gambia (Rowland, 1983) and from Keneba, a rural village in The Gambia (Whitehead *et al.*, 1978). In this graph, mean weight is expressed as a per cent of the NCHS reference values for age and as a per cent of the Cambridge weights-for-age observed in the babies that were initially breast-fed. It is apparent that the peri-urban babies gained more rapidly than their rural counterparts, that the rural babies begin to fall behind during the second six months of life, but that weight gain in both groups is generally comparable to the NCHS standards and even more like the pattern observed in the Cambridge study. Whitehead and Paul proposed that since the Cambridge babies were reared in a clean and safe environment, exclusively

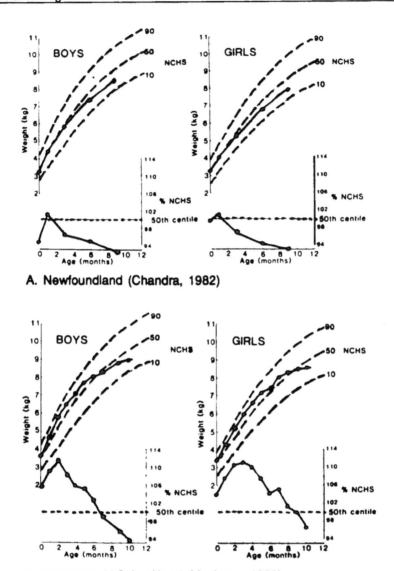

A. Newfoundland (Chandra, 1982)

B. Baltimore, U.S.A. (Ahn & MacLean, 1980)

Figure 2. A. Mean weights, by month, and mean weight expressed as a percentage of expected weight for age (NCHS 50th percentile), in exclusively breast-fed boys and girls in Newfoundland (Data from Chandra, 1982). Similar data from Baltimore, USA (Data from Ahn and MacLean, 1980). Graphs re-drawn from Whitehead and Paul, 1984.

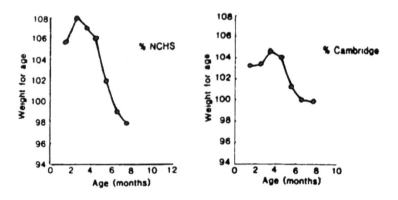

A. Bakau, The Gambia [peri-urban], (Rowland, 1983)

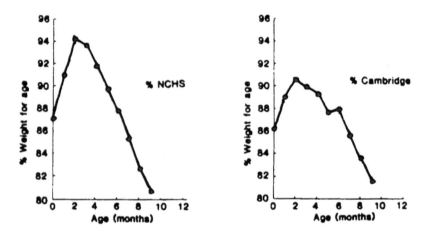

B. Keneba, The Gambia [rural], (Whitehead et al, 1977)

Figure 3. A. Mean weights of a population of breast-fed peri-urban infants in the Gambia expressed as percentage of expected weight for age according to the NCHS 50th percentile levels and as a percentage mean weights of breast-fed Cambridge infants (Data from Rowland, 1983). B. Similar data from a population of breast-fed rural infants in the Gambia (Whitehead et al., 1977) Graphs re-drawn from Whitehead and Paul, 1984.

breast-fed and generally healthy, they might provide a more appropriate standard for breast-fed babies in the Third World. Most important of all is that increased risks of mortality associated with serious malnutrition appear only when weight is below 80 percent (Kielmann and McCord, 1978), or even 65 per cent (Chen *et al.*, 1980) of expected weight for age, then it is clear that the exclusively breast-fed babies in those studies were at no significant risk because of inadequate nutrition.

Lopez Bravo and her colleagues in Santiago have reported a study from a population in transition that is also worth noting (1984). They followed the growth of infants in an urban slum, where they observed that mothers had received little schooling, fathers were usually unskilled or casual laborers, and houses were crowded, all of which indicated a low socioeconomic status, although 85 per cent had "drinking water and sewerage."

They calculated the cumulative monthly weight gain for infants on different types of feeding and produced the results shown in Figure 4, which are of interest not only because they show the difference in mean weight gain between infants that were exclusively breast-fed and those that were partially or wholly bottle-fed, but also because they show that even under those conditions exclusive breast-feeding can sustain normal growth well beyond the sixth month.

What must be remembered finally, however, is that no matter how well nourished the mother, no matter how much mammary tissue she has, sooner or later a healthy baby outgrows her ability to meet their total nutrient needs. When studies report that infants that are still exclusively breast-fed at or beyond one year of age are not doing well, this is the result of physiologic limitations, not because of some defect or qualitative inadequacy of breast milk. Exclusive breast-feeding can be nutritionally completely adequate until around six months and, as we have seen, for many babies it suffices well beyond the sixth month. In some situations, however, where mothers may be seriously undernourished, growth faltering may appear before the sixth month. In those babies, and in all babies sooner or later, the mother's milk must be supplemented if growth is to continue at a satisfactory pace (Brakohaipa *et al.*, 1988).

The growth faltering that commonly appears when breast milk is not supplemented adequately, is aggravated by infections that begin to increase in frequency in most infants at about the same age (Gordon *et al.*, 1963; Mata, 1978). Those who are familiar only with industrialized countries today must keep in mind that growth faltering beginning at around the sixth month is, in fact, the statistically average, or "normal," pattern in many, if not most traditional cultures to this day (as it was in most industrialized countries until

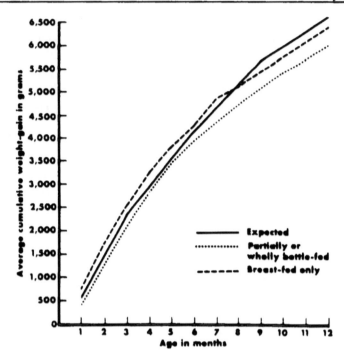

Figure 4. Cumulative mean monthly weight gain of exclusively breast-fed and partially or wholly bottle-fed infants in a low-income population in Santiago, Chile, plotted against norms based on Stuart and Smith. Graph re-drawn from Lopez Bravo *et al.*, 1984.

well into this century). It is important to understand that in these societies growth faltering occurs because culturally determined weaning practices are simply inadequate. That is to say, the foods that the mother is taught by her particular culture to provide, as a supplement to or replacement for her own milk, in the process of weaning, do not provide enough calories and nutrients to sustain adequate growth. The situation is even more complex; Underwood (1989) recently described what she called the "weaning's dilemma:"

> "When complementary food is introduced too early the child is vulnerable to contaminated foods which can cause diarrheal disease. If breast milk complements are offered too late, the infant suffers from inadequate nutrient intake. This is the weanling's dilemma. The unfortunate result -- undernutrition,

> slow growth and retarded development -- is well documented."

What we know is that the average values for height and weight (as well as any other anthropometric parameters that are measured) among breast-fed infants in these cultures are close to the North American or European 50th percentile values until around the sixth month. At that point mean values begin to fall behind and by the end of the first year of life, they are typically around the third percentile levels as a result of the poor weaning diets and repeated infections. Thus, when studies reveal growth faltering and morbidity or mortality in such infants, it should be remembered that these are almost always due to a combination of undernutrition and infection, rather than to some consequence of breast-feeding *per se*. It is important to keep in mind, however, that in these same cultures the babies that *do* receive breast milk beyond six months of age, in addition to whatever else they are receiving, are going to be better off than those receiving only the culturally prescribed weaning diet. On the basis of what we know about the diets of infants in Third World settings, we can assume that the protein they receive in breast milk is going to be especially important, since the supplements commonly used are unlikely to provide protein that is adequate in quantity or quality. What matters is that the protein in breast milk can be used for growth energy if the baby gets enough calories from supplements; if the supplementary calorie intake is insufficient, then the protein in breast milk is metabolized to produce needed calories. In addition, as we will see below, breast-fed babies are less likely to have infections. Field studies have indeed shown that children that are still receiving breast milk in their second year grow better and have fewer infections than their peers that are fully weaned (Wray and Aguirre, 1969; Antrobus, 1971; Briend *et al.*, 1988).

The Breast Milk Immunologic Context

As we examine what has been learned from clinical and epidemiological studies of the "protective" value of breast-feeding, it is important to keep in mind what is now known about the biological basis for a protective effect. As a matter of fact, the cumulative knowledge concerning humoral and cellular factors, highly concentrated in the colostrum but continuing as long as breast milk is secreted, is considerable. Perhaps the first scientific study was carried out by Paul Ehrlich in the 1890s, when he showed, in a very cleverly designed study, that newborn mice had received antibodies trans-placentally, and continued to receive them, for several weeks, *via* the mammary glands in breast milk (Ehrlich, 1892). Gerrard (1974) pointed out that farmers have known for centuries, it seems, that newborn calves, piglets and lambs simply will not survive without a dose of colostrum to protect them from infection, and a host of studies of all kinds have shown a remarkable and varied array of protective factors that operate similarly to protect the human newborn.

Among the more recent of such studies, Gillin *et al.*, (1983) showed, for example, that antiparasitic factors in breast milk kill *Giardia lamblia* as well as *Entamoeba histolytica*. In the former case, 50 percent of the *Giardia* were killed in less than 30 minutes by 3 percent human milk; and in approximately 60 minutes by 1 percent milk. Glass *et al.* (1983) described antibodies in human milk against *V. cholerae* and the findings of Gillin *et al.* and of Glass *et al.* were abundantly documented in the longitudinal field studies that were carried out by Mata (1978) when these organisms simply could not be found in the intestines of breast-fed infants in Guatemalan villages. Infectious diseases aside, failure to breast-feed may be a factor in the development of allergies (Goldman, 1977; Gerrard, 1974), and such conditions as Crohn's disease (Koletzko *et al.*, 1989) or necrotizing enterocolitis (Jelliffe and Jelliffe, 1978; Santulli, 1974). The immunologic factors were reviewed comprehensively by Jelliffe and Jelliffe (1978), Chandra (1978) and more recently by Hanson (1982). Hanson, as well as Walker and Isselbacher (1977), have reviewed the evidence that lymphocytes, stimulated by antigens in the gut, migrate *via* the entero-mammary circulation to the mammary glands where they are responsible for the production of specific IgA antibodies that appear in the mother's milk within hours of the arrival of a pathogen in the mother's gut mucosa. He summed up the role of the mammary gland as follows:

> "In addition to specific antibodies and leukocytes, human milk contains several other factors of major importance in the host defense of the infant. Lactoferrin which binds iron, a growth factor for most aerobic bacteria, has already been mentioned, but lysozyme, interferon, complement factors, anti-staphylococcal factor(s), lactoperoxidase, bifidus factor, various antiviral factors, glucoproteins and oligosaccharides preventing bacterial attachment to mucosae have also been reported." (Hanson, 1982).

The sum of this evidence suggests that there are innumerable and incontrovertible reasons to believe that breast milk can protect infants from infection.

The Nutrition-infection Context

In addition to protective factors associated directly with breast milk, there is the well known, abundantly documented effect of nutrition *per se* on immunity and the human organism's ability to resist infection, especially in children. Our understanding of these issues goes back to the original WHO monograph by Scrimshaw *et al.* (1968), amplified in many other reviews (*e.g.*, Suskind, 1977; Keusch and Katz, 1979). The consequence of this is that, as many studies have shown, malnourished infants and children are at much greater risk both of morbidity (*e.g.* Wray and Aguirre, 1969), and also of mortality (Kielmann and McCord, 1978; Chen *et al.* 1979). For this reason, when excessive morbidity or mortality is found to be associated with certain types of feeding of infants or young children, it is important to try to determine whether or not the effect observed is due to some influence of breast-feeding, or to the effect of nutritional status *per se*. In the West, 75 or a hundred years ago, the substitutes for breast milk available to poor mothers were usually nutritionally inadequate -- seriously so; this is true to this day in the Third World. The baby therefore that is not breast-fed not only fails to receive the immunologic benefits, but is also very likely to be receiving food that is nutritionally inadequate *and* contaminated. Thus the baby has impaired resistance to infection because of malnutrition and has increased exposure to infections.

The Environmental Context

A final caveat concerns the interaction between the environment and feeding methods. A number of the studies discussed below, both old and recent, deal directly with this issue, but it is so important that a summary statement is in order at the outset. What will be seen is that as the standard of living improves, and the environment becomes less hostile, the protective effect of breast milk becomes less crucial. This translates into the fact that studies carried out in benign environments may show lower mortality in bottle-fed infants than has been observed in breast-fed infants in less favorable environments. The significance of such a finding can therefore be interpreted properly only by taking the environment into account.

EVIDENCE CONCERNING THE SUPERIORITY OF BREAST-FEEDING

Some Historical Evidence

It is in the various contexts described above that the evidence both from the older and more recent studies must be examined. The validity of some of the older evidence has been questioned; the research methods have been challenged. We must therefore examine the evidence carefully to determine whether or not it is acceptable today. The Kovar *et al.* review mentioned above excluded studies carried out before 1970; the Jason *et al.* review was limited to studies in the developing world that were carried out in the last 25 years. Can we learn from 19th century studies or from those carried out in the first half of this century? The assumption here that such studies *can* provide information that is useful, even today, is based on the fact that both the mortality rates and also the leading causes of death among infants in Europe and the US were, until well into this century, similar to those today in many Third World countries (For example, see McDermott, 1966, or Rohde, 1983). Similarly, the desperate poverty, the appalling environmental and sanitary conditions, the illiteracy and ignorance, and the many other risks to which infants were exposed in the West, were also quite comparable to those that are still to be found in much of the Third World. Thus, although pre-1950 studies of the effect of feeding practices on morbidity or mortality in western countries may have limited relevance to the situation in those countries today, they undoubtedly have implications for the Third World. They are also a thought-provoking reminder that the problems that concern us today are not new, that physicians have been aware of them for over a century and carried out basically sound, comprehensive and revealing studies.

All the evidence cannot be examined in detail, but a brief review and a few examples of the findings of some of the more thought-provoking studies are in order. European physicians became critically concerned about the differences between mortality rates observed in breast- and artificially-fed babies in the 1860s and a number of interesting studies were carried out between that time and the mid-20th century, first in Europe and later in the US. Although some of these studies can be criticized for methodologic flaws, they are quite remarkably consistent in revealing higher mortality rates in artificially-fed infants (Wray, 1978; Wray, 1979; Cunningham, 1981). As early as 1865, Denis-Dumont studied 6,407 breast-fed and 3,204 artificially-fed infants in the *departement du Calvados* of France and found a three-fold difference in infant mortality, with a rate of 108.9 per 1,000 in breast-fed infants and of 307.7 in artificially-fed infants (cited in Rollet, 1978). Studies

Table I. Number of infants, number of deaths, and mortality rates per thousand live births, by type of feeding, in the first year of life, Derby, England, 1900-1903.

Type of Feeding	Number Fed	Deaths	Rate/1000
Breast milk	5278	368	69.8
"Hand-fed", total	1626	321	197.5
Diluted cow's milk only	895	158	177
Condensed milk only	149	38	255
"Bread, rusks, oatmeal, arrowroot, cornflour, sago, tapioca, and mixed foods"	159	40	252
"Patent foods"	482	85	202

Source: Howarth, 1905. Adapted from Tables I and III.

of the mortality rates per 1,000 survivors each month from birth to 12 months, by type of feeding, were carried out in Berlin in 1885-86, 1895-96 and 1906 (Thiemich and Bessau, 1930) and revealed four- to seven-fold higher mortality rates in bottle-fed babies during the period studied.

Among the many studies that followed, several are noteworthy for the insights that they provide. One of the first prospective studies was carried out by Howarth, in Derby, England, at the turn of the century (1905). He followed all live born infants through the first year of life and compared mortality rates by type of feeding, and distinguished among the different kinds of artificial foods then in use, as shown in Table I. He noted that the highest death rates were in infants fed sweetened condensed milk, a source of continued excess mortality in the Third World to this day. Table II shows his findings concerning the rates from various causes by type of feeding. Even then, it was assumed that diarrheal diseases were most strongly associated with artificial feedings, but Howarth also noted that mortality from respiratory infections was higher in artificially-fed babies. His conclusion, cast in turn-of-the-century terms, clearly anticipates contemporary ideas:

> "It is not easy to associate an increase of 12 per thousand, or nearly 100% in the mortality from bronchitis and pneumonia with the manner of feeding ... the probable reason is to be found in the production of children suffering from what might be termed 'lessened powers of resistance' or 'diminished vitality.' ... It is more probable that these enfeebled constitutions are the direct result of improper feeding, for when food constituents are not given to a child in their

Table II. Mortality rates per thousand live births, by diagnosis and by type of feeding, in the first year of life, Derby, England, 1900-1903. Data from Table II, Howarth, 1905.			
Diseases	Mortality Rates Per Thousand		
	"Breast-fed"	"Mixed"	"Hand-fed"
"Bronchitis and pneumonia"	14.4	12.6	26.5
"Diarrhoea and zymotic enteritis"	10.0	25.1	57.9
"Marasmus, atrophy and debility"	12.6	18.9	39.4
"Convulsions"	15.0	20.9	25.9
All other diseases	18.4	21.7	48.3
Total	69.8	98.7	197.5
Source: Howarth 1905. Adapted from Table II.			

> proper proportions, or the substances ... are un-
> suitable, it requires very little imagination to suggest
> the evolution of a child who will show ... diminished
> resistance to attacks of the common zymotic ail-
> ments." (Howarth, 1905,)

Almost twenty years later a prospective study of over 22 thousand infants, followed through the first year of life in eight cities in the northeastern US, was reported by Woodbury (1922). Records included the type of feeding and mortality at each month of age. This study too provided clear-cut evidence of the protective effect of breast-feeding. In his analysis Woodbury took advantage of the size of his sample and the fact that he had the relevant data on a monthly basis and produced one of the most interesting sub-sets of data of all of these studies. He calculated the cumulative mortality, month-by-month, among those who were breast-fed exclusively through the first year, and for the cohorts of infants that were weaned from the breast entirely in each succeeding month. He was struck by the fact that the earlier breast-feeding was abandoned and bottle-feeding was begun, the worse the mortality. He wrote,

> "In each month of life the mortality rate was higher
> the longer the period of previous artificial feeding.
> For example, among infants whose artificial feeding
> commenced in the first month, the rate in the fifth
> month was 24, as compared with rates in the fifth
> month of 18.7 among those whose artificial feeding
> commenced in the second month, 18.3 in the third,
> 13.6 in the fourth, and only 3.8 in the fifth. The

comparison is even more striking when the rates
among the artificially fed are compared with those
among the exclusively breast-fed infants. Thus the
mortality in the fifth month prevailing among infants
who had been artificially fed from the first month, or
from birth, was seven times as high as among the
breast-fed; the mortality among the infants who had
been artificially fed from the second month was nearly six times, from the third month over five times and
from the fourth month four times, as high as among
infants who had been breast-fed from birth, while the
rates among infants whose artificial feeding com-
menced in the fifth month was only slightly greater
than that among the breast-fed infants." (Woodbury,
1922).

In Figure 5 these differences are shown graphically (Wray, 1978). The
variation in mortality, by the age in months at which breast milk was abandoned entirely, is clear from the slope of the curves. In fact, Knodel and
Kintner (1977) have proposed, on the basis of such findings, that the type and
timing of infant feeding can be predicted by comparing the slope of the
cumulative mortality rates during the first six months with that of the second
six months. Where the slope is steeper in the second six months, the infants
were almost certainly artificially-fed from an early age. Another point that is
apparent in Figure 5 is worth noting: the rates show that the child who was
breast-fed exclusively was more likely to survive than the child who was
changed to artificial feeding at any time up to the seventh month of life. From
the eighth month on, the bottle-fed child was about as likely to survive as the
exclusively breast-fed infant.

Closely related, but somewhat different findings were reported in a study
of much older data by Rollet, who analyzed French government records of
infant feeding and mortality in late 19th century France (1978). She found two
regions of high mortality: in a number of *departements* in the north, a relatively small proportion of infants were breast-fed and the duration of breast-feeding was brief; in the *Midi* and in several southeastern *departements*, infants
were exclusively breast-fed for long periods. She postulated that mortality
was highest in the first few months in the north because of the inadequacy of
artificial feeding early in life and that the higher rates *after* six months of age
in the south were due to the progressively increasing inadequacy of exclusive
breast-feeding during the second six months of life. Both of these historical

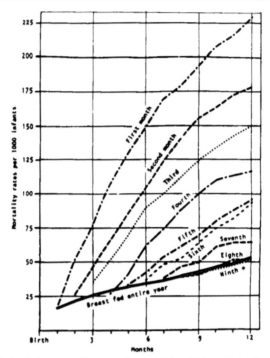

Figure 5. Cumulative infant mortality rates, by month in which artificial feeding was initiated, compared with rates in infants breast-fed exclusively for the entire year. Eight cities in the USA, 1920s. Re-drawn from Wray, 1978, based on data from Woodbury, 1922.

studies have been confirmed in the contemporary Third World by the observations of Wyon and Gordon (1971) in the Punjab of India. Punjabi village babies that were artificially fed from birth almost always died (although Wyon and Gordon acknowledged that the conditions that caused them to be artificially-fed undoubtedly contributed to the mortality); beyond six months of age babies who were receiving some sort of supplementary weaning food were more likely to survive than those who were still exclusively breast-fed.

Among the first prospective studies to examine both morbidity and mortality from different causes, was that of Grulee and his colleagues in Chicago (1934), who followed over 20 thousand infants enrolled in "infant welfare clinics" in Chicago, US, between 1924 and 1929. Robinson carried out a similar study, though with a smaller sample, between 1936 and 1942 in Liverpool, England (1951). Both studies confirmed the findings of Howarth many years earlier: breast-fed babies were more likely to survive regardless of diagnosis. They also showed that the difference in morbidity rates between

Table III. Morbidity and mortality rates per thousand infants age 1 to 9 months, and case fatality rates (deaths per 100 cases), by diagnosis and type of feeding, Chicago, U.S.A., 1924-1929.

Diagnosis	Breast-fed	Partially Breast-fed	Artificially Fed	Ratios Bottle:breast
Respiratory				
Morbidity	279.9	339.9	389.6	1:1.4
Mortality	0.4	5.1	53.9	1:134.7
Case fatality	0.15	1.5	13.8	1:92
Gastro-intestinal				
Morbidity	51.8	120.4	158.8	1:3.1
Mortality	0.2	0.7	8.2	1:41.0
Case fatality	0.4	0.6	5.2	1:13.0
"Unclassified"				
Morbidity	33.0	59.9	81.4	1:2.5
Mortality	0.7	2.9	19.3	1:27.6
Case fatality	2.2	4.9	23.7	1:10.8
Infants at risk	9,749	8,605	1,707	

Source: Grules, *et al.* 1935. Adapted from Tables I and II.

breast-fed and artificially-fed infants was appreciably less than the difference in mortality rates. The findings showed that breast-feeding offers some protection from infection, but that the protection is by no means complete; on the other hand, as the data from Grulee *et al.* in Table III show, breast-fed babies seem to be very effectively protected from dying.

In their follow-up paper (1935) they too noticed differences in mortality during the second six months which they attributed to feeding practices. Although Robinson's findings in Liverpool differed in absolute numbers, differences were qualitatively similar, with much greater relative risk of mortality than of morbidity among artificially-fed children.

Finally, Mannheimer's study (1955) provided a variety of insights that were new at the time. He obtained data concerning all deaths in the first year of life among infants born in Stockholm between 1943 and 1947 as well as information concerning feeding practices at that time from a sample survey of the total infant population. It is altogether likely that conditions in Stockholm during the mid-1940s were comparable to those in some developing countries today and better than those in many; overall infant mortality was around 50 per 1000 live births -- the level now promulgated by UNICEF and the WHO as a goal to be achieved throughout the world by the year 2000. Like the investigators cited above, Mannheimer limited his analysis to the post-neona-

Income	Type of Feeding		
(Swedish Crowns)	Breast-fed	Mixed	Bottle-fed
≤5000	8.31	4.32	16.78
5000-10,000	4.20	2.35	9.21
≥10,000	1.94	2.71	7.29

Table IV. Death risk per thousand among infants aged 2 to 12 months, by parents' annual income and by type of feeding, Stockholm, 1943-1947.

Data from Mannheimer, 1955, p. 156.
Source: Mannheimer, 1955, p. 156

tal period in order to eliminate deaths in the early days of life that might have been caused by complications unrelated to type of feeding. He estimated death risks per thousand infants by age, by birth weight, by cause of death, and by family income, according to type of feeding. Risks were consistently, and significantly, higher in bottle-fed babies in all of these analyses. Interestingly, the lowest risks at times were in the babies that received mixed feeding. The risks associated with family income, shown in Table IV, are of special interest. The data show that mortality among bottle-fed infants in the highest income families was slightly lower than that among breast-fed infants in the poorest families. The relative motality risks among bottle-fed infants in the higher income group were, however, almost four times greater than in breast-fed babies in that income group, while only twice as high in the low income group. It is of interest that Goldberg *et al.* found the same thing in North-eastern Brazil (1984). Although absolute infant mortality rates were higher, as would be expected, among infants born to mothers with no schooling, the relative risk of mortality among non-breast-fed infants born to mothers who had completed primary school was 3.3; among those born to mothers who had no schooling, it was only 2.0.

In spite of criticism that might be offered of older studies, there were features that can be seen to offset the deficiencies. First of all, the sample sizes in many of them were quite large, so large (22,000 babies) that they would be prohibitively expensive today, and several included regular and frequent follow-up visits that would be almost impossible today. Not only were the sample sizes sufficient to reveal clearly the differences in mortality rates associated with different types of feeding, but the numbers also allowed examination of differences in morbidity and mortality rates by cause, and in some of them it was possible to control for a number of other important factors. Perhaps even more impressive is the fact that in Woodbury's study the numbers were so large that he could examine the differences in mortality on a month-by-month basis, and reveal the striking patterns seen in Figure 5. The authors of the studies had no doubt whatsoever about the significance of their findings. Given the basically sound design of most of the studies (even if some details might be questioned), the power of the numbers and the size of the differences observed, and, finally, the quite remarkable consistency of the findings among all of them, there is surely no valid reason that we should doubt them; we must, instead, learn from them.

The Twentieth Century Transition

After a review of these studies and several others, the graph shown in Figure 6 was prepared as a device to summarize the findings (Wray, 1978). It must be stressed that the curves are simply estimates and are not based on biostatistics; they are intended only to provide a visual impression of trends. What the curves show is the cumulative evidence that during the latter half of the 19th century, infant mortality rates in the West were very high, regardless of type of feeding, but that the rates in artificially-fed infants were consistently at least twice as high as those in breast-fed infants. Around the turn of the century, varying in time from country to country, infant mortality rates began to fall, regardless of type of feeding. As is clear, however, from the time-series data from Berlin mentioned earlier, shown in Table V (Thiemich and Bessau, 1930), the fall was generally more rapid in artificially-fed infants. The declines in both groups continued on into the mid-20th century. Unfortunately, no comparable studies of mortality have been carried out since the late 1940s; by that time mortality rates in both groups were very low, although still at least twice as high in the artificially-fed babies (Douglas, 1950; Mannheimer, 1955).

Overall, then, the data suggest a process of transition somewhat comparable to the "demographic transition" -- with very high but significantly different mortality rates in the two groups during the pre-transition stage, when data first became available. During the transition to low motality rates, which lasted roughly 50 years, rates declined steadily in both groups. Finally, as the post-transition is approached, rates were quite low in absolute terms, but they still revealed at least two-fold differences in mortality between breast- and artificially-fed infants.

If we are concerned with the "superiority" of breast-feeding, however, it is important to consider the role of breast-feeding in the demographic transition. In a comprehensive review of evidence concerning the factors associated with the rapid infant mortality decline in England Wales between 1861 and 1921, Woods and colleagues (1989) looked carefully for reasons to explain the decline. Among other things, they paid particular attention to contem-

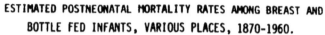

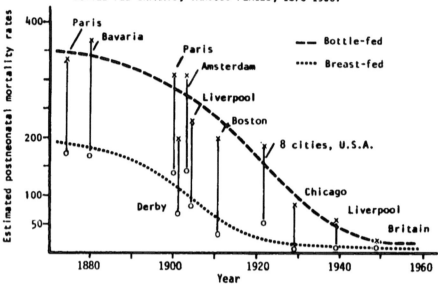

Figure 6. Changes in postneonatal mortality rates among breast-fed and bottle-fed infants in various places in Europe and the USA, between 1870 and 1960. Re-drawn from Wray, 1978.

Table V. Mortality rates per thousand infants surviving each month, from 1 month through 12 months, Berlin, 1885-86, 1895-96, and 1906. Data from Thiemich and Bessau, 1932, p. 72.					
	Breast Fed Infants			**Bottle Fed Infants**		
	1885-86	1895-96	1906	1885-86	1895-96	1906
1 Month	22.4	19.6	22.4	142.0	111.9	59.1
2 Months	9.0	7.3	7.9	82.7	58.7	31.3
3 Months	6.8	4.3	4.3	72.2	49.7	27.3
4 Months	6.4	3.6	2.4	61.8	46.6	22.1
5 Months	5.3	2.6	1.7	57.1	37.0	18.5
6 Months	4.9	2.5	2.2	50.7	31.0	16.1
7 Months	4.7	2.5	1.4	46.5	27.7	14.1
8 Months	4.5	2.3	1.8	40.8	24.1	12.2
9 Months	5.3	2.0	2.1	33.3	21.3	10.2
10 Months	5.4	3.8	1.5	29.5	19.1	9.2
11 Months	6.3	3.1	1.3	24.9	16.7	8.0
12 Months	-	3.6	1.5	-	14.6	8.0
Average	8.1	6.0	6.3	54.1	35.8	23.6
Source: Thiemich and Bessau, 1930, p. 72						

porary analyses of the problem and reviewed a number of the studies cited here. They were especially interested in the possible contribution of breast-feeding to the decline and they noted,

> "... there is good reason to accept Newsholme's view that the breastfeeding norm among working-class mothers must have helped to reduce infant mortality where poverty, environment and sanitation would otherwise have resulted in higher rates ... [but] there is little reason to suppose that either the incidence or duration of breastfeeding increased during the first decade of this century in the towns for which we have data; yet infant mortality rates declined everywhere, especially the post-neonatal rates and rates from diarrhoea. Breastfeeding practices helped to keep infant mortality down, they do not appear to have made it decline further during the early years of the twentieth century ..." (Woods *et al.*, 1989,)

While considering the protective effects of breast-feeding, they still could not attribute the decline in infant mortality to it since neither prevalence nor duration were increasing at the time mortality rates were falling. Instead, they attributed the declines to a number of other factors including improved "domestic and municipal sanitation, [and] housing," which we might describe today as improved standard of living. They also believed that reduced fertility was an important factor. Their proposal that environmental factors contributed to lowered infant mortality, and that these factors interacted with breast-feeding, derived in part from the observations of social class differences in mortality that had been described by Newsholme:

> "... probably 80 per cent of the mothers of infants in wage-earning populations suckle their infants partially or entirely and that the proportion of mothers in the well-to-do classes who are able and willing to continue to give their infants this immensely important start in life is believed, I think rightly, to be much smaller. There must be reasons of great potency, enabling the infants of the well-to-do to survive in much higher proportions to the end of the first year of life, notwithstanding this heavy handicap against them.

> "And it is the ability to obtain skilled guidance in the
> preparation of infants' food, to spend sufficient
> money in purchasing it, and to prepare such food
> under the safest conditions that explains in large
> measure the lower infant mortality among the non-in-
> dustrial classes." (Newsholme, 1910, quoted in
> Woods *et al.*, 1989,)

Implicit in the findings of the older studies, then, and in the analysis by Woods and colleagues, as suggested in the transition theory, is that our interpretation of the results of contemporary studies must take into account the socioeconomic and environmental circumstances of the infants being studied. If mortality rates are relatively low, because of such factors, and absolute differences in mortality rates by type of feeding are small, the results must be interpreted carefully and extrapolated with care, if at all. Within-country differences in the standard of living can also be substantial and we can no longer assume that the findings reported in a study from a so-called developing country represent *all* of that country, or others like it. Instead, as we will see in several studies mentioned below, the findings need to be considered in the context of the situation of the specific population that has been studied. Only when we have some idea of where they are in the socioeconomic and environmental transition can we be sure of the significance of the findings that have been obtained.

Evidence from the Third World

Evidence from Third World countries is relatively recent although British Colonial Medical Officers attributed high infant mortality to failure to breast-feed in such places as Jamaica as early as 1920 (Crook, 1924). Dr. Cicely Williams, working in what was then called The Gold Coast, in West Africa, in the 1930s, described a syndrome called "kwashiorkor," which meant "the sickness of the deposed baby" in the local language -- *i.e.*, the child deprived of its mother's breast milk by the next child (Williams, 1953). Her ideas about the importance of breast-feeding had progressed to the point that in 1939 she delivered an address to the Rotary Club of Singapore entitled "Milk and murder," in which she recognized the same social class differences in the effect of breast-feeding that Newsholme had noted thirty years earlier. She said,

> "There is no possible doubt, and every sentient being
> in the world agrees, that the best possible food for a
> baby is its mother's milk. Nothing has as yet been

invented that provides a satisfactory substitute. Statistics have been collected to show that the death rate among artificially fed babies is much greater than among breast-fed babies. And this is a death rate that shows a very marked class prejudice.

Among the *tuan besars*, the *taipans* and the *tokays*[1], the death rate among artificially fed babies is only slightly higher than among breast-fed babies.

Among the *kranis*, the small shopkeepers and the middle-class population, the death rate is distinctly higher.

But among the coolie population, the really poor people of Chinatown and the kampongs, the death rate among artificially fed babies is at least twice as high as that of the breast-fed babies." (Williams, 1939, p.1)

Wyon and Gordon (1971) included infant feeding among the things they investigated in the Punjab in what was probably the first prospective longitudinal study of the health of villagers in the Third World. They paid particular attention to mortality in infants and young children and to the factors that affected it. As noted earlier, they found that babies artificially-fed from birth almost always died, while those that were exclusively breast-fed too long were also at a disadvantage. One of their many interesting analyses, which is of particular relevance here, was based on the relation between month of birth and mortality. Noting that the annual peak incidence of diarrheal disease occurred during May and June, the hot dry season, and that weaning commonly began from the sixth to the eighth month of life, they examined mortality from diarrhea by season and observed:

"Children born in spring and during the hot dry season, shortly before and at the height of diarrhea prevalence, had the lowest death rates for diarrheal disease during the first year of life. They were predominantly breast-fed at the time of major risk.

1   *tuan besar, taipan,* and *towkay* are Malay and chinese words used in Singapore for "big bosses;" *kranis* are clerks.

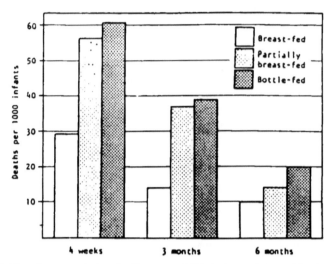

Figure 7. Mortality rates during the first year of life in breast-fed, partially breast-fed and bottle-fed infants, among those surviving at 4 weeks, and at 3 and 6 months, rural Chile, 1969-1970. Re-drawn from Wray, 1978, based on data from Plank and Milanesi, 1973.

> Children born in autumn, with weaning beginning in the hot dry season at the time of greatest risk, had the highest death rates of any cohort determined by month of birth." (Gordon *et al.*, p 368, 1963).

Plank and Milanesi carried out one of the earliest studies designed to investigate specifically the impact of type of feeding on infant mortality in a developing country 1973). Their findings are shown in Figure 7, where the death rates per thousand infants surviving at age four weeks, three months and six months are compared by type of feeding. It is clear that the protective effect of breast-feeding on the infants observed in this study was comparable to that observed in more developed countries a few decades earlier.

At about the same time, Puffer and Serrano were directing the Pan American Health Organization (PAHO) study of mortality in childhood in 15 cities of 10 countries of the Western Hemisphere, including three each in Colombia and Brazil and two in Argentina (1973). Among other things, they were able to ascertain the proportion of infants that had been breast-fed for less than, or more than, six months among infants that died during the second six months of life. They showed that mortality rates were much higher among those breast-fed less than six months than among those breast-fed longer.

Table VI. Percentage of infants breast-fed for less than 6 months and more than six months, in the total population and among infants dying between 6 and 12 months of age, in four of the Pan American Health Organization study areas, around 1970, and the relative risk of mortality in the two feeding groups.

Study Area	Percent Breast-fed				Ratio of mortality risk for breast-feeding < 6 mos. : ≥ 6 mos.
	Total Infant Population		Infants Dying (58) At 6-11 Months		
	< 6 mos.	≥ 6 mos.	< 6 mos.	≥ 6 mos.	
El Salvador	20	80	78.0	22.0	14.2:1
Kingston, Jamaica	51	49	87.4	12.6	7.1:1
Medellin, Columbia	61.8	31.2	91.3	8.8	6.4:1
Sao Paolo, Brazil	77.2	22.8	95.9	4.1	6.8:1

Based on data from Puffer and Serrano, 1973; other sources cited in Wray, 1978.

Subsequently, studies of the prevalence of breast-feeding in the total population in four of the PAHO study sites were found. Thus, it was possible to combine these findings with the PAHO data and calculate the relative risk of mortality for those breast-fed less than and more than six months in the four sites, as shown in Table VI (Wray, 1978), where it may be seen that the risk ranged from 6.4 to over 14.

Since a comprehensive review (Wray, 1979) carried out ten years ago concerning mortality, morbidity and feeding in the Third World, the number of studies has increased substantially. Several recent reviews (Jason et al., 1984; Feachem and Koblinsky, 1984; Popkin et al., 1989) reveal the variety of approaches, including prospective surveys, cross-sectional surveys, cohort studies, and hospital-based case control studies, as well as the wide range of socioeconomic and ecological conditions covered. As with the older studies, there are wide variations in methodological rigor and a generic problem with defining precisely just what is meant by breast-feeding and bottle-feeding. As might be expected there was overlap among the studies reviewed, but the number was surprisingly limited.

Jason et al. were specifically concerned with developing countries, but included a few studies from affluent ones that related to specific pathogens or organ systems. They found useable data in 28 studies from developing countries; 14 of those included mortality data. The Feachem and Koblinsky review was part of a WHO-supported series of reviews of interventions for the control of diarrheal diseases among young children; thus, they included all studies that were considered reasonably sound and reflected the association between diarrheal disease and infant feeding, including ten studies from Third World countries. Popkin et al. were also concerned primarily with diarrheal disease and divided the studies reviewed into those from "higher income" and from "lower income" countries; there were 19 of the latter. All three reviews presented calculations of relative risk, or odds ratios, for morbidity or mortality associated with different modes of feeding and most of their findings were presented in tabular form, thus facilitating a comparison of findings in the different studies.

With few exceptions the studies from the Third World showed significant increases in the relative risk associated with partial or complete bottle-feeding. The increased risk varied from country to country. As had been observed by Grulee and Robinson 50 years or more earlier, the relative risk of mortality associated with bottle-feeding was greater than the relative risk of morbidity, whether from diarrhea or other infections. A decrease in the relative risk with increasing age was observed almost everywhere. All of these differences are most easily conveyed by the figures prepared by Feachem and Koblinsky. Figure 8 shows the median relative risk of *morbidity* in infants under six months of age.

Median relative risk of diarrhea *mortality* by feeding mode and age, through five months, is shown in Figure 9. Thus it is clear that the observations of Grulee *et al.* (1934) and Robinson (1951) that the relative risk of mortality is much greater than the relative risk of morbidity have been amply confirmed. Breast-feeding provides babies with some protection against infections, but it provides much more protection against dying if they do acquire an infection.

The Third World Transition

As infant mortality fell in industrialized countries early in this century because living standards and the environment were improving, the dangers associated with bottle feeding diminished, although relative differences in mortality remained substantial. The protective effect of breast-feeding was less necessary in the more affluent families, as Newsholme observed, than in the poorer families. The same phenomenon has been observed recently in the Third World and it is apparent that absolute levels of mortality, regardless of feeding, depend on the environment. A study of Pakistani immigrants living in Bradford, England, reported by Aykroyd and Hossain (1967), illustrates this point beautifully. Although basic patterns of life had changed little, with families relying heavily, for example, on foods imported from Pakistan, the men were well employed and standards of living were much higher than those they had left behind in Pakistan. In addition, however, the mothers had easy access to modern health care and "as a result of the instruction and supervision provided by the clinics and health personnel, the immigrant mothers had

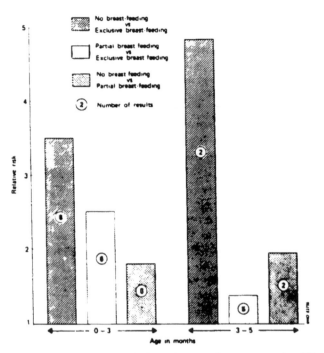

Figure 8. Median relative risks of morbidity from diarrheal disease, comparing different types of feeding, in infants under six months of age. Based on estimates prepared by Feachem and Koblinsky (1984) from studies carried out in various parts of the world and re-drawn from their Figure 2.

adopted an 'artificial' infant feeding regimen similar to that of English infants in Bradford." In spite of the fact that the Pakistani infants weighed an average of 300 grams less than English infants at birth, they grew well and differences in weight at one year were minimal. Interestingly, however, infant mortality among the bottle-fed Pakistani infants was 47.2, more than twice that of non-Asian infants in Bradford, but only about one third of the then current rate in the part of Pakistan from which they came, where the vast majority of babies were still breast-fed. Bottle-fed babies in a benign environment were clearly more likely to survive than breast-fed babies in a hostile environment.

Since that time, conflicting reports have emerged. In a study of a transitional population in Malaysia, Dugdale reported that "the type of feeding had no statistically significant effect on the frequency of minor respiratory or alimentary illnesses" (1971). Similarly, Zeitlin et al., studied children in a "depressed urban area" of Manila, in the Philippines, where, however, the

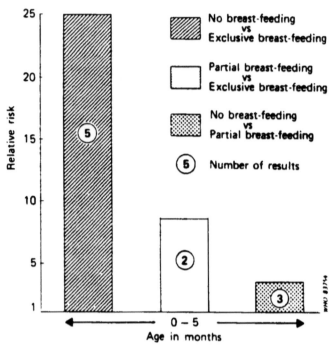

Figure 9. Median relative risks of mortality from diarrheal disease during the first six months of life, comparing various types of feeding, and showing that relative risk of *mortality* is substantially higher than relative risk of *morbidity*. Based on estimates prepared by Feachem and Koblinsky (1984) from studies carried out in various parts of the world and re-drawn from their Figure 4.

average mother had at least six years of education and 90 per cent of the households had piped water (1978). They found little impact of bottle- or breast-feeding on the nutritional status of children and they concluded that "bottle-feeding was not a statistically significant cause of malnutrition in a sample of 513 six to forty-eight month old children."

On the other hand, Hermelo *et al.* found in Cuba that "infants breast-nursed were less affected by diarrheal fits and their nutritional status was better, exactly the contrary to those nursed artificially since birth" (1968). More recently, similar findings have been reported from children born in urban hospitals in Cairo, Egypt (Janowitz *et al.*, 1981), from peri-urban communities around Santiago, Chile (Lopez Bravo *et al.*, 1984), from Porto Alegre and Pelotas, in southern Brazil (Victora *et al.*, 1987 and Barros *et al.*, 1986) and from Lima, Peru, (Brown *et al.*, 1989) where, for example, the authors concluded that "Regardless of the explanatory mechanisms, exclusive breast-feeding during the first 6 months of life and continuous breast-feeding for a least 1 year were clearly associated with a reduced incidence and prevalence of infections in this setting." Tu examined the role of breast-feeding and birth interval in child survival in Shaanxi province and in Shanghai, China (1989). Shanghai, as is well known, is one of the most prosperous, industrialized and generally well developed cities in China; Shaanxi is an inland province, not so prosperous, with a large proportion of its population living in rural areas. His study showed that breast-feeding and birth interval did significantly affect child survival in Shaanxi, but had essentially no discernible effects in Shanghai.

One of the most enlightening explorations of this particular issue was based on a study of the correlates of mortality among 5471 Malaysian infants, reported by Butz et al. (1984), in which they were able to analyze mortality rates by type of feeding and by household sanitation. They concluded that

> "... Breastfeeding is more strongly associated with infant survival in homes *without piped water or toilet sanitation. In homes with both modern facilities, supplemented breastfeeding has no significant effect, and unsupplemented breastfeeding is statistically significant only for mortality in days 8-28.* Presence of modern water and sanitation systems appears unimportant for mortality of infants who are breastfed without supplementation for six months." (Butz et al., 1984, emphasis added.)

Table VII shows some of the data from one of their detailed analyses. Using mortality estimates of breast- and non-breast-fed infants from homes with and without toilets or piped water, or both, they calculated the *increase* in mortality that might be expected if unsupplemented breast-feeding were reduced to zero at various times during the first year, and made similar calculations for the effect of reducing partial breast-feeding to zero. In a subsequent paper they reported further analyses of their data in which they estimated the *increase* in mortality associated with the introduction of different types of foods, compared with mortality in fully breast-fed babies (Habicht et al., 1986). These estimates led them to conclude that "The use of powdered infant formula did not appear to offset the detrimental effects of early weaning and supplementation." Victora et al., in their population-based case-control study in southern Brazil, reached a similar conclusion. They found that the relative risks of mortality from diarrhea and respiratory infec-

Table VII. Estimated increases in mortality rates per thousand infants, if exclusive and partial breast-feeding were stopped altogether at various ages during the first year of life, by presence or absence of toilets and or piped water in the home, among a national sample of Malaysian infants, 1970s.

Toilet	Piped Water	Changes in mortality in:		
		Days 0-28	Months 2-6	Months 7-12
		When exclusive breast-feeding reduced to zero from:		
		1 Week	28 days	6 Months
No	No	43.6	90.2	43.0
No	Yes	37.1	75.5	29.0
Yes	No	16.0	22.1	25.2
Yes	Yes	9.6	7.5	11.2
		When partial breast-feeding reduced to zero from:		
		1 Week	28 days	6 Months
No	No	29.7	55.6	22.2
No	Yes	33.6	48.6	11.0
Yes	No	1.0	10.7	14.8
Yes	Yes	5.0	3.7	3.6

Data from Butz *et al.*, 1984.

tions to be 14.2 and 3.6, respectively, in completely weaned compared with exclusively breast-fed infants, but they observed that "Cow's and formula milk seemed to be equally hazardous." Barros *et al.* in discussing other aspects of the same study (1986) noted that the environments where the protective effects of breast-feeding are most needed, are also the environments where women are most likely to be poor, to produce low birth weight babies, to have difficulties with lactation, and also to have difficulties in affording or preparing alternative food for their babies.

Finally, Popkin *et al.* in their review of breast-feeding patterns in low-income countries based on World Fertility Survey data (1982), report that, aside from within- and between-country differences, there was a "very large difference in breast-feeding patterns between the two major regions studied. Breast-feeding ... seems to be the norm in most Asian countries, but not in most Latin American countries." They went on to discuss the implications of this, as follows:

> "A stronger statement about the negative consequences of reduced breast-feeding can be made about rural Latin America. Even though overall income levels are

generally much higher in this region, income distribution is so unequal -- especially as between urban and
rural areas -- that the fairly early ages of weaning in
rural Latin America almost certainly contribute to
demographic and health problems. These problems
are likely to be much more serious than the consequences of the very low levels of breast-feeding in
urban Latin America, given the urban availability of
potable drinking water and the much higher levels of
income and education (hence capacity and ability to
administer alternative foods satisfactorily)." (Popkin
et al.. p 1082, 1982)

Breast-feeding and the Control of Diarrheal Diseases

Aside from promoting the use of oral rehydration therapy (ORT) to
prevent deaths from diarrheal dehydration, The Programme for Control of
Diarrhoeal Diseases of the World Health Organization has sponsored a careful
review and evaluation of possible interventions for the control of diarrheal
diseases. Given the evidence reviewed here showing that breast-feeding is
associated both with lower morbidity rates from diarrhea, and thus has a
preventive effect, and also with lower mortality rates, it is hardly surprising
that breast-feeding was one of the interventions selected for review. That of
Feachem and Koblinsky as mentioned earlier, was carried out for this purpose.
Their estimates of the relative risk of diarrhea morbidity and mortality, when
infants that were exclusively breast-fed were compared with partially breast-
fed and with bottle-fed infants, are shown in the figures. Having concluded
that the evidence shows that breast-feeding provides a significant protective
effect, primarily in infants under 6 months of age, they then examined the
evidence concerning the effectiveness of programs intended to promote
breast-feeding. They found that results of such efforts vary considerably,
depending on the pre-existing prevalence and duration of breast-feeding, on
the mothers' education level and many other factors. Not only did they
recommend that such efforts be included in diarrhea control programs, but
also they estimated the impact that might reasonably be expected. Their
results, expressed as potential percentage reduction, and based on carefully
qualified assumptions about pre-existing levels of breast-feeding as well as
the effectiveness of breast-feeding promotion programs, have been adapted
and are presented in Table VIII, where it is apparent that the effect is greater
where the pre-existing prevalence and duration of breast-feeding was lower.

Table VIII. Estimated percentage reduction in diarrheal mortality rates produced by breast-feeding promotion programs of varying levels of effectiveness, and by pre-existing patterns of breast-feeding, among 0 to 5 month infants, and in total under-5 year population. Data from Feachem and Koblinsky, 1984.

Pre-intervention Pattern of Breast-feeding	Age Group (mos.)	Percent reduction in diarrhea mortality rate, by effectiveness of breast-feeding promotion		
		High Impact	Medium Impact	Low Impact
Traditional				
High Prevalence	0-5	44	24	14
Long Duration	0-59	14	8	4
Transitional	0-5	54	27	16
	0-59	18	9	5
Modernizing				
Lower Prevalence	0-5	56	28	13
Shorter Duration	0-59	17	8	4
Source: Adapted from Feachem and Koblinsky, 1984.				

Even though the predicted reduction was limited essentially to the first six months of life, there was a non-trivial impact on overall under-five mortality from diarrhea. They also concluded that breast-feeding is a preventive measure that is economically feasible and recommend that it be included as a major element in programs to control diarrhea. In fact, both the promotion of breast-feeding in general, as well as stress on the continuation of breast-feeding during diarrhea, are now well recognized as important components of our armamentarium against diarrhea (See, *e.g.*, Schroeder *et al.*, 1989).

BREAST-FEEDING AND FERTILITY

Women in most cultures have probably known "forever" that breast-feeding had something to do with fertility. McCann *et al.* (1981) noted that a contraceptive effect of lactation has been recognized "at least since the ancient Egyptians" and Thapa *et al.* (1988) wrote that "Aristotle pointed out that 'while women are suckling children menstruation does not occur according to nature, nor do they conceive; if they do conceive, the milk dries up'." The relationship between breast-feeding, postpartum amenorrhea, and fertility merits consideration in a review of the superiority of breast-feeding because sound understanding of the physiologic mechanisms by which birth interval is affected is rather recent, and because we now have good estimates of the impact of breast-feeding on the total fertility (the number of children ever born) for a number of countries.

Ancient folk knowledge of the contraceptive effects of breast-feeding must have been combined with awareness that it was not dependable. Breast-feeding surely made a difference, but a woman could not depend upon it. In some cultures, at least, frequent breast-feeding was combined with postpartum sexual abstinence to enhance its effectiveness. A variety of studies have shown that in many African cultures the combination provides effective birth-spacing (Page and Lestheaghe, 1981). In the chapter by Schoenmaeckers *et al.* (1981), for example, their review of the Human Relations Area files and other comparable sources, showed that in the 171 African tribal groups for which data were adequate, the duration of postpartum sexual abstinence ranged from 0 to 40 days in 22 groups, from 40 days up to a year in 37, and for a year or more in 72. In these cultures the birth interval was rarely less than two years and was occasionally as much as four years. Today in many of these same tribal groups, the polygyny that probably made prolonged postpartum abstinence acceptable to husbands, is becoming steadily less common. At the same time the practice of breast-feeding is declining, especially in urban areas, while utilization rates for modern contraceptives remain low. As a consequence birth intervals are becoming shorter and total fertility is increasing. The consequences of these changes are not trivial, either at the family level or at national or global levels.

Physiologic Mechanisms

The physiologic basis for the delay of ovulation associated with breast-feeding, as described by Short (1984), among many others, is the physical stimulation of the mother's nipple by the nursing infant which results in neural inputs to the hypothalamus. These inputs, as described by Thapa *et al.* (1988),

> "... seem to cause a local release of beta-endorphin, which in turn inhibits hypothalamic secretion of gonadotrophin-releasing hormone and dopamine, thereby suppressing gonadotrophin secretion and ovarian activity while stimulating the secretion of prolactin.

> "The key to the short-term and long-term success of lactation as a contraceptive is therefore the frequency with which afferent neural inputs generated by the baby's stimulation of the mother's nipple reach the hypothalamus. Not only do these neural inputs regulate fertility, but elevated prolactin levels stimulate the long-term synthesis and secretion of milk in the

> breast, while the sucking-induced discharge of
> oxytocin from the posterior pituitary causes contrac-
> tion of the myo-epithelial cells around the mammary
> alveoli, leading to milk ejection. If the alveoli are not
> repeatedly emptied in this manner, milk production
> will be inhibited, and eventually lactogenesis will
> cease altogether..." (Thapa *et al.* 1988, p 679)

These physiologic details are repeated here, not only for their scientific fascination, but also because they help to explain many of the previously confusing differences in postpartum amenorrhea that have been observed. Frequency, as noted above, is the key. Tyson *et al.* have suggested, in fact, that the maximum interval between feeds that will maintain the suppression of ovulation is from three to four hours (1976). Thus, the modern urban mother, who wants to breast-feed her baby, but also wants the baby to sleep through the night as soon as possible, may provide other foods at night in order to discourage nursing then. The effect is to satisfy the baby with something other than breast milk, and reduce the frequency and vigor of nipple stimulation. The inhibition of ovulation and stimulation of lactation described above are quickly affected and ovulation soon resumes while breast milk production is gradually decreased. All too often this may lead the mother to believe that she is incapable of providing sufficient milk for her baby.

The Impact on Fertility

Bonte *et al.* carried out a study in Rwanda that provides a beautiful illustration of the fertility effects of these processes in a traditional African population in a state of transition (1974). They followed populations of postpartum urban and rural Rwandan women, including lactating and non-lactating women in both groups, and observed the pregnancy rate, by months postpartum in the four sub-groups. Their findings are shown in Figure 10, which was prepared for a previous review of this topic (Wray, 1978). The figure shows clearly that among the non-lactating women in both urban and rural areas the postpartum conception rate was high and quite similar -- over 80 percent were pregnant within a year. The cumulative rates in the lactating mothers, on the other hand, were much lower, but there were substantial differences between the urban and rural mothers. Roughly 50 per cent of the urban women were pregnant by the end of the first year, while fewer than 20 per cent of the rural women were pregnant within the first year and barely 50 per cent by the 24th month.

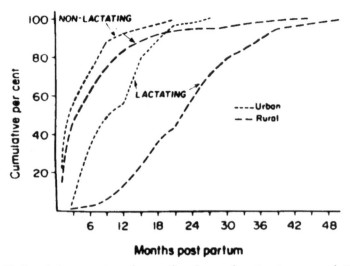

Figure 10. Cumulative percentage of conceptions, by month post partum, among lactating and non-lactating urban and rural women in Rwanda, during the 1970's. Based on data from Bonte *et al.*, 1974, and re-drawn from Wray, 1978.

Why these differences? It has been postulated that the duration of postpartum amenorrhea may be affected by the nutritional status of the mothers (*e.g.*, Chavez *et al.*, 1975). That the cumulative pregnancy rates observed by Bonte *et al.* were essentially the same in the non-lactating urban and rural women strongly suggests that in Rwanda, at least, this was not the case. Instead, the clear differences they found in the pregnancy rates of urban and rural mothers who were lactating can be explained by the newer understanding of mechanisms. Bonte and her colleagues found that there were important differences in the nursing practices of the rural and urban women. Rural mothers kept their babies constantly on their backs and nursed them frequently, day and night, for prolonged periods of time. Urban women were much less likely to keep their babies on their backs, they did not nurse them frequently on demand and they initiated supplementary feeds earlier. In the light of present knowledge the effect of these different practices on frequency of nipple stimulation and the resulting neural effects on the inhibition of ovulation, can explain the different conception rates quite well. Kolata has reported both similar differences in nursing among urban and rural !Kung people and also similar changes in postpartum conception patterns (1974).

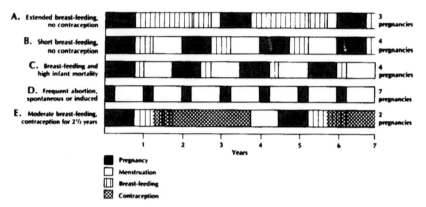

Figure 11. Diagramatic representation of the effects of different patterns of breast-feeding and contraception on fertility. Model A depicts a traditional society where breast-feeding lasts two years, postpartum amenorrhea for approximately 18 months resulting in about three pregnancies in seven years, even in the absence of contraception. Models B, C, and D show the increased number of pregnancies likely to occur with different patterns of breast-feeding, infant mortality or abortions. Model E shows the effect of a combination of breast-feeding and contraception. From McCann *et al.*, 1981.

National and Global Implications

The impact of breast-feeding on postpartum amenorrhoea has implications that go far beyond family or tribal levels. Bongaarts and colleagues (1983a; 1983b) have estimated that 96 per cent of the variance in duration of postpartum amenorrhoea is due to the duration of breast-feeding and that in populations without access to effective contraception the interval between births is the primary determinant of total fertility. In their extensive review of this subject, McCann *et al.* produced Figure 11, which shows the impact of various patterns of breast-feeding on fertility. Thapa *et al.* have used the Bongaarts model and current World Fertility Survey data from 29 developing countries to examine the impact of current breast-feeding practices on total fertility. The total fertility rates observed in the WFS data, their estimates of the number of births that are inhibited by breast-feeding, as well as estimates of the number of births averted by current levels of contraception, are shown in Figure 12. The figure includes estimates for Africa, the Americas and Asia, as well as the individual countries in each continent for which data were available. The figure shows clearly that currently breast-feeding has a far greater impact on fertility than contraception does in all the African and most of the Asian countries for which data are available. The impact obviously varies from continent to continent and country to country, but it is important almost everywhere: In Africa breast-feeding probably inhibits an average of four births per woman; in Bangladesh, with its huge population, an average of 6.5 children per woman are inhibited and in Indonesia the number is almost as great.

Breast-feeding, Fertility, and Maternal Mortality

Thapa *et al.* cite the fact that there is now evidence "that breast-feeding can nearly halve the risk of breast cancer relative to that of a parous woman who bottlefeeds her babies; the longer a woman breastfeeds, the greater the protection" (1988). They note that effect will be more pronounced in affluent countries. In poor countries there is another connection between breast-feeding and maternal mortality that is probably more important. It derives from an important difference between infant mortality and maternal mortality: an infant is exposed to the risk of infant mortality only once; a mother is subject to the risk of maternal mortality with every pregnancy. Thus, although the absolute rates for maternal mortality are much lower than the rates for infant mortality, the cumulative effect of repeated exposure to the risk of mortality associated with repeated pregnancies is serious. This cumulative effect may be defined as lifetime risk (R), and calculated by using the maternal mortality ratio (MMR) and the total fertility rate (TFR), where $R = 1 - (1 - MMR)(1.2TFR)$. Lettenmaier *et al.* have estimated that, excluding China, the average woman in the Third World faces a lifetime risk of one in 33 that she will die of a complication of pregnancy or childbirth.

If we consider the impact of breast-feeding on the TFR, it is easy to estimate the potential impact of breast-feeding on the lifetime risk of mortality of women. Bangladesh is perhaps an extreme example, but it illustrates the issue clearly. The Population Reference Bureau estimates that the population of Bangladesh is around 114.7 million, with a birth rate of 43 per thousand (Haub and Kent, 1989), producing a total of around 5 million births per year. Estimates of the national maternal mortality rate was estimated to be as high as 3000 per 100,000 both in 1981 and in 1983 (WHO, 1985), but in Matlab Thana, a large rural population that has been under careful surveillance for vital events for 20 years, the estimate at the same time was as low as 510 per 100,000. If we accept a compromise estimate of 700 to 1000, then we can calculate that the total number of maternal deaths per year is between 34,000 and 49,000 per year. Given the same maternal mortality rate and an estimated TFR of around 6, we can estimate that the lifetime risk of mortality for women in Bangladesh is roughly one in 30. We can also take the Thapa *et al.* estimates of the impact of breast-feeding on the TFR in Bangladesh and calculate that in the absence of breast-feeding, the number of maternal deaths per year might reach 90,000 or more and the lifetime risk would be on the order of one in 15!

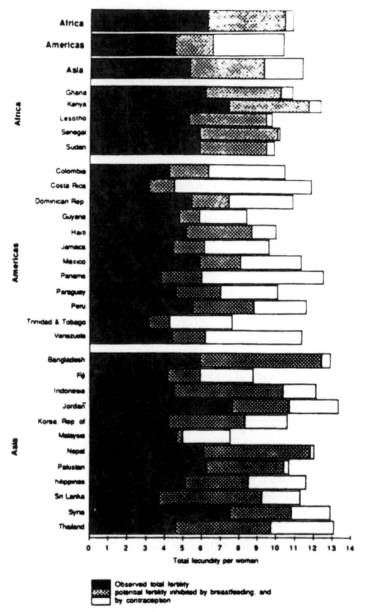

Figure 12. Total fertility rates of women (based on estimates of the number of children that would be born to a woman during her lifetime if she were to live through all her childbearing years and conform to the current age-specific fertility rates), and the estimated number of births currently inhibited by breast-feeding and by modern forms of contraception, in the three major regions of the world and in countries for which World Fertility Survey data were available. From Thapa *et al.*, 1988, their Figure 2.

Breast-feeding, birth interval, and infant mortality.

The same World Fertility Survey data that have made it possible to estimate the impact of breast-feeding on maternal mortality, through its effect in reducing maternal "exposure" to the risk of dying during pregnancy or childbirth, have also provided evidence of the impact of birth interval on infant and young child mortality. Maine and McNamara (1985) as well as Murphy (1986) have provided comprehensive reviews of the increased mortality associated with birth intervals of less than two years. In the light of current knowledge of the effect of breast-feeding on birth intervals, as summarized graphically in Figure 11, there is no doubt that in many countries the birth spacing effect of breast-feeding is an important aspect of its superiority. Thus it can be asserted confidently that the direct effects of breast-feeding on infant mortality that are produced by the immunologic benefits of breast milk, the "bifidus factor," the absence of contamination, and the improved overall nutrition, are substantially enhanced by the reduction in mortality that is associated with longer birth intervals. Figure 13 shows the differences in the mortality rates between infants born after a long or short birth interval as estimated by Maine and McNamara (1985), while Figure 14 shows their estimates of the reduction in infant mortality that might be expected in the same countries if all infants were born after an interval of at least two years. Thapa et al. estimated that if, the world around, all births were at least two years apart, we might expect a fall of 20 per cent in infant mortality -- saving half a million lives. If breast-feeding declines, in the absence of substantial increase in the use of effective contraception, or of improvement in other conditions affecting infant mortality, we can expect that number to increase.

Some appreciation of the global importance of breast-feeding and fertility, and its effectiveness as a contraceptive, may be obtained from a report prepared by a multidisciplinary group of researchers convened by the WHO and the Rockefeller Foundation at Bellagio, Italy, in 1988 (Kennedy et al., 1989). They concluded that,

> "The consensus of the group was that the maximum birth spacing effect of breastfeeding is achieved when a mother 'fully' or nearly fully breastfeeds and remains amenorrheic. When these two conditions are fulfilled, *breastfeeding provides more than 98% protection from pregnancy in the first six months.*"
> (Kennedy et al., 1989, emphasis added)

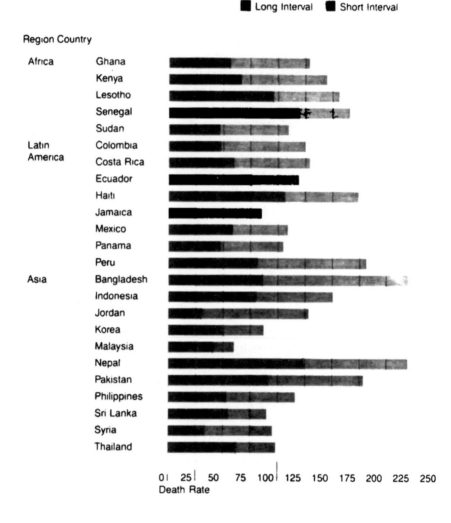

Figure 13. Death rates per thousand live births among infants born after intervals of less than two years and greater than two years in various countries for which World Fertility Survey data were available. From Maine and McNamara, 1985, their Figure 2.

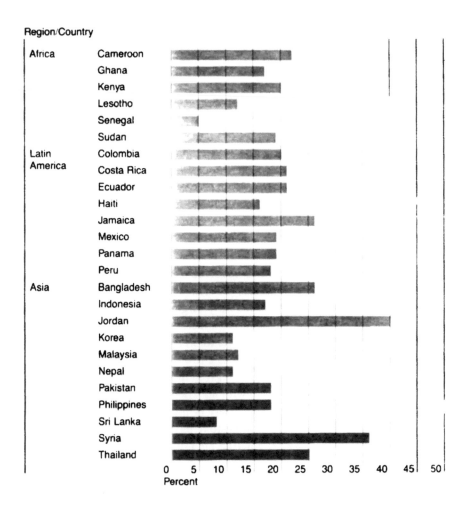

Figure 14. Estimates of the percentage reduction in infant death rates that might be expected if all children were born after an interval of at least 2 years. Based on estimates from World Fertility Survey data of the proportion of infants currently born after an interval of less than two years in various countries. From Maine and McNamara, 1985, their Figure 6.

BREAST-FEEDING TRENDS AND THEIR CAUSES

There have been a number of in depth studies of the prevalence and duration of breast-feeding, and the factors that affect both (*e.g.*, W.H.O., 1981; Winikoff *et al.*, 1988) as well as a number of reviews of trends (*e.g.*, Popkin *et al.*, 1982; Brown, 1986; Millman, 1987; Williamson, 1989). What they show is that patterns and trends vary, that in some places the incidence is declining, while in others there are significant increases, both in the prevalence and the duration of breast-feeding. The consensus, in general, is that the trend to more and longer breast-feeding is on the rise in much of the world.

Differences associated with social class or education are especially interesting. In affluent countries the prevalence and duration of breast-feeding among women with limited education is catching up with the rates among better educated women. In much of the Third World, rates are highest in the rural women and those with least education (Popkin *et al.* 1982, for example), but in Singapore, this trend has reversed (Chua *et al.*, 1989). Almost everywhere, as might be expected, women who work find it difficult to breast-fed their babies; China is the only large country that has created an extensive network of on-site creches -- in factories, schools, communes, etc., -- that make it easy for working mothers to breast-feed (Wray, 1975).

"... It may be appropriate to analyze a few of the reasons responsible for the large number of babies, that are not given the tremendous advantage as to health and resistance always allied with maternal nursing. As deplorable as it may seem, the medical profession itself is probably more at fault in this connection than any other group, and among physicians in the highly specialized branches of obstetrics and pediatrics are found the worst offenders." Thus wrote Sedgwick and Fleishner almost fifty years ago (1921) and they also wrote, "These authors do not absolve their brother physicians from responsibility in the high infant mortality through bottle feeding and note that medical schools spend hours teaching artificial feeding against a casual attitude in discussing maternal nursing."

There is considerable evidence that health personnel are still a "part of the problem" (*e.g.*, Hull *et al.*, 1989; Labbok and Simon, 1988; Winikoff and Baer, 1980). Sometimes this takes the form of resisting specific practices such as demand feeding or rooming-in; at other times it has been found that health professionals are simply poorly- or mis-informed. Labbok and Simon, (1988) in their study of low income mothers in the U.S., found that encouragement to breast-feed from other women -- friends or siblings -- was, in fact, more effective than advice from health personnel. Winikoff and Baer (1980) stressed the importance of changing hospital procedures and Clavano (1981) reported the dramatic effects of instituting rooming-in and eliminating early bottle-feeding. Popkin *et al.* (1990) recently reported that changing national regulations on the hospital promotion of infant formula in the Philippines had more effect on hospital practice than did the World Health Organization Code (1981) on the marketing of breastmilk substitutes.

One of the main targets of that Code was the practice of providing infant formula "samples" to mothers at the time of their discharge from hospital. The effects of this practice have been investigated recently in industrialized countries. Feinstein *et al.* (1986) studied a low-income urban population in Chicago and found that duration of breast-feeding was not affected by formula samples, but initiating breast-feeding within the first 16 hours, and minimization of formula supplementation in the nursery, correlated positively with improved breast-feeding rates. On the other hand, Bergevin *et al.* (1983) and Frank *et al.* (1987) found that "discharge packs" did have a negative effect. Frank *et al.* concluded "that in high risk maternity populations, commercial discharge materials for breast-feeding women should be replaced by materials consistent with the WHO Code."

One fascinating current aspect of the infant-formula-promotion controversy is that many years ago, the industry made a conscious and explicit choice to market infant formula products only by advertising through the medical profession (Apple, 1980). Very recently, some industry leaders appear to want to reverse that decision (Oski, 1989). The outcome of this approach remains to be seen.

No less important is the fact, as noted in the Feachem and Koblinsky review, that efforts to promote breast-feeding can be effective. Winikoff and Baer (1980) provided a comprehensive review of studies of the impact of breast-feeding promotion activities on the prevalence or duration of breast-feeding, largely in industrialized countries, but also in a few Third World countries. Fourteen of those were based on providing information or support, mainly to midwives or other health personnel; eleven were based on changes in hospital routines and three of them combined both. There was, as might be expected, considerable variation in the results, but, with few exceptions, the increases in prevalence or duration, or both, were positive. Various approaches to promotion have been reviewed by Huffman and Combest (1988), and by Jelliffe (1988). Just as important as the fact that promotion can be effective, is that improvements in breast-feeding practices have an effect on the health of infants. There are clear and convincing examples that when such efforts are carried out, and the practice of breast-feeding improves, whether in the hospital (Clavano, 1981) or in the community (Mata *et al.*, 1982), there can be dramatic improvements in morbidity and mortality.

OVERVIEW AND CONCLUSIONS: "BREAST IS STILL BEST"

The variety and the contradictions that can be found in the evidence reviewed here, which represents only a fraction of the total available, pose a challenge. For some issues there is an abundance of evidence; for others, no less important, there may be very little. There are problems of method, of definition, of sample size, of ecology, and so on; many of the reviews cited above make specific and numerous recommendations concerning research needs and there are monographs devoted to such matters (Millman and Palloni, 1984; W.H.O. Regional Office for Europe, 1987). There is no doubt of the need for more and better information.

However, for those concerned with the immediate welfare of infants and young children -- whether the concern is with policy, planning, or program implementation -- there is an equally important need to take the range of available evidence, examine it carefully in the context of what we do know, and, without too much equivocation or confusing qualification, use that information to make the best possible decisions, and then take action -- always recognizing that it may become necessary to modify that action as new or better information becomes available. If such is the case, what can be concluded with reasonable confidence and what are the implications of those conclusions?

The Context

Whatever is said about the nutritional value of breast-feeding, about its effects on morbidity and mortality, or on fertility and birth-spacing, it is essential to keep in mind that the effects depend upon, or vary with:

- The environment into which the infant is born, the standard of living and the socioeconomic status of its family, and this must include the adequacy of the mother's diet. For the purposes of this discussion, we will speak of poor, transitional (urban slum), and affluent environments.

- The age of the infant or young child under consideration; the effects we are concerned with generally become less pronounced with increasing age. Here we need to consider the effects on infants during the first six months, during the second six months, and during the second year of life.

- The interaction between nutrition and infection. We are concerned with the effects of breast-feeding on the nutritional status of the child, as manifest by growth, and on the incidence and severity of infections, as manifest by morbidity and mortality. The interaction between these two factors must, however, be kept in mind. Poor nutrition impairs resistance to infection; repeated infections impair nutrition.

Breast-feeding and Nutrition

- During the first six months, in poor, transitional and affluent families mothers that are reasonably well nourished can produce sufficient milk to meet all the nutrition requirements of their babies. In a few very poor communities, or in times of famine or other dislocations, where and when mothers may be severely undernourished, the milk supply may not be adequate for the full six months unless the mothers' diets are supplemented.

- During the second six months, in most environments, well nourished mothers can produce enough milk to sustain normal growth well into this period. In all environments, however, there comes a point sometime after six months when it becomes essential to supplement breast-feeding with additional calories, and, somewhat later, other nutrients.

- During the second six months, and beyond, in poor environments, babies that are breast-fed exclusively will gradually become undernourished and fall behind in their growth (as well as be more susceptible to infection).

- During the second six months, and well into the second year, in poor and transitional environments, babies that are receiving supplements, will benefit from continued breast-feeding -- they will grow better (and be less susceptible to infection).

Breast-feeding and Infection

- During the first six months, in poor and transitional environments, in exclusively breast-fed babies the relative risk of infection is less, and the relative risk of mortality is far less; in partially breast-fed babies the difference is not so great, but is still significant. The protective effect decreases gradually during this period. In affluent environments, absolute rates of morbidity and mortality, regardless of feeding method, are far lower, but relative risks are still significantly higher in bottle-fed babies..

- During the second six months, in poor and transitional environments, the benefits though lessening, are still significant. They are less apparent in affluent environments.

- During the first six months, and later, in transitional environments, where certain factors make the environment safer -- water supply and toilets, for example -- the protective effects of breast-feeding may be less apparent, and less essential.

- Beyond six to nine months, and into the second year, in poor and transitional environments, the protective effect of exclusive breast-feeding gradually disappears.

Breast-feeding and Fertility

- Among the millions of people who live where modern contraceptives are not available, or are not acceptable, breast-feeding is the most important determinant of the interval between births.

- For the women in those populations, breast-feeding increases the interval between births and thus reduces total fertility. That, in turn, reduces the risk of maternal mortality, simply by decreasing their exposure to that risk.

- For the infants and young children in those populations, higher mortality rates are associated with birth intervals of less than two years, whether the interval precedes or follows, and breast-feeding is the most important determinant of that interval.

THE WHO/UNICEF TEN STEPS TO SUCCESSFUL BREAST-FEEDING

In recognition of the superiority of breast-feeding, and of the fact that something can be done about it, the World Health Organization and UNICEF are requesting the participation of every facility providing maternity services and care for new-born infants to observe the Ten Steps to Successful Breast-feeding. The importance of each of these steps has been established in recent years and, as noted in The State of the World's Children 1990 (Grant *et al.*,

1989), the "ten points are universal in nature and apply equally to health facilities in the industrialized and the developing nations of the world ... Every mother who gives birth in a hospital or maternity clinic anywhere in the world should have the right to a '10 out of 10' breast-feeding service from doctors, midwives and nursing personnel." The Ten Steps are:

- Have a written breast-feeding policy that is routinely communicated to all health care staff.
- Train all health care staff in the skills necessary to implement this policy.
- Inform all pregnant women about the benefits and management of breast-feeding.
- Help mothers initiate breast-feeding within a half-hour of birth.
- Show mothers how to breast-feed and how to maintain lactation even if they are separated from their infants.
- Give new-born infants no food or drink other than breast milk unless medically indicated.
- Practice rooming-in -- allow mothers and infants to stay together -- 24 hours a day.
- Encourage breast-feeding on demand.
- Give no artificial teats or pacifiers (also called dummies and soothers) to breast-feeding infants.
- Foster the establishment of breast-feeding support groups and refer mothers to them on discharge from hospital or clinic. (Grant *et al.*, p 31, 1989).

REFERENCES

Ahn, C. H., and MacLean, W. C.: Growth of the exclusively breast-fed infant. *Am. J. Clin. Nutr.*, 33:183-192 (1980).

Akin, J. S., Bilsborrow, R. E., Guilkey, D. K., and Popkin, B. M.: Breastfeeding patterns and determinants in the Near East: An analysis of four countries. *Population Studies*, 40:247-262 (1984).

Antrobus, A. K. C.: Child growth and related factors in a rural in St. Vincent. *J. Trop. Peds.*, 17:188-210 (1971).

Apple, R. D.: "To be used only under the direction of a physician:" Commercial infant feeding and medical practice, 1870-1940. *Bull. Hist. Med.*, 54:402-417 (1980).

Aykroyd, W. R., and Hossain, M. A.: Diet and state of nutrition of Pakistani infants in Bradford, Yorkshire. *Brit. Med. J.* 1:42-45 (1967).

Bailey, K. V.: Quantity and composition of breast milk in some New Guinean populations. *J. Trop. Peds.*, 11:35-49 (1965).

Barros, F. C., Victora, C. G., Vaughan, J. P., and Smith, P. G.: Birth weight and duration of breast-feeding: Are the beneficial effects of human milk being overestimated? *Pediatrics*, 78:656-661 (1986).

Bauchner, H., Leventhal, J. M., and Shapiro, E. D.: Studies of breast-feeding and infections: How good is the evidence? *JAMA*, 256:887-892 (1986).

Baumslag, N., and Putney, P. J.: *Infant Feeding Patterns, Practices and Trends; Selected Asia/Near East Countries*. ANE Bureau, USAID, Washington and Office of International Health, DHHS, Rockville, MD (1989).

Bergevin, Y. C., Dougherty, and Kramer, M.: Do infant formula samples shorten the duration breastfeeding? *Lancet*, I:1148-1153 (1983).

Bongaarts, J.: The proximate determinants of natural marital fertility. In: *Determinants of fertility in Developing Countries*. vol. I, pp 103-138. RA Bulatao and RD Lee (eds). Academic Press, New York (1983).

Bongaarts J., and Potter, R. G.: *Fertility, Biology and Behavior: An Analysis of the Proximate Determinants*. Academic Press, New York (1983).

Bonte, M., Akingeneye, E., Gashakamba, M., Mbarutsa, E., and Nolens, M. Influence of the socio-economic level on the conception rate during lactation. *Int. J. Fert.*, 19:97-102 (1974).

Brakohiapa, L. A., Bille, A., Quansah, E., Kishi, K., Yartey, J., Harrison, E., Armar, M. A., and Yamamoto, S.: Does prolonged breastfeeding adversely affect a child's nutritional status? *Lancet*, I:416-418 (1988).

Briend, A., Wojtyniak, B., and Rowland, M. G. M.: Breast-feeding, nutritional state, and child survival in rural Bangladesh. *Brit. Med. J.*, 296:879-881 (1988).

Brown, K. H., Black, R. E., Lopez de Romana, G. and Creed de Kanashiro, H.: Infant-feeding practices and their relationship with diarrheal and other diseases in Huascar (Lima), Peru. Pediatrics, 83:31-40 (1989).

Brown, R. E.: Breastfeeding trends. *Am. J. Public Health*, 76:238-240 (1986).

Butz, W. R., Habicht, J-P, and DaVanzo, J.: Environmental factors in the relationship between breastfeeding and infant mortality: The role of sanitation and water in Malaysia. *Am. J. Epidiol.*, 119:516-525 (1984).

Chandra, R. K.: Immunological aspects of human milk. *Nutr Reviews*, 36:265-272 (1978).

Chandra, R. K.: Physical growth of exclusively breast-fed infants. *Nutr. Res.*, 2:275-276 (1982).

Chavez A., and Martinez, C.: Nutrition and development in infants of poor rural areas. *Nutr. Rep. International*, 7:1-8 (1973).

Chavez, C., Martinez, C., Bourges, H., Coronado, M., Lopez, M., and Basta, S.: Child nutrition problems during lactation in poor rural areas. In: *Proceedings of the 9th International Congress of Nutrition*, Mexico, 1972. Karger, Basel, Switzerland (1975).

Chen, L. C., Alauddin, A. K. M., Chowdhury, and Huffman, S. L.: Anthropometric assessment of energy-protein malnutrition and subsequent risk of mortality among pre-school age children. *Amer. J. Clin. Nutr.*, 33:1836-1845 (1980).

Chua, S., Viegas, O. A. C., Counsilman, J. J., and Ratnam, S. S.: Breastfeeding trends in Singapore. *Soc. Sci. Med.*, 28:271-274 (1989).

Clavano, N.: The results of a change in hospital practices. *Assignment Children*, 55/56:139-165 (1981).

Crooks, L. A.: Report on the sanitary conditions of the city and parish of Kingston for the year 1919. (Colonial Medical Reports). *J. Trop. Med. and Hyg.*, 25:67-68 (1922).

Cunningham, A. S.: Breastfeeding and morbidity in industrialized countries: An update. In: *Advances in International Maternal and Child Health*, D. B. Jelliffe, (Ed.), Oxford University Press, Oxford (1981).

Douglas, J. W. B.: The extent of breast-feeding in Great Britain in 1946 with special reference to the health and survival of children. *J. Ob. Gyn. Brit. Emp.*, 57:335-361 (1950).

Dugdale, A. E.: The effect of the type of feeding on weight gain and illnesses in infants. *Brit. J. Nutr.*, 26:423-432 (1971).

Edozien, J. C., Rahim, M. A., Khan, and Waslien, C. I.: Human protein: Results of a Nigerian village study. *J. Nutrition*, 106:312-328 (1976).

Ehrlich, P.: Ueber Immunitat durch vererhung und Baugaung. *Zeitshr fur Hyg u Infectionskr*, 12:183-203 (1892).

Feachem, R., and Koblinsky, M.: Interventions for the control of diarrhoeal diseases among young children: Promotion of breast-feeding. *Bull WHO*, 62:271-291 (1984).

Feinstein, J., Berkelhamer, J., Gruszka, M., Wong, C., and Carey, A.: Factors related to early termination of breast-feeding in an urban population. *Pediatrics*, 78:210-215 (1986).

Frank, D. A., Wirtz, S. J., Sorenson, J. R., and Heeren, T.: Commercial discharge packs and breast-feeding counseling: Effects on infant-feeding practices in a randomized trial. *Pediatrics*, 80:845-854 (1987).

Gerrard, J. W.: Breast-feeding: Second thoughts. *Pediatrics*, 54:757-764 (1974).

Gillin, F. D., Reiner, D. S., and Wang, C-S: Human milk kills parasitic intestinal protozoa. *Science*, 221:1290-1292 (1983).

Glass, R. I., Svennerholm, A. M., Stoll, B. J. et al.: Protection against cholera in breast-fed children by antibodies in breast milk. *N. Engl. J. Med.*, 308:1389-1392 (1983).

Goldberg, H. I., Rodriques, W., Thome, A. M. T., Janowitz, B. and Morris, L.: Infant mortality and breast-feeding in North-eastern Brazil. *Population Studies*, 38:105-115 (1984).

Goldman, A. S.: Cow milk sensitivity: A review. In: *Food and Immunology*, pp 99-118, L. Hambraeus, L. Hanson, and H. Macfarlane (Eds). Almquist and Wiksell, Stockholm (1977).

Gopalan, C.: Studies on lactation in poor Indian communities. *J. Trop. Peds.*, 4:87-97 (1958).

Gordon, J. E., Chitkara, I. D., and Wyon, J. B.: Weanling diarrhea. *Am. J. Med. Sci.*, 245:345-377 (1963).

Grant, J. G., Adamson, P., and Adamson, L.: *The State of the World's Children.* Oxford University Press for UNICEF, London (1989).

Grulee C. G., Sanford, H. N., and Herron, P. H.: Breast and artificial feeding: Influence on morbidity and mortality of twenty thousand infants. *JAMA*, 103:735-738 (1934).

Grulee, C. G., Sanford, H. N., and Schwartz, H.: Breast and artificially fed infants: A study of the age incidence in the morbidity and mortality in twenty thousand cases. *JAMA*, 104:1986-1989 (1935).

Habicht, J-P, DaVanzo, J., and Butz, W. P.: Does breastfeeding really saves lives, or are apparent benefits due to biases? *Am. J. Epid.*, 123:279-290 (1986).

Hanson, L. A.: The mammary gland as an immunological organ. *Immunology Today*, 3:168-172 (1982).

Haub, C., and Kent, M. M.: *1989 World Population Data Sheet.* The Population Reference Bureau, Washington, DC (1989).

Hermelo, M., Amador, M., Hernandez, P., Gonzalez, M. E., Gonzalez-Celaa, F., and Tudela, J.: Los tipos de lactancia y al destete como factores determinantes de diarrea aguda y des-nutricion en el lactante menor de seis meses. *Rev Cubana de Ped.*, 40:299-318 (1968).

Howarth, W. J.: The influence of feeding on the mortality of infants. *Lancet.*, ii:210-213 (1905).

Huffman, S. L., and Combest, C.: *Promotion of breastfeeding: Yes, it works!* Center to Prevent Childhood Malnutrition, Bethesda (1988).

Hull, V. J., Thapa, S., and Wiknjosastro, G.: Breast-feeding and health professionals: A study in hospitals in Indonesia. *Soc. Sci. Med.*, 28:355-364 (1989).

Janowitz, B., Lewis, J. H., Parnell, A., Hefnawi, F., Younis, M. N., and Serour, G. A.: Breast-feeding and child survival in *Egypt. J. Biosoc. Sci.*, 13:287-297 (1981).

Jason, J. M., Nieburg, P., and Marks, J. S.: Mortality of infectious disease associated with infant-feeding practices in developing countries. *Pediatrics*, 74(Suppl):702-727 (1984).

Jelliffe, D. B. (Ed.): *Programmes to Promote Breast-feeding.* Oxford University Press, London (1986).

Jelliffe, D. B., and Jelliffe, E. F. P.: *Human Milk in the Modern World.* Oxford University Press, London (1984).

Karmarkar, M. G.: Studies on Human lactation, *Indian. J. Med. Res.*, 47:344-351 (1959).

Kennedy, K. I., Rivera, R., and McNeilly, A. S.: Consensus statement on the use of breastfeeding as a family planing method. *Contraception*, 39:477-496 (1989).

Keusch, G. T., and Katz, M.: Malnutrition and infection. Chapter 10, pp 307-332. In: *Nutrition, Pre- and Postnatal Development*. M. Winick (Ed.). Plenum Press, New York (1979).

Kielmann, A. A., and McCord, C.: Weight-for-age as an index of risk of death in children. *Lancet*, i:1247-1250 (1978).

Killien, M. G., Evans, C., and Lyons, N.: The effect of infant formula samples on breastfeeding practice. *JOGNN*, 15:401-405 (1986).

Knodel, J., and Kintner, H.: The impact of breast-feeding patterns in the biometric analysis of infant mortality. *Demography*, 14:391-409 (1977).

Kolata, G. B.: !Kung hunter-gatherers: Feminism, diet, and birth control. *Science*, 185:932-934 (1974).

Koletzko, S., Sherman, P., Corey, M., Griffiths, A., and Smith, C.: Role of infant feeding practices in development of Crohn's disease in childhood. *Brit. Med. J.*, 298:1617-1618 (1989).

Kovar, M. G. , Serdula, M. K., Marks, J. S., and Fraser, D. W.: Review of the epidemiologic evidence for and association between infant feeding and infant health. *Pediatrics*, 74(Suppl):615-638 (1984).

Labbok, M. H., and Simon, S. R.: A community study of a decade of in-hospital breast-feeding: Implications for breast-feeding promotion. *Am. J. Prev. Med.*, 4:62-67 (1988).

Lettenmaier, R. N., Liskin, L., Church, C. A., and Harris, J. A.: Mother's lives matter: Maternal health in the community. *Population Reports Series*, L-7:1-31 (1988).

Leventhal J. M., Shapiro, E. D., Aten, C. B., Berg, A. T., and Egerter, S. A.: Does Breast-feeding protect against infections in infants less than 3 months of age? *Pediatrics*, 78:896-903 (1986).

Lopez Bravo, I., Cabiol, C., Arcuch, S., Rivera, E., and Vargas, S.: Breast-feeding, weight gains, diarrhea and malnutrition in the first year of life. *Bull Pan Am. Health Organ.*, 18:151-163 (1984).

Maine, D., and McNamara, R.: *Birth Spacing and Child Survival*. Center for Population and Family Health, Columbia University, New York (1985).

Mannheimer, E.: Mortality of breast fed and bottle fed infants: A comparative study. *Acta. Genet. Med.*, 5:134-163 (1955).

Mata, L.: *The Children of Santa Maria Cauque: A Prospective Field Study of Health and Growth*. The MIT Press, Cambridge, Mass. (1978).

Mata, L.: Breast-feeding: Main promoter of infant health. *Amer. J. Clin. Nutr.*, 31:2058-2065 (1978).

Mata, L., Allen, M. A., Jimenez, P., Garcia, M. E., Vargas, W., Rodriquez, M. E., and Valerin, C.: Promotion of breast-feeding, health, and growth among hospital-born neonates, and among infants of a rural area of Costa Rica. In: *Diarrhea and Malnutrition: Interactions, mechanisms, and Interventions*. pp 177-202. LC Chen and NS Scrimshaw (eds). Plenum Press, New York (1982).

McCann, M. F., Liskin, L. S., Piottow, P. T., Rinehart, W., and Fox, G.: Breast-feeding, fertility, and family planning. *Population Reports, Series*, J-24:525-575 (1981).

McDermott, W.: Modern medicine and the demographic disease pattern of overly-traditional societies: A technologic misfit. *J. Med. Educ.*, 41(Supplement):137-162 (1966).

Millman, S.: Trends in Breastfeeding in a dozen developing countries. *Int. Fam. Plann. Persp.*, 12:91-95 (1986).

Millman, S., and Palloni, A.: *Breastfeeding and Infant Mortality: Methodological Issues and a Research Strategy*. (CDE Working Paper 84-10). Center for Demography and Ecology, University of Wisconsin-Madison (1984).

Murphy, E.: *Family Planning Saves Lives: A Strategy for Maternal and Child Survival*. Population Reference Bureau, Inc., Washington, DC (1986).

Oski, F.: Formula for profits: Heating up the bottle battle. *The Nation*, 249:655,683-684, (Dec 4, 1989).

Palloni, A., and Tienda, M.: The effects of breastfeeding and pace of childbearing on mortality at early ages. *Demography*, **23**:31-52 (1986).

Plank, S., and Milanesi, L.: Infant feeding practices, breast-feeding and the prevention of infant malnutrition. *Bull WHO*, **48**:203-210 (1973).

Popkin, B. M., Bilsborrow, R. E., and Akin, J. S.: Breast-feeding patterns in low-income countries. *Science*, **218**:1088-1093 (1982).

Popkin, B. M., Adair, L., Akin, J. S., Black, R., Briscoe, J., and Flieger, W.: *Breast-feeding and diarrhea morbidity*. Paper prepared for and circulated by the Evaluation Office of UNICEF, New York (May, 1989).

Popkin, B. M., Fernandez, M. E., and Avila, J. L.: Infant formula promotion and the health sector in the Philippines. *Am. J. Pub. Hlth.*, **80**:74-75 (1990).

Puffer, R. T., and Serrano, C. A.: *Patterns of Mortality in Childhood*. Pan American Health Organization, Washington (1973).

Report of the Task Force on the Assessment of the Scientific Evidence of Problems of Infant Feeding. *Pediatrics* 74 Supplement (1984).

Robinson, M.: Infant morbidity and mortality. A study of 3266 infants. *Lancet.*, i:788-794 (1951).

Rohde, J. E.: Why the other half dies: The science and politics of child mortality in the Third World. (Leonard Parsons Lecture at the University of Birmingham.) *Assignment Children*, **61/62**:35-67 (1983).

Rollet, C.: Allaitement, mise en nourrice et mortalite infantile en France a la fin du XIXe Siecle. *Population*, **33**:1189-1202 (1978).

Rowland, M. G. M.: *Growth in young breastfed Gambian infants and some nutritional implications* (1983). Cited in Whitehead and Paul (1984).

Saarinen, U. M., and Siimes, M. A.: Role of prolonged breast-feeding in infant growth. *Acta. Pediatr. Scand.*, **68**:245-250 (1979).

Santulli, T. V.: Acute necrotizing enterocolitis: Recognition and management. *Hospital Practice*, **9**:129-135 (1974).

Schoenmaeckers, R., Shah, I. H., Lesthaeghe, R., and Tambashe, O.: The child-spacing tradition and the postpartum taboo in tropical Africa: anthropological evidence. In: *Child Spacing in Tropical Africa: Traditions and Change*. Page, H. J., and Lesthaeghe, R. (Eds.) Chapter 2, pp 25-71. Academic Press, New York (1981).

Schroeder, D. G., Piwoz, E. G., Black, R. E., and Kirkwood, B. R.: *Improving Infant Feeding Practices to Prevent Diarrhea and Reduce its Severity*. (Occasional Paper No. 8). Institute for International Programs, Johns Hopkins University, Baltimore, Md (1989).

Scrimshaw, N. S., Taylor, C. E., and Gordon, J. E.: *Interactions of Nutrition and Infection*. (Monograph Series No. 57) World Health Organization, Geneva (1968).

Sedgwick, J. C., and Fleischner, E. C.: Breast-feeding in the reduction of infant mortality. *Am. J. Public Health*, **11**:153-157 (1921).

Senecal, J.: Alimentation de l'enfant dans les pays tropicaux et subtropicaux. *Courrier*, **9**:1-22 (1959).

Short, R. V.: Breastfeeding. *Scientific American*, **250**:35-41 (1984).

Suskind, R. M. (Ed.): *Malnutrition and the Immune Response*. Raven Press, New York (1977).

Thapa, S., Short, R. V., and Potts, M.: Breast-feeding, birth spacing and their effects on child survival. *Nature*, **335**:679-682 (1988).

Thiemich, M., and Bessau, G.: *Allgemeiner Teil in Lehrbuch der Kinderheilkunde (10th Edition)*, Feer, E. (Ed.) Berlin (1930).

Tu, P.: The effects of breastfeeding and birth spacing on child survival in China. *Stud. Fam. Plan.*, **20**:332-342 (1989).

Tyson, J. E., Freedman, R. S., Perez, A., Zacur, H. A., and Zanartu, J.: Significance of the secretion of human prolactin and gonadotropin for puerperal lactational infertility. In: *Breast-Feeding and the Mother*. (Ciba Foundation Symposium, New Series, 45) K Elliot (ed), pp 49-71. Elsevier/Exerpta Medica, Amsterdam (1976).

Underwood, B. A.: The weanling dilemma. *Worldview*, 1:8 (1989).

Victora, C. G., Vaughan, J. P., Lombardi, C., Fuchs, S. M. C., Gigante, L. P., Smith, P. G., Nobre, L. C., Teixeira, A. M. B., Moreira, L. B., and Barros, F. C.: Evidence for protection by breast-feeding against infant deaths from infectious diseases in Brazil. *Lancet.*, ii:319-322 (1987).

Walker, W. A., and Isselbacher, K. J.: Intestinal antibodies. New J. Med., 297:767-773 (1977).

Whitehead, R. G., and Paul, A. A.: Infant growth and human milk requirements: a fresh approach. *Lancet*, ii:161-163 (1981).

Whitehead, R. G., and Paul, A. A.: Review article: Growth charts and the assessment of infant feeding practices in the western world and in developing countries. *Early Human Development*, 9:187-207 (1984).

Whitehead, R. G., Coward, W. A., Lunn, P. G., and Rutishauser, I. H. E.: A comparison of the pathogenesis of protein-energy malnutrition in Uganda and The Gambia. *Trans. R. Soc. Trop. Med. Hyg.*, 71:189-195 (1977).

Williams, C. D.: Kwashiorkor. *JAMA*, 153:1280-1285 (1953).

Williamson, N. E.: Breastfeeding trends and patterns. *Int. J. Gynecol. Obstet.*, (Suppl)i:145-152 (1989).

Winikoff, B., and Baer, E. C.: The obstetricians's opportunity: Translating "breast is best" from theory to practice. *Am. J. Obs. and Gyn.*, 138:105-117 (1980).

Winikoff, B., Castle, M. A., and Laukaran, V. H. (Eds.): *Feeding Infants in Four Societies: Causes and Consequences of Mothers' Choices.* Greenwood Press, New York (1988).

Winikoff, B., and Laukaran, V. H.: Breast-feeding and bottle feeding controversies in the developing world: Evidence from a study in four countries. *Soc. Sci. Med.*, 29:859-868 (1989).

Woodbury, R. M.: The relation between breast and artificial feeding and infant mortality. *Am. J. Hyg.*, 2:668-687 (1922).

Woods, R. I., Watterson, P. A., and Woodward, J. H.: The causes of rapid infant mortality decline in England and Wales, 1861-1921. Part II. *Population Studies*, 43:113-132 (1989.

World Health Organization: *International code of marketing of breastmilk substitutes.* Resolution 34.22, adopted May 21, 1981. World Health Assembly, Geneva (1981).

World Health Organization: Contemporary Patterns of Breast-feeding. *Report on the WHO Collaborative Study on Breast-feeding.* The World Health Organization, Geneva (1981).

World Health Organization: *Maternal mortality rates: A tabulation of available information.* (FHE/85.2) The World Health Organization, Geneva (1985).

World Health Organization Regional Office for Europe: *Infant Morbidity-Infant Mortality: Recommendations for Research.* (ICP/NUT 102/s03). The WHO Regional Office for Europe, Copenhagen (1987).

Wray, J. D.: Child care in the People's Republic of China (Parts I and II). *Pediatrics*, 55:539-559; 723-734 (1974).

Wray, J. D.: Maternal nutrition, breast-feeding and infant survival. In: *Nutrition and Human Reproduction*, W. H. Mosley (Ed.) pp. 197-229. Plenum Press, New York (1978).

Wray, J. D.: *Feeding and survival: Historical and contemporary studies of infant morbidity and mortality.* Unpublished background paper prepared for the WHO/UNICEF Conference on Infant Feeding held in Geneva (1979).

Wray, J. D., and Aguirre, A.: Protein-calorie malnutrition in Candelaria Colombia. I. Prevalence: Social and demographic factors. *J. Trop. Peds.*, 15:76-98 (1969).

Wyon, J. B., and Gordon, J. E.: *The Khanna Study.* Harvard University Press, Cambridge, Mass (1971).

Zeitlin, M., Masangkeny, Z., Consolacion, M., and Nass, M.: Breast-feeding and nutritional status in depressed urban areas of Greater Manila, Philippines. *Ecol. Food Nutr.*, 7:103-113 (1978).

5

Science and Lactation

Frank Hytten

Emeritus
Division of Perinatal Medicine
Clinical Research Centre
Harrow, England

A joint meeting between WHO and UNICEF held in October 1979, "The International Year of the Child," issued, *inter alia*, the following statement:

"Breast-feeding is an integral part of the reproductive process, the natural and ideal way of feeding the infant and a unique biological and emotional basis for child development. This, together with its other important effects, on the prevention of infections, on the health and wellbeing of the mother, on child spacing, on family health, on family and national economics, and on food production, makes it a key aspect of self-reliance, primary health care and current development approaches."

That impressive claim is political rather than scientific, and like all oracular pronouncements disregards the possibility of exceptions and individual variability.

When breast-feeding and lactation are discussed it is important to keep a scientific perspective. The intention of this chapter is to maintain an impartial position between breast-feeding and its alternatives, while examining some evidence for the propositions embraced by the WHO/UNICEF statement:

In this chapter, then, I propose to examine some evidence for the propositions embraced by that WHO/UNICEF statement:

Is breast-feeding an integral part of the reproductive process -that is to say does every woman producing a baby also produce and deliver enough milk for the infant's continued growth and development?

Is breast milk always the ideal food for the infant? and is its "uniqueness" important?

Is breast-feeding a unique emotional basis for child development?

Does breast milk prevent infections?

Does breast-feeding promote health and well-being in the mother?

Does breast-feeding have a beneficial effect on child spacing?

What is the basis for suggesting that breast-feeding is economical for the family or for a nation, and how does it affect food production?

CAN EVERY MOTHER BREAST-FEED?

It is likely that every woman can produce at least some milk after giving birth to a baby. This is not the issue; what we need to know is whether every woman is capable of producing, and delivering to her infant, enough milk of sufficient quality to sustain normal growth and development for, say, at least 3 months.

Prevalence of Breast-feeding

The prevalence of breast-feeding is considered in detail elsewhere in his volume. Here it is only necessary to discuss some aspects in the context of the claim that every woman is capable of breast-feeding (as the advocates[1] have it "if she wants to)." Lactation, which is the proper subject of this chapter should not be confused with breast-feeding. Lactation involves the physiological aspects of milk production, and is of course an essential component of breast-feeding, but breast-feeding is a complex behavioural activity with many socio-cultural and psychological features.

It is generally assumed that breast-feeding was universal in primitive man (for example Jelliffe, 1976), as it is in all other mammalian species, and yet there is evidence from prehistoric times of infant graves containing infant feeding vessels of a type which continued until the relatively recent past. That does not necessarily suggest that alternative feeding techniques were very successful, but it does suggest that there was an apparent need for them. In most, perhaps all other mammals an individual female's inability to produce sufficient milk will automatically condemn her offspring to death, so that the trait would be eliminated in one generation. The social organization associated with *Homo sapiens* could avoid that: the young of a woman who was unable to breast-feed could be fed by some other lactating woman in the tribe, and no doubt wet-nursing has been available in human society almost since such a society evolved. In that way the inability to breast-feed will become as recognizable an individual characteristic as hair colour. It is a small step from needing an alternative mother to having an alternative method of feeding.

Therefore, we cannot say that breast-feeding in human society has ever been universal. Nor is it possible to assert that complete and successful breast-feeding is universal anywhere in the world now, although there are many reports from such continents as Africa that it is. The most recent survey by WHO (1981) of mothers with children under 2, found that breast-feeding had been universal in Nigeria, Zaire and rural India. But if children who had not been successfully breast-fed had died they would not have been included in the survey. What is needed is a prospective study of a population of infants from birth to answer the question: is there a place where all children born alive and able to suck survive and thrive for 3 months on only their own mother's milk?

---

1   Since Science considers breast-feeding to be the ideal, the term "advocate," as used here, merely refers to those proponents who feel, perhaps, even more strongly.

Quantity and Quality of Breast Milk

The estimation of a woman's capacity to produce milk is complex, and sufficiently intrusive often to affect the result; few published data are satisfactory or even comparable.

The amount of milk which the baby takes from the breasts depends on at least three fundamentals: 1. the secretory capacity of the breast, which is dependant in part upon 2. the vigour of the infant in demanding milk; and 3. the capacity of the breast to store milk. Thus a perfectly satisfactory inherent capacity to produce milk may appear as an inadequate supply if infants are lethargic in their sucking. Further, breasts with a small capacity for storage may produce inadequate amounts of milk if they are emptied only 4 or 5 times a day, but perfectly adequate amounts to a baby who is allowed to suckle frequently throughout the 24 hours.

Most estimates of breast milk output do not examine these three aspects separately, but only attempt to answer the more practical question: how much does the baby get in 24 hours?

There are many such studies, of which a good example is the report by WHO (1985a) of measurements by test-weighing in contrasting socio-economic groups in 5 countries. The studies were cross sectional and showed a big variation in patterns of feeding and milk taken, but the extremes of milk output were not defined and it is not possible to say what proportion of women appeared to produce an inadequate supply. What is clear is that a proportion of infants were growing poorly even in the first few months, and in no country, even rural Zaire, were all the babies of any age exclusively breast-fed. From these data, therefore, it is not possible to assert that every woman of whatever community can fully breast-feed satisfactorily.

The measurement of milk quality, from analysis of samples, is similarly unsatisfactory. Because there is great variation in milk composition during a feed, from feed to feed during the day, and even between breasts (Hytten, 1954a,b; 1956), a proper estimate can only be achieved from a complete 24 hour sample, and that is almost never possible. The WHO study, which used highly standardized single feed samples, showed wide variation particularly in fat content, which suggested that a proportion of milks were of low caloric density.

There was no attempt to estimate what proportion of women were incapable of feeding their infants satisfactorily entirely on breast milk, but calculations based on quantities and composition from two of the countries surveyed by WHO - Hungary and Guatemala - suggested "...that only a small proportion of mothers could satisfy the needs of a 7kg baby. This implies the advisability of supplementation from about 4 - 6 months of age...." Another review by Underwood and Hofvander (1982) came to a similar conclusion, but suggested further that in ill-nourished women insufficiency is likely to be apparent before 4 months

So far as it is possible to judge from the data available it seems likely that, at least in Western countries, about one third of women are probably unable to produce enough milk, or milk of sufficient quality, to breast-feed an infant for more than a comparatively short time, at least with the 5 or 6 feeds per day schedule employed in these communities.

That estimate is based on three kinds of data. There is a huge quantity of epidemiological evidence from many parts of the world showing that up to 40% of women seem unable to breast-feed satisfactorily; there is evidence of milk output and composition; and there is the very compelling anatomical evidence of Engel (1941; 1947). Engel examined histologically cross sections of breasts removed at autopsy from 80 recently delivered women. Only 20 - 30% of the breasts "contained glandular tissue in the same abundance as animals such as cows, dogs, guinea pigs and others which were examined for comparison." Another 30 - 40% were grossly deficient; they consisted largely of fibrous tissue and fat.

Why do women display such a wide variation in their capacity to produce milk? There are probably two main reasons. One is genetic: it may never have been necessary for a woman to produce milk in order that her infant should survive. The other is the effect of age. In a study of complete 24-hour milk samples obtained on the 7th day of lactation from 500 primiparae (Hytten, 1955) there was a continuous decline both in milk volume and fat content with age, although in each age group there was the expected wide individual variation. Thus 93 primiparae of under 20 years of age had a mean milk output of 441 ml with a fat content of 3.25g/100ml, compared to amounts of 313ml and 2.83g/100ml for 68 primiparae over 30. We can only speculate about what changes, analogous to disuse atrophy, occur if the mammary glands are not used for milk production for many years after sexual maturity, but it is likely that delays of this length are uniquely human.

The breasts enlarge in pregnancy much more in young women than older women, and that is obvious clinically. The degree of enlargement presumably reflects the amount of glandular tissue present; it correlates closely with milk output (Hytten, 1954c).

There is an interesting genetic footnote to be added: the relation between the size of the breast before pregnancy and the eventual milk output is very weak, whereas there is an extremely high correlation between the size of the udder and milk output in goats. The human breast seems, perhaps, to have been bred for size rather than for function.

Maternal Undernutrition

An additional impediment to milk production may be maternal malnutrition, but the data are generally unsatisfactory. Where there is serious undernutrition there are usually more pressing problems than the estimation of milk yield, and associated circumstances usually make it difficult to judge the possible contribution of inadequate milk supply to diminished infant growth. Famine conditions undoubtedly lead to reduced lactation, and in poorly nourished populations women usually have a somewhat smaller milk yield (Jelliffe, 1976). On the other hand maternal dietary supplementation in these circumstances has been shown to have little or no beneficial effect on milk yield or composition (Prentice *et al.*, 1983a; WHO, 1985a).

In general, it is probable that the breast has a high priority for nutrients and that moderate maternal undernutrition will have little effect on milk production. But severe malnutrition, which rarely exists without associated ill-health and other adverse circumstances, may reduce milk yield.

IS BREAST MILK UNIQUELY SUITED TO THE HUMAN INFANT?

When breast milk is compared to the milk of other mammals its average gross composition is obviously suited to the mature human infant. Fat content is relatively low so that the caloric density of breast milk is also comparatively low; protein content is perhaps the lowest of all milks, and the lactose content is the highest. It has been suggested that galactose is an important structural sugar, particularly needed by the central nervous system, so that, in general terms, average human milk is appropriate for the average inactive, slow-growing, big brained human infant. That does not of course imply that other milks of different overall composition are necessarily inappropriate; nor that human milk whose composition deviates from the average, with for example a low fat content, is always suitable.

That gross picture conceals a large number of detailed differences in human milk; many have been described but their biological significance is generally a matter for speculation.

Energy

Energy requirements for the normally growing young infant are low, and probably lower than have been recommended. A recent study by Lucas *et al.* (1987) used the doubly labelled water method and found intakes at 5 and 11 weeks to be about 0.4MJ/Kg/day compared to the 0.49 MJ recommended by WHO (1985b).

Proteins

Much used to be made of the large differences between human and cow's milk in the constituents of milk protein with the major fraction in cow's milk being casein which formed hard "indigestible" curds in the infants stomach. That is not necessarily a disadvantage. Yorston and Hytten (1957) found that in some well-nourished babies who cried excessively after feeding, the gut appeared to be hypermotile; breast milk feeds passed rapidly from the stomach leaving it empty, and the baby presumably hungry, whereas cow's milk feeds left the stomach much more slowly and the baby appeared more content. More rapid transit for breast milk has also been shown by Cavell (1981).

More recently, interest has been focused on the many other proteins in milk such as enzymes and antibodies which may have important specific functions. Lactoferrin is an iron-binding protein with bacteriostatic properties (Bullen et al., 1972) and lysozyme and the immunoglobulins, particularly secretory IgA, contribute to a battery of anti-infective agents. IgA is not degraded by the infant and is able to prevent bacterial attachment at the intestinal surface (Hansen et al., 1982). There is a tendency for ill-fed women to have lower concentrations of IgA in their milk (Prentice et al., 1983; Cruz et al., 1982), but individual variation is large and concentrations tend to fall during the course of lactation.

Lipids

Total lipid concentration is much the most variable component of breast milk, and much the most susceptible to sampling errors, so that the majority of published studies, which have used small samples of breast milk for analysis, are uninterpretable. But complete 24 hour samples from the 7th day of lactation have been shown to have fat contents varying from under 1.5g/100ml to more than 5g/100ml (Hytten, 1955).

The large rise in concentration which occurs during the course of emptying the breast is probably a physical phenomenon, with fat globules adhering to the sides of the alveoli and ducts and only being squeezed out as these structures empty (Hytten, 1954a); but Hall (1975) developed a theory that the change in composition played a regulatory role in infant appetite. The theory has been tested in a number of ways and refuted (for example Drewett, 1982).

The composition of lipids reflects to some extent maternal dietary lipids with a weak association between the ratio of saturated to polyunsaturated fatty acids in the diet and in milk (Aitchison *et al.*, 1977). Cholesterol in milk is little affected by maternal intake or plasma level, but Mellies *et al.* (1979) cite the case of one woman, homozygous for familial hypercholesterolaemia, where milk cholesterol was 16 times the usual level.

It is claimed that fat from human milk is particularly well absorbed by the human infant, partly because of the presence in milk of a bile salt-stimulated lipase, which, together with a lingual lipase released by the infant during suckling, potentiates the action of pancreatic lipase (Jensen *et al.*, 1982).

Carbohydrates

Lactose, the predominant carbohydrate, occurs in remarkably constant amounts in human milk at around 7g/100ml, but there are a number of other carbohydrates present in very small amounts. Of most importance may be the nitrogen-containing oligosaccharides which help promote the growth of *Lactobacillus bifidus* in the infant gut (Bezkorovainy *et al.*, 1976) which produces an acid environment that helps suppress the growth of pathogens, and may assist calcium absorption.

Minerals

The relatively recent ability to measure small quantities of minerals in biological fluids has led to a spate of studies and a confusing mass of published data.

Of the more important metals, iron occurs in concentrations of rather less than 1mg/l, falls somewhat with the progress of lactation, and is not apparently related to maternal diet (Feely *et al.*, 1983a). Zinc levels are high in colostrum, but fall rapidly and continue to decline throughout lactation to levels of a little above 1mg/l in mature milk. There appears to be no relation to maternal diet or plasma levels (Moser & Reynolds, 1983).

Calcium levels also tend to decline somewhat with the progress of lactation but average around 250mg/l (Feely *et al.*, 1983b).

It would be reasonable to assume that all the minerals in breast milk, which seem to be regulated by the breast and are little subject to vagaries of maternal diet, are present in adequate amounts for the average infant. Whether they are enough for the needs of an infant after the first few months is unclear, but it is probable that iron intake from breast milk alone is insufficient, and unless the baby has established good fetal iron stores *in utero*, it is likely to become iron deficient.

The minerals in human milk are much more readily available for absorption than those from cow's milk, so that a direct comparison between mineral levels in the two milks is unhelpful. The difference appears to be due to different binding characteristics and ligands (Casey *et al.*, 1981; Fransson & Lonnerdal, 1983).

Vitamins

Fat soluble vitamins in milk appear to be almost independent of maternal diet, although massive intakes can be shown to have a small effect. Vitamin D has been the subject of controversy since the suggestion by Lakdawala & Widdowson (1977) that there was a considerable quantity available as the water soluble sulphate. That has now been refuted and it seems that total Vitamin D activity in milk is about 40-50IU/l, mostly as Vitamin D itself and as the more potent 25-hydroxy Vitamin D3 (Reeve *et al.*, 1982).

The water soluble vitamins in milk all seem to reflect current dietary intake although folate appears to be less susceptible (Cooperman *et al.*, 1982). Milk from vitamin deficient mothers will itself be deficient, but it responds quickly to supplementation of the mother's diet.

How Reliable Are Data on the Composition of Breast Milk?

What has been said above refers to average milk from healthy mothers and it can not be assumed that all breast milk is therefore nutritionally adequate. A proportion of women, perhaps a considerable proportion in some societies, do not have sufficient fat in the milk to satisfy the energy needs of their infant, and other specific deficiencies are on record. Inadequate quantities of water soluble vitamins will occur if the mother is deficient, and this can occur even in the absence of overt deficiency. For example, Vitamin B_{12} deficiency has been described in a 5-month old baby breast-fed by an apparently healthy mother with latent pernicious anaemia; zinc deficiency, due to low levels in breast milk unresponsive to large maternal supplements, has now also been described for a number of infants (for example Connors *et al.*, 1983) together with deficiency of chloride in milk (Hill & Bowie, 1983).

Does Colostrum have Special Value?

Colostrum, a somewhat ill-defined term used to describe milk during the first few days of lactation, is often claimed to have special nutritional merit. It is a concentrated milk with a high but variable content of protein and sometimes of fat, with high levels of some vitamins and minerals. In young ruminants the very high content of immune globulins is necessary for their survival, but human infants obtain their passive immunity from the mother through the placenta and colostrum does not have that role in man.

Although in general it "...provides all the nutrients, including water, that are needed by the infant in this early period" (DHSS, 1988), it certainly does not appear to have any special function, and in many African societies it is deliberately discarded (Ebrahim, 1976).

Is Breast Milk Suitable for the Low Weight Pre-term Baby?

It is often claimed that the milk produced by women who have delivered a pre-term infant differs from that produced after a full-term birth, and, by implication, is more appropriate for them. A general finding of higher contents of protein, sodium and chloride, and lower lactose, suggests the more concentrated colostral-type milk which would be expected if the breasts were producing low volumes because they were, of necessity, emptied by hand. Anderson *et al.* (1983) concluded that if the breasts are emptied completely, pre-term milk has no nutritional differences compared to term milk, and Forbes (1978) argued that the particular needs of the rapidly growing low birth weight baby cannot be supplied by breast milk alone.

Is Breast Milk Free from Dangerous Chemical Contaminants?

The breast-fed infant is not protected from dangerous chemicals in the environment and there are many reports of pesticide residues in breast milk (WHO, 1985a); and concern has recently been expressed about the widespread exposure of infants in Africa to aflatoxin present in breast milk (Lamplugh *et al.*, 1988). Most drugs taken by the mother will appear in her breast milk, though not usually in important amounts, but some radioactive isotopes, notably halides, are concentrated in milk.

Conclusions

While it is true in the most general terms that breast milk is particularly suitable for the human infant, there are many provisos. A substantial proportion of women will be unable to produce enough milk, or milk of sufficient quality, to support the growth and health of a full term infant, and it is at least doubtful whether breast milk is the ideal food for the small pre-term infant. Moreover, specific deficiencies of micronutrients can occur in milk which is otherwise adequate, and there is a growing problem of contamination of breast milk with environmental toxins.

IS BREAST-FEEDING A UNIQUE EMOTIONAL BASIS FOR CHILD DEVELOPMENT?

The hypothesis behind this question has been widely held and has an obvious appeal. The belief is this: that if an infant is breast-fed, rather than bottle-fed, then it is in more intimate contact with the mother, which is more emotionally satisfying for both of them, and that this, in turn, leads to better "bonding" -a more affectionate attachment -and in the long run to better emotional health and intellectual development in the child. It would be hard to think of anything more difficult to prove.

There is an underlying assumption that there is less intimacy and close contact associated with the act of bottle-feeding, and yet apart from the obvious absence of infant mouth-to-nipple contact the difference is not self-evident. It would be surprising if, other things being equal, the long term development of the child depended on whether it had sucked a nipple or a rubber teat, but other things are seldom equal. Women who choose to breast-feed are likely to be from higher socioeconomic groups, better educated, and probably better able to devote more time to contact with their infant, to child care and education.

Bonding

The strong attachment between mother and child is claimed to depend on the mother's prolonged, intimate (skin-to-skin), and private contact with the baby immediately after birth. Mothers allowed this opportunity appear more likely to breast-feed successfully than those where the baby is removed for some hours after birth (Sosa et al., 1976). Whether or not the early contact promotes breast-feeding, if bonding is itself important then there is no reason why all infants should not have that experience, however they are to be fed.

But the evidence seems to be that "bonding" is of little longterm importance. In Sweden, Hwang (1981) showed that early behavioural differences between babies who had either prolonged, or limited early contact with their mothers had disappeared by 6 weeks. And Lamb (1982) in a review of over 20 studies, claims that few have shown any positive advantage of bonding, and that in these other circumstances could have explained the difference. Lozoff (1983) from an examination of the anthropological literature, found that in 186 traditional societies early skin-to-skin contact and immediate suckling was uncommon, although contact between mother and infant was generally very close in the early months of life. On anthropological ratings there was no increase in maternal affection in societies which fostered skin-to-skin contact.

A prospective study of 1037 children in New Zealand showed no difference at 3 years in such developmental characteristics as coordination, verbal ability, intelligence and behavioural problems, between those who were breast-fed and those who were not when matched for such maternal characteristics as education and socio-economic status (Silva *et al.*, 1976). Further follow up to ages 5 and 7 showed a marginally higher score in those breast-fed, which the authors attributed to subtle differences in the quality and nature of the home environment, rather than to differences in feeding (Fergusson *et al.*, 1982).

In short, breast-fed infants will often be found to have developmental advantages, but these are almost certainly due to upbringing in the kind of family where breast-feeding is practiced rather than to the method of feeding itself.

DOES BREAST-FEEDING PROTECT AGAINST INFECTIONS AND OTHER DISEASES IN THE CHILD?

A great deal of discussion, based on many studies, revolves around whether or not breast-feeding protects the infant against a number of diseases, mostly infections. But it should be remembered that at times when the prevalence of breast-feeding has been declining, both in Britain and in the United States, the infant mortality rates have also declined (Hytten, 1958; American Academy of Pediatrics, 1984). Nobody would suggest a causal relation, but the appeal to the safety of breast-feeding, which was so cogent earlier in this century, is no longer easy to sustain, at least in industrialised countries.

Infections

Ogra and Greena (1982) have reviewed many components of breast milk, including immune globulins, lactoferrin, lysozyme, oligosaccharides and lymphocytes, and these could well contribute to the protection of the breast-fed infant from infection. But in spite of that persuasive theoretical background, numerous studies have been unable to demonstrate that the infant enjoys that advantage.

Because it would clearly be unethical, even if possible, to conduct a randomized control trial of exclusive breast-feeding against bottle-feeding, the evidence must rest on cohort and case control studies, almost all of which suffer from serious design faults. They have been discussed in detail by Bauchner *et al.* (1986). Some of the more obvious pitfalls involved biased ascertainment of cases. For example, the evidence in several studies is based on hospital admissions, but it is probable that breast-fed and non-breast-fed infants with the same degree of illness are not equally likely to be admitted, which might lead to the erroneous conclusion "...that breast-feeding protects against infections, when, in fact, breast-feeding is protecting against hospitalization." Also the stools of breast-fed infants are normally both looser and more frequent than those of bottle-fed infants, so that diarrhoea is much more readily detected in non-breast-fed infants. Even the definition of what constitutes breast-feeding is often unclear. Bauchner *et al.* concluded that most of the studies they assessed had major methodological flaws, but that they "...do not allow a definitive conclusion about the possible protective effect of breast milk against infectious illnesses to be reached. However, the studies that met the methodological standards ... and controlled for confounding variables suggest that breast-feeding has at most a minimal protective effect against infections among infants in industrialized countries.

The report of the American Academy of Pediatrics (1984) also assessed the evidence and noted the major shortcomings of most studies, but concluded that the best studies did demonstrate a positive effect in favour of breast-feeding against gastroenteritis and diarrhoea, particularly three investigations based on American Indian and Inuit populations.

For respiratory tract infections, most of the studies that showed a protective effect of breast-feeding did not eliminate such important confounding variables as maternal smoking, maternal respiratory infection, the presence of other children, and overcrowding in the home. Fergusson *et al.* (1981) concluded that "... the apparent correlation between duration of breast-feeding and rates of lower respiratory illness [in the first 2 years] arose because both prolonged breast-feeding and reduced risks of lower respiratory illness were symptomatic of a superior child-rearing environment rather than being causally related."

There appears to be some protection offered by breast-feeding against otitis media (for example, Saarinen, 1982), but it is not clear whether this is due to some protective effect of breast-feeding itself, or whether the tendency for bottle-fed babies to be fed lying on their backs may not allow milk to enter the middle ear through the eustachian tubes (Gordon, 1981).

Whether the sudden infant death syndrome (SIDS) has an infective basis is uncertain but claims have been made for a protective effect of breast-feeding against this not uncommon cause of infant death. Publications have been for and against the proposition, but a review by the American Academy of Pediatrics (1984) concluded that the association was unproven.

In summary, the evidence that breast-fed infants in an industrialised society suffer less infective morbidity than bottle-fed infants is weak, so that any protection offered by breast-feeding is likely to be no more than marginal.

The position is quite otherwise in non-industrial countries where hygiene is likely to be poor and the level of education among mothers low. An extensive review of the literature in the report of the American Academy of Pediatrics shows persuasively that breast-feeding is associated with a considerable advantage in terms of overall mortality, mortality and morbidity associated with diarrhoeal diseases, and with mortality and morbidity in the high risk newborn infant. What is not clear is whether the protective effect is due to some aspect of breast milk, or whether at least some is due to the avoidance of contact with pathogenic organisms. In babies who are bottle-fed, the contamination of feeds by dirty water supplies and general lack of hygiene must play a conspicuous part, and this is likely to be the primary difference between developing countries and more sophisticated societies where cleanliness can very often be taken for granted.

On the other hand, Briend *et al.* (1988) showed that breast-fed Bangladeshi infants aged 18-36 months, even though breast milk was by then supplemented by a variety of other foods, still had protection against diarrhoeal diseases compared to those who were no longer breast-fed. The effect was particularly apparent in malnourished infants and suggests that there may be a specific and direct effect of breast milk itself.

Similarly, randomly selected infants in a Delhi special care nursery, at high risk of infection, obtained considerable protection if given expressed breast milk rather than bottle feeds (Narayanan *et al.*, 1981).

It is often assumed that breast milk is bacteriologically "clean" in that it carries no pathogenic organisms. But if the mother has an infection, particularly if it is viral, then the organisms may well be present in the milk. Cytomegalovirus and hepatitis B antigen are well known examples, and there are fears that human immunodeficiency virus (HIV) could be a growing threat.

Allergies

Breast milk has been claimed to protect against allergic disease in later life, both by preventing gut infection which would allow the entry of allergens through the gut, and by avoiding exposure to large amounts of foreign protein in cow's milk. Several studies on the subject were reviewed in the American Academy of Pediatrics report. Eczema appears to be no more common in bottle-fed infants; nor is allergic rhinitis and food allergy. But there is some moderately convincing evidence (for example, Hide & Guyer 1981; Blair, 1977) that asthma may be less prevalent in children who were breast-fed. Moreover it would seem that even a very short period of breast-feeding may be protective.

In this context the possibility should be noted that breast-feeding may protect against the development of coeliac disease. In 3 Italian cities 216 coeliac children were compared with their healthy siblings. Early introduction of gluten to the diet was not apparently responsible but those breast-fed for more than 30 days had only one quarter the risk of developing the disease compared to those breast-fed for shorter periods (Auricchio *et al.*, 1983). The mechanism is unknown.

Obesity

Two English studies (Eid, 1970; Taitz, 1971) were probably responsible for suggesting that "excessive" weight gain in the first six months of life led to later obesity. And overnutrition in infants was generally blamed on over-generous bottle-feeds and the practice of introducing solids in the first few months of life. This led some advocates of breast-feeding to assert that breast-feeding protected against obesity.

The published information is muddled and contradictory. Fomon (1980) found that indices of fatness at 8 years were not related to the type of feeding in infancy, but Kramer (1981), who studied adolescents, found that breast-feeding did protect against subsequent obesity. There is so much variance in nutritional experience, environment and genetic factors that occurs between infancy and 8 years, or adolescence, that no acceptable conclusion is possible.

DOES BREAST-FEEDING PROMOTE MATERNAL HEALTH AND WELL BEING?

Many women enjoy breast-feeding. They derive considerable sensual, even erotic pleasure from the suckling and a sense of pride and satisfaction when the baby is obviously thriving.

Such a picture is held up by enthusiasts for breast-feeding as the norm, yet for the majority of women breast-feeding offers no such pleasures. If it did then it would seem curious that a constant stream of advocacy on behalf of breast-feeding should require being directed by public health and other health professionals at those who should know best: the mothers themselves.

The Cost in Well-being

In a detailed personal study of women with young babies (Hytten *et al.*, 1958) breast-feeding was seen to exact a considerable cost. The most common complaint was fatigue, often associated with backache or headache, and sometimes with persistent minor infections such as boils or styes. The general impression conveyed was of impaired vitality and well being.

For the mother with a first baby the first few months represent the most constant work and the longest hours in her experience. Unless she lowers her domestic standards, which few seem willing to do, the ordinary work of shopping, cleaning and preparing meals is undiminished, and now she has the tyranny of a small baby demanding frequent attention which cannot be delegated as she is breast-feeding. She can seldom depend on more than four hours continuous sleep.

In addition, fatigue is accentuated by worry, and worry is more characteristic of the breast-feeding mother who often lacks confidence and is emotionally labile compared to her bottle-feeding sister.

These defects are not attributable to breast-feeding itself, but to the environment is which it is practiced. No doubt is less sophisticated societies, living under the extended family system, the puerperal woman is allowed to concentrate her energies on the baby, unconcerned by many of the worries which afflict the woman living in Western society. But whatever the cause, in modern industrialised countries well being is not the most obvious characteristic of the breast-feeding woman.

In addition to that, local pain from tender nipples and the more severe pain of an engorged or inflamed breast, which may attend some women, does little to emphasize the feeling of good health.

Weight Loss and Undernutrition

Weight loss occurs normally in puerperal women as they lose the fat store accumulated in pregnancy. It is lost whether or not the woman breast-feeds, so that the argument that breast-feeding gives back the schoolgirl figure is misleading. But it more weight is lost, as it may be from the demands of breast-feeding, then this will accentuate the general feeling of fatigue.

Breast-feeding is an efficient process physiologically, perhaps as high as 80-90% (Thomson *et al.*, 1970), so that if the baby is taking 500 kcal (2.1MJ) daily in breast milk, the mother will require some extra 600 kcal (2.5MJ) in her diet. If she is busy then her total energy needs for the day will be substantial and a tired mother may not have the appetite to eat such a diet. Weight loss will result. That will be particularly true of women, such as those in rural Africa, who perform hard agricultural work and it is worth noting that while supplementation of the diet of lactating Gambian women had no effect on their milk output, they felt less fatigued and their general health improved (Prentice *et al.*, 1983a,b).

The Effect of Breast-Feeding on Maternal Disease

There is no evidence that breast-feeding exacerbates any disease, and in general maternal disease is not a contraindication to breast-feeding providing the mother is in reasonable overall condition. Obviously a woman debilitated, for example, by congestive cardiac failure would be foolish to attempt breast-feeding.

The only exception may be severe depressive illness which can worsen in the puerperium and is perhaps potentiated by breast-feeding. In that case, although the mother's condition may deteriorate, the baby is at even greater risk from disturbed maternal behaviour and should be separated on those grounds.

A more sinister association, which is sometime used as an argument for breast-feeding, is that it protects against breast cancer. There is good evidence that there is no such link (Kvale & Heuch, 1988).

DOES BREAST-FEEDING HAVE A BENEFICIAL EFFECT ON CHILD SPACING?

The Effect of Breast-Feeding Itself

In a normal puerperal woman who is not lactating the secretion of gonadotrophins by the pituitary gland, which is suppressed during pregnancy, resumes within about 4-6 weeks. That leads to the resumption of ovulation and fecundity, so that conception is possible, at least for some women, within about 2 months of a previous pregnancy. Salber *et al.* (1966) found 91% of non-lactating Boston women to be menstruating by the end of the third month *post-partum*.

In women who are breast-feeding that interval is prolonged and the current theory to explain it is that the suckling stimulus causes the release of prolactin from the pituitary gland, which together with a neural stimulus suppresses the hypothalamic release of gonadotrophin releasing hormone (GnRH). Thus, gonadotrophins are not released from the pituitary and ovulation does not occur (McNeilly *et al.*, 1985).

That account greatly simplifies a very complex process which is subject to numerous other influences. Prolactin secretion, for example, may be increased by many things including physical exertion, stress and perhaps food intake (Robyn *et al.*, 1985). But in general it seems clear that the longer the breast is suckled the longer will be the period of amenorrhea and infecundity. Anovulation is generally accompanied by amenorrhea, but anovulatory menstrual cycles are also common.

It would appear that the most potent single influence on lactational anovulation is the amount of suckling. McNeilly *et al.* (1985) calculated that with less than 65 minutes per day of suckling, ovulation is likely to resume, and the attenuation of suckling which occurs when the infant is given supplementary feedings is often held to be responsible. Thus breast-feeding in Western society, which is seldom the exclusive method of feeding, is seen to be less effective as a means of inhibiting ovulation than the exclusive and much more intensive breast-feeding seen in less sophisticated societies where suckling occurs on demand throughout the 24 hours. For example, New Guinea infants may enjoy more than 30 breast-feeding episodes per day (Jenkins & Heywood, 1985).

Howie *et al.* (1981) showed that the introduction of supplements by 27 lactating Edinburgh mothers led to a fall in basal prolactin levels and a return of ovulation, which was more rapid if weaning was abrupt, and Indian women who supplemented their breast-feeding have similarly been shown to have lower basal prolactin levels than those who were breast-feeding exclusively (Shatrugna *et al.*, 1982). Another study of poor Indian women showed that if supplements were introduced before 12 months, then menstruation resumed within 1-3 months, but after the first 12 months of lactation, menstruation resumed regardless of supplementation (National Institute of Nutrition, 1981).

Huffman (1983) has pointed out that malnourished infants suckle more frequently than those who are better nourished, and during illness they maintain or increase the amount of suckling. He therefore argues that a high prevalence of infant ill-health in developing countries may contribute to reduced fertility. That poses something of a dilemma: if a child is undernourished on exclusive breast-feeding it should be supplemented and yet that is likely to lead to an earlier return of ovulation and a further pregnancy which, under the circumstances, would by highly undesirable.

The Effect of Maternal Undernutrition

The fact that breast-feeding appears to be much more effective in suppressing ovulation in developing countries than in more affluent communities has suggested that there may be another element involved.

The difference may be due to undernutrition. There is an undoubted link between low body weight and amenorrhea, not only in situations such as anorexia, but also in healthy women in athletic training (Frisch, 1985). The effect is reversible (Knuth *et al.*, 1977).

The importance of this extra ingredient in promoting child spacing in ill-nourished communities is hard to assess. In almost all societies where the women tend to be underweight from poor nutrition and the need to do hard physical work, exclusive breast-feeding is also practiced. Corsini (1979) showed a convincing relation between daily energy intake and the duration of *post-partum* amenorrhea in lactating women from a number of countries, but it is obvious that those countries with a low energy intake also practice prolonged on-demand breast-feeding. Such women also suffer other disadvantages, including a greater load of disease, so that the part played by undernutrition is unclear.

It should also be remembered that in many underdeveloped areas of the world there are still taboos on sexual intercourse during lactation - a much more effective contraceptive.

In summary,there is no doubt that suckling an infant has an inhibitory effect on ovulation, and the longer breast-feeding occurs, the longer will be the effect. The phenomenon is much more evident in disadvantaged communities which suggests that such factors as undernutrition and disease may have an additive inhibitory effect.

Thus, while the desirability of child spacing makes a compelling argument in favour of breast-feeding, it may be better for the public health if the mother were better fed, the infants supplemented if such is needed, and alternative contraception arranged.

IS BREAST-FEEDING AN ECONOMIC ADVANTAGE TO THE MOTHER AND TO THE COMMUNITY?

An early argument in favour of breast-feeding was that it cost nothing. That was of course absurd and it is possible to calculate the cost with some precision. If the baby is growing well on breast milk then its energy intake can be calculated and the energy cost to the mother of producing that milk is a matter of simple arithmetic (Thomson *et al.*, 1970). And because the food the mother will eat is expensive compared to the grass the cow eats the production costs of human milk are greater than those of cow's milk. The mother can, of course, choose not to eat the extra food in which case she will lose weight and the costs will be in terms of general health.

The U.S. Department of Agriculture estimated in 1976 that the cost of breast-feeding an infant in the early months of life was between $3.50 and $5.50 per week, whereas whole or evaporated cow's milk would cost under $3.00 per week (Consumer Reports, 1977).

By contrast, the cost of feeding an infant on prepared commercial formulas is very much greater. Gueri (1980) calculated the cost of Trinidad women to be 4 or 5 times the cost of extra diet to support lactation, and similar calculations have been made for a number of countries (Jelliffe, 1976).

The equation is complex. For the Western woman who is unable or unwilling to breast-feed, the cost of prepared substitutes is not an economic problem. But in poor communities a number of aspects must be considered. Since the cost of breast milk substitutes is high, it encourages their overdilution, often with contaminated water, which leads to a great deal of ill-health in the children. That in turn leads to high costs for treatment, added to which are the costs of a contraceptive service if prolonged breast-feeding is no longer available to provide it (Jelliffe, 1976).

The extra costs of bottle feeding may be offset to some extent in some countries by the fact that the mothers are better able to work.

The economic argument for breast-feeding is unfortunate. While it cannot be denied that prepared formula feeds are relatively expensive in the poorer countries, it also cannot be denied that many young infants and children will need supplementary and weaning foods for their optimum growth and health. The solution, surely, is not to assert that breast-feeding must be promoted to the exclusion of alternatives, but that affordable safe substitutes and weaning foods must be developed. And if these cost more than breast-feeding alone, then it is probably a small price to pay for a healthy child population.

GENERAL CONCLUSIONS

The WHO/UNICEF statement with which this chapter began is a half-truth. For women who lactate well, and who find breast-feeding easy and enjoyable there are advantages: it gives considerable self satisfaction to the mother, and the baby has undoubted protection from some infective organisms.

But a substantial minority of women, perhaps a third in Western societies and an unknown proportion elsewhere, are not able to lactate satisfactorily or for various reasons choose not to breast-feed. For them, it is both cruel and dishonest to cause feelings of guilt and to suggest that they have compromised themselves, their babies and their country by not breast-feeding.

Properly formulated breast milk substitutes are at least as good as breast milk nutritionally, and in some cases may be better. And properly bottle-fed babies can enjoy as close an emotional attachment to their mothers as breast-fed infants, with no evidence of any disadvantage in somatic or intellectual development. The extra vulnerability of the bottle-fed baby to some infections must be faced by the vigilance with hygeine which is taken for granted in modern society.

That clean breast milk substitutes and supplementary and weaning foods are essential to health and good growth in the infant population is inescapable; developing countries must find ways of providing them within their economic resources. It seems more reasonable to take the line that well-grown and healthy children are an economic asset, than that the provision of clean supplementary weaning food is an economic burden.

If child spacing is important, and for many communities it is, then breast-feeding is an inefficient way of achieving it, except in ill-nourished societies where other methods of preventing conception are available.

REFERENCES

Aitchison, J. M., Dunkley, W. L., Canolty, N. L., and Smith, L. M. Influence of diet on trans-fatty acids in milk. *Am. J. Clin. Nutr.*, 30:2006-2015, (1977).

American Academy of Pediatrics, Report of the Task Force on the Assessment of the Scientific Evidence relating to Infant-Feeding Practices and Infant Health. *Pediatrics*, 74 Supplement 579-761, (1984).

Anderson, D. M., Williams, F. H., Mercatz, R. B., Schulman, P. K., Kerr, D. S., and Pittard, W. B. Length of gestation and nutritional composition of human milk. *Am. J. Clin. Nutr.*, 37:810-814, (1983).

Auricchio, S., Follo, D., DeRitis, G., Giunta, A., Marzorati, D., Prampolini, L., Levi, P., Dall'-Olio, D., and Bossi, A. Does breast-feeding protect against the development of clinical symptoms of coeliac disease in children? *J. Pediatr. Gastroenterol. Nutr.*, 2:428-433, (1983).

Bauchner, H., Leventhal, J. M., and Shapiro, E. D. Studies of breast-feeding and infection. How good is the evidence? *J.A.M.A.*, 256:887-892, (1986).

Bezkorovainy, A., Nichols, J. M., and Shy, D. A. Proteosepeptone fractions of human and bovine milk. *Int. J. Biochem.* 7:639-645, (1976).

Blair, H. Natural history of childhood asthma: A twenty year follow-up. *Arch. Dis. Childh.*, 52:613-619, (1977).

Briend, A., Wojtyniak, B., and Rowlands, M. G. M. Breast-feeding, nutritional state and child survival in rural Bangladesh. *Brit. Med. J.*, 296:879-882, (1988).

Bullen, J. J., Rogers, H. J., and Leigh, L. Iron-binding proteins in milk and resistance to Escherichia coli infection in infants. *Brit. Med. J.*, 1:69-75, (1972).

Casey, C. E., Walravens, P. A., and Hambidge, K. M. Availability of zinc: loading tests with human milk, cow's milk and infant formulas. *Pediatrics*, 68:394-396, (1981).

Cavell, B. Gastric emptying in infants fed human milk or infant formula. *Acta. Pediatr. Scand.*, 70:639-641, (1981).

Connors, T. J., Czarnecki, D. B., and Haskett, M. I. Aquired zinc deficiency in a breast-fed premature infant. *Arch. Dermatol.*, 119:319-321, (1983).

Consumer Reports, *Is breast-feeding best for babies?* March, 152-157, (1977).

Cooperman, J. M., Dweck, H. S., Newman, L. J., Garbarino, C., and Lopez, R. The folate in human milk. *Am. J. Clin. Nutr.*, 36:576-580, (1982).

Corsini, C. A. Is the fertility reducing effect of lactation really substantial? In: *Natural Fertility* (H. Leridon & J. Menkin, Eds.) Liege, Ordina Editions, (1979).

Cruz, J. R., Carlsson, B., Garcia, B., Gebre-Medhin, M., Hofvander, Y., Urrutia, J. J., and Hanson, I. A. Studies on human milk III Secretory IgA quantity and antibody levels against *Escherichia coli* in colostrum and milk from underprivileged and privileged mothers. *Pediatr. Res.* 16:272-276, (1982).

D.H.S.S. *Present day practice in infant feeding: third report.* Reports on Health and Social Subjects, 32. London, H.M.S.O., (1988).

Drewett, R. F. Returning to the suckled breast: a further test of Hall's hypothesis. *Early Hum. Develop.*, 6:161-163, (1982).

Ebrahim, G. J. Cross-cultural aspects of breast-feeding. In: *Breast-Feeding and the Mother.* Ciba Foundation Symposium No. 45, Amsterdam, Elsevier, (1976).

Eid, E. E. Follow-up study of physical growth of children who had excessive weight gain in the first six months of life. *Brit. Med. J.,* 2:74-76, (1970).

Engel, S. Anatomy of the lactating breast. *Brit. J. Child. Dis.,* 38:14-18, (1941).

Engel, S. Discussion on some recent developments in knowledge of the physiology of the breast. *Proc. Roy. Soc. Med.,* 40:899-900, (1947).

Feeley, R. M., Eitenmiller, R. R., Jones, J. B., and Barnmart, H. Copper iron and zinc contents of human milk at early stages of lactation. *Am. J. Clin. Nutr.,* 37:443-448, (1983a).

Feely, R. M., Eitenmiller, R. R., Jones, J. B., and Barnmart, H. Calcium, phosphorus and magnesium contents of human milk during early lactation. *J. Pediatr. Gastroenterol. Nutr.,* 2:262-267, (1983b).

Fergusson, D. M., Horwood, L. J., Shannon, F. T., and Taylor, B. Breast-feeding, gastrointestinal and lower respiratory illness in the first two years. *Aust. Padiatr. J.,* 17:191-195, (1981).

Fergusson, D. M., Beautrais, A. L., and Silva, P. A. Breast-feeding and cognitive development in the first seven years of life. *Soc. Sci. Med.* 16:1705-1708, (1982).

Foman, S. J. Factors in influencing food consumption in the human infant. *Int. J. Obes.,* 4:348-350, (1980).

Forbes, G. B. Is human milk the best food for low birth weight babies? *Pediatr. Res.,* 12:434, (1978).

Fransson, G. B., and Lönnerdal. Distribution of trace elements and minerals in human and cow's milk. *Pediatr. Res.,* 17:912-915, (1983).

Frisch, R. E. Maternal nutrition and lactational amenorrhea: perceiving the metabolic costs. In: *Maternal Nutrition and Lactational Infertility* (J. Dobbing, Ed.) New York, Raven Press, (1985).

Gordon, A. G. Breast is best, but bottle is worst. *Lancet,* ii:151, (1981).

Gueri, M. Some economic implications of breast-feeding. *Cajanus,* 13:85-94, (1980).

Hall, B. Changing composition of human milk and early development of appetite control. *Lancet,* i:779-781, (1975).

Hanson, L. Å., Carlsson, B., Fällström, S. P., Mellander, L., Porras, O., and Söderström, T. Food and immunological development. *Acta. Pediatr. Scand.,* Suppl., 299:38-42, (1982).

Hide, D. W., and Guyer, B. M. Clinical manifestations of allergy related to breast and cow's milk feeding. *Arch. Dis. Childh.,* 56:172-175, (1981).

Hill, I. D., and Bowie, M. D. Chloride deficiency syndrome due to chloride deficient breast milk. *Arch. Dis. Childh.,* 58:224-226, (1983).

Howie, P. W., McNeilly, A. S., Houston, M. J., Cook, A., and Boyle, H. Effect of supplementary food on suckling patterns and ovarian activity during lactation. *Brit. Med. J.,* 283:757-759, (1981).

Huffman, S. L. Maternal and child nutritional status: its association with the risk of pregnancy. *Soc. Sci. Med.,* 17:1529-1540, (1983).

Hwang, C-P. Aspects of the mother-infant relationahip during nursing, 1 and 6 weeks after early extended *post partum* contact. *Early Hum. Dev.,* 5:279-287, (1981).

Hytten, F. E. Clinical and chemical studies in human lactation II Variations in major constituents during a feeding. *Brit. Med. J.,* i:176-179, (1954a).

Hytten, F. E. Clinical and chemical studies in human lactation III Diurnal variation in major constituents of milk. *Brit. Med. J.,* i:179-182, (1954b).

Hytten, F. E. Clinical and chemical studies in human lactation VI The functional capacity of the breast. *Brit. Med J.,* i:912-914, (1954c).

Hytten, F. E. Infant feeding. Etudes Neonat. 4:155-164, (1955).

Hytten, F. E. Differences in yield and composition of the milk from right and left breasts. *Proc. Nutr. Soc.,* 15:vi, (1956).

Hytten, F. E. Some theoretical and practical difficulties in neonatal feeding. *Proc. Nutr. Soc.*, 1757-63, (1958).

Hytten, F. E., Yorston, J. C., and Thomson, A. M. Difficulties associated with breast-feeding. A study of 106 primiparae, *Brit. Med. J.*, 1310-315, (1958).

Jelliffe, D. B. Community and sociopolitical considerations of breast-feeding. In: *Breast-Feeding and the Mother*. Ciba Foundation Symposium, 45:231-245, Amsterdam, Elsevier, (1976).

Jelliffe, E. F. P. Maternal Nutrition and Lactation. In: *Breast-Feeding and the Mother*. Ciba Foundation Symposium, 45:119-130, Amsterdam, Elsevier, (1976).

Jenkins, C. L., and Heywood, P. F. In: *Breast-Feeding, Child Health and Child Spacing*, pp. 11-34, (V. Hill and M. Simpson, Eds.) Beckenham Kent, Croom Helm, (1985).

Jensen, R. G., Clark, R. M., DeJong, F. A., Hamosh, M., Liao, T. H., and Mehta, N. R. The lipolytic triad: human lingual, breast milk and pancreatic lipases: physiological implications of their characteristics in digestion of dietary fats. *Pediatr. Gastroenterol. Nutr.*, 1243-255, (1982).

Knuth, U. A., Hull, M. G. R., and Jacobs, H. S. Amenorrhea and weight loss. *Brit. J. Obstet. Gynaec.*, 84:801-807, (1977).

Kramer, M. S. Do breast-feeding and delayed introduction of solid foods protect against subsequent obesity? *J. Pediat.*, 98883-887, (1981).

Kvåle, G., and Heuch, I. Lactation and cancer risk: is there a realtion specific to breast cancer? *J. Epidemiol. Comm. Health*, 42:30-37, (1988).

Lakdawala, D. R., and Widdowson, E. M. Vitamin D in human milk. *Lancet*, 1:167-168, (1977).

Lamb, M. E. Early contact and maternal-infant bonding: one decade later. *Pediatrics*, 70:763-768, (1982).

Lamplugh, S. M., Hendrickse, R. G., Apeagyei, F., and Mwanmut, D. D. Aflatoxins in breast milk, neonatal cord blood and serum of pregnant women. *Brit. Med. J.*, 296:968, (1988).

Lozoff, B. Birth and 'bonding' in non-industrial societies. *Develop. Med. Child. Neurol.*, 25:295-600, (1983).

Lucas, A., Ewing, G., Roberts, S. B., and Coward, W. A. How much energy does the breast-fed infant consume and expend? *Brit. Med. J.*, 29575-77, (1987).

McNeilly, A. S., Glasier, A., and Howie, P. W. Endocrine control of lactational infertility I. In: *Maternal Nutrition and Lactational Infertility* (J. Dobbing, Ed.) New York, Raven Press, (1985).

Mellies, M. J., Burton, K., Larson, R., Fixler, D., and Glueck, C. J. Cholesterol, phytosterols and polyunsaturated fatty acid ratios during the first 12 months of lactation. *Am. J. Clin. Nutr.*, 32:2383-2389, (1979).

Moser, P. B., and Reynolds, R. D. Dietary zinc intake and zinc concentrations of plasma, erythrocytes and breast milk in ante partum and post partum lactating and non-lactating women: a longtitudinal study. *Am. J. Clin. Nutr.*, 38:101-108, (1983).

Narayanan, I., Prakesh, K., and Gujral, V. V. The value of human milk in the prevention of infection in the high-risk low-birth-weight infant. *J. Pediatr.*, 99496-498, (1981).

National Institute of Nutrition, Hyderabad, Annual report, pp. 110-113, (1981).

Ogra, P. L., and Greene, H. L. Human milk and breast-feeding: an update on the state of the art. *Pediatr. Res.*, 16:266-271, (1982).

Prentice, A., Prentice, A. M., Cole, T. J., and Whitehead, R. G. Determinants of variations in breast milk protective factor concentrations of rural Gambian mothers. *Arch. Dis. Childh.*, 58:518-522, (1983).

Prentice, A. M., Roberts, S. B., Prentice, A., Paul, A. A., Watkinson, M., Watkinson, A. A., and Whitehead, R. G. Dietary supplementation of lactating Gambian women I Effect on breast milk volume and quality. *Hum. Nutr. Clin. Nutr.*, 37C:53-64, (1983a).

Prentice, A. M., Lunn, P. G., Watkinsom, M., and Whitehead, R. G. Dietary supplementation of lactating Gambian women II Effect on maternal health, nutritional status and biochemistry. *Hum. Nutr. Clin. Nutr.*, 37C:65-74, (1983b).

Reeve, L. E., Chesney, R. W., and DeLuca, H. F. Vitamin D of human milk: identification of biologically active forms. *Amer. J. Clin. Nutr.*, 36:122-126, (1982).

Robyn, C., Meuris, S., and Hennart, P. Endocrine control of lactational infertility II. In: *Maternal Nutrition and Lactational Infertility* (J. Dobbing, Ed.) New York, Raven Press, (1985).

Saarinen, U. M. Prolonged breast-feeding as prophylaxis for recurrent otitis media. *Acta. Pediatr. Scand.*, 71:567-571, (1982).

Salber, E. J., Feinleib, M., and MacMahon, B. the duration of post partum amenorrhea. *Am. J. Epidemiol.*, 82:347-358, (1966).

Shatrugna, V., Raghuramulu, N., and Prema, K. Serum prolactin levels in undernourished Indian lactating women. *Brit. J. Nutr.*, 48:193-199, (1982).

Silva, P. A., Buckfield, P., and Spears, G. F. Some maternal and child developmental characteristics associated with breast-feeding. A report from the Dunedin Multidisciplinary Development Study, *Aust. Pediatr. J.*, 14:265-268, (1978).

Sosa, R., Kennell, J. H., Klaus, M., and Urrutia, J. J. The effect of early mother-infant contact on breast-feeding, infection and growth. In: *Breast-Feeding and the Mother*. Ciba Foundation Symposium 45, Amsterdam, Elsevier, (1976).

Taitz, L. S. Infantile overnutrition among artificially fed infants in the Sheffield region. *Brit. Med. J.*, 1:315-316, (1971).

Thomson, A. M., Hytten, F. E., and Billewicz, W. Z. The energy cost of human lactation. *Brit. J. Nutr.*, 24:565-572, (1970).

Underwood, B. A., and Hofvander, V. appropriate timing for complementary feeding of the breast-fed infant: a review. *Acta. Pediatr. Scand.*, Suppl, 294:1-32, (1982).

WHO. *Contemporary patterns of breast-feeding. Report on the WHO collaborative study on breast-feeding*, Geneva, WHO, (1981).

WHO. *The quantity and quality of breast milk*. Report on the WHO collaborative study on breast-feeding, Geneva, WHO, (1985a).

WHO. *Energy and protein requirements*. WHO Technical Report Series No. 724, Geneva, WHO, (1985b).

WHO/UNICEF. *Joint WHO/UNICEF meeting on infant and young child feeding*. Geneva, WHO, (1979).

Yorston, J. C., and Hytten, F. E. Rapid gastric emptying time as a cause of crying in breast-fed babies, *Proc. Nutr. Soc.*, 16:vi, (1957).

6

Contemporary Feeding Practices in Infancy and Early Childhood in Developing Countries

Jean King

Cancer Research Campaign
2 Carlton House Terrace
London, England

Ann Ashworth

Centre for Human Nutrition
London School of Hygiene & Tropical Medicine
London, England

In this chapter we describe contemporary methods of feeding young children in a number of developing countries: Kenya, Nigeria, Zaire, India, Malaysia, Mexico and the English-speaking Caribbean. Since breast-feeding patterns are discussed elsewhere in the book, we focus on foods other than breast milk, first considering traditional practices and then the changes that have taken place over recent years and the probable determinants of these practices. Finally we discuss the problems of dietary bulk and contamination which have important nutritional implications.

DEFINITIONS

There is inconsistency in the literature in the use of some expressions associated with infant feeding. Terms that we have for this reason avoided are: 'bottle-feeding', since a variety of substances may be fed by bottle; 'mixed feeding', since this does not specify whether breast milk is being given; and 'weaning', which is used by some to indicate termination of breast-feeding and by others the introduction of supplementary foods. Terms that are used in the text are defined as follows:

Exclusive breast-feeding includes breast-feeding with or without supplements of water, fruit juice or vitamins. This is the most commonly used definition in the literature.

Supplementation refers to the use of other milk and/or other food together with breast milk. Although not usually specified, regular supplementation rather than the casual offering of 'titbits' is inferred.

Sevrage indicates the total replacement of breast milk with other milk and/or other food.

Other milk refers to processed milk, specified where known as infant formula (IF), sweetened condensed milk (SCM), or dried milk powder (DMP - skimmed or whole), and fresh animal milk.

FEEDING PATTERNS AND PRACTICES

In this chapter, the feeding of infants and young children will be considered under four broad headings: pre-lacteal feeds; 'exclusive' breast-feeding; supplemented breast-feeding; and sevrage. In non-traditional cultures, breast milk may be totally replaced by other milks.

Pre-lacteal Feeds

The feeding of various substances prior to the first breast-feed has been reported in many communities around the world. A common reason for giving pre-lacteal feeds is the rejection of colostrum as unclean or unwholesome. A further reason in some cultures is the belief that the meconium is harmful. Pre-lacteal feeds thus include colostrum-substitutes (*e.g.* diluted animal milks) and substances with a purgative action (*e.g.* oil, butter). Examples of traditional pre-lacteal feeds are shown in Table I.

Until the mid-eighteenth century, the recommended practice in Britain was to give newborn infants a purge of honey and oil followed by a bread pap or cereal broth; alternatively, a surrogate nursemaid was found (Wickes, 1953). Fildes (1980) suggests that it was the subsequent medical denouncement of purging and recommendation of colostrum that led to the decline in neonatal mortality witnessed in Britain after 1750. In India, purging with honey and butter has also been recommended since ancient times (Agarwal *et al.*, 1982) and recent studies show that the rejection of colostrum persists, although the most common substitutes are now diluted animal milk or water sweetened with sugar, honey, glucose or jaggery (crude brown sugar) (Wijga *et al.*, 1983; Nutrition Foundation of India, undated; Karnawat *et al.*, 1987).

The practice of giving pre-lacteal medicinal teas to newborn infants is common in both western Nigeria and the Caribbean, where teas made from herbs, known as *agbo* and *bush tea* respectively, traditionally formed the first supplement. Some teas may have a purgative action but are considered to give strength and maintain health (Jelliffe, 1953) or to be more digestible than milk as the first and last feed of the day (Landman *et al.*, 1976). A tea made commonly with camomile or oregano, often with added sugar, is also still given to neonates in central Mexican villages in order to remedy colic (Millard *et al.*, 1985); here again colostrum is considered unhealthy.

In some cultures, large quantities of plain water are given, both as pre-lacteal feeds and continuing into lactation. For example, in a study in western Nigeria, 95% of mothers gave only water for an average of 13 hours after birth, and up to 3 months of age, water contributed more than half the infants' fluid intake (Omololu, 1982). In the Caribbean, water and glucose-water are now common pre-lacteal feeds. Reports from Nigeria, India and Malaysia indicate a small but increasing use of IF as a pre-lacteal feed, especially in hospital deliveries. Although many health workers continue to stress the value of colostrum, old beliefs often persist among traditional birth attendants, for example in Nigeria (Akenzua *et al.*, 1981). By contrast, among the Kikuyu of Kenya no prejudice against colostrum exists and breast-feeding is usually initiated within 24 hours of birth (Esterik *et al.*, 1986). Similarly, among tribal groups in India, colostrum is universally accepted as beneficial (Vimala *et al.*, 1987).

Table 1. Early traditional practices related to infant feeding in Britain, Malaysia, the Caribbean, Nigeria and Zaire

Traditional Practice	Britain[1]	Malaysia[2]	Caribbean[3]	Nigeria[4]	Zaire[5]
1. Postpartum confinement and special diet.		Malay women-44 days' confinement. Given 'heating' foods.	Nine days' confinement.	Varying periods of confinement. Wealthy women in SE Nigeria stayed in 'fattening' house for several months. In south, women given yam, pepper soup and palm wine.	A few days only. Some tribes given luxury foods, e.g. meat.
2. Rejection of colostrum and giving of prelacteal feeds.	Common until 1750. New born gives oil/honey purge, then pap or panada, or fed by another woman.	Colostrum considered 'dirty'. Mashed banana given until lactation established.	In Jamaica-new born given castor oil, then bush tea. In Trinidad, new born given sugar/honey water.	Igbos-rejected colostrum, gave water. Yoruba-gave agbo, a herbal infusion, or diluted.	Some tribes rejected colostrum. Others put baby to breast immediately.
3. Prolonged lactation.	16th century-18 months. 18th century-seven months.	18 months-three years (Malays).	Up to 18 months.	South-two to three years (relactation by grandmothers). North-two years. Wet-nursing in cases of lactation failure.	Two to four years.
4. Early supplementation with foods or beverages.	Bread, pap or panada given in first weeks.	Rice or banana pap with added sugar, hand-fed from first days of life.	Breadkips, pap of arrowroot/cornstarch/wheatflour, sweetened with sugar. Bush teas given throughout the region.	Eket (SE), mashed plantain given at two to three months. Igbo-two to four months, maize pap. Yoruba-gave agbo (herb tea) and water from birth.	Many tribes gave a pap of cassava, banana, sorghum, millet, cassava-maize flour in first weeks of life. Others from four to six months.
5. Reported reasons for early supplementation.		Rice considered 'strength-giving', breast-milk not a sufficient food for a baby. Also, women working in plantations; lactation failure reported.	Mothers' return to work on plantations. Arrowroot believed to be fattening. One report that breast-milk not a sufficient food.	Yoruba-agbo believed to be nutritious. Hausa-lactation failure reported.	Breast-milk not a sufficient food. Mother had to return to farm. Child crying, not satisfied with breast-milk.
6. Postpartum abstinence/belief in contraceptive properties of lactation.		Lactation believed to prevent conception.	Lactation believed to prevent conception. Immediate sevrage if pregnant.	Abstinence usually for 18-24 months. Some northern tribes-40 days. Immediate sevrage if pregnant.	Abstinence common, but some tribes continued breast-feeding during pregnancy.

[1] See text. [2] King et al., 1987b, [3] King et al., 1987c, [4] King et al., 1987d, [5] King et al., 1987e.

Social Group	Age Group								
	0-1 Months			1-2 Months			2-3 Months		
	Kenya	Mexico	Malaysia	Kenya	Mexico	Malaysia	Kenya	Mexico	Malaysia
Urban Elite	16	19	13	2	5	7	3	0	0
Urban Poor	23	34	22	15	13	7	11	21	0
Rural	31	32	12	28	31	16	17	26	2

Table II. The percentage of breast-fed infants in 3 social groups who were exclusively breast-fed in early infancy.

(Data taken from Dimond et al., 1987)

In traditional societies such as India and West Africa, the use of pre-lacteal feeds is compatible with prolonged lactation. However, in societies which have been exposed to western methods of infant feeding, there may be a negative effect on the duration of breast-feeding (Gueri et al., 1977). In Jamaica, infants given supplementary milk-feeds after delivery were rarely exclusively breast-fed on leaving hospital; however other factors such as prematurity, low birth weight and abnormal delivery were also found to influence breast-feeding performance (Grantham-McGregor et al. 1970). Similar detrimental effects have been shown in Brazil (Martines, 1989). Other hazards of pre-lacteal feeds include the probable contamination of the fluids and occasional solids given at such a young age as well as the traditional feeding methods used, such as allowing the infant to suck a cloth soaked in the preparation (Kushwaha et al., 1987). The risk of contamination is coupled with the loss of the rich supply of protective agents found in colostrum. A highly significant correlation between the discarding of colostrum and the incidence of infections was shown in Indian neonates (Bhandari et al., 1983).

Exclusive Breast-feeding

This topic is dealt with in Chapters 4 and 5, so we will only touch on it in relation to the degree of 'exclusiveness' involved. It is increasingly evident that infants are rarely fed only breast milk; frequently this description has been loosely applied to situations where water, fruit juices and perhaps herb teas, tonics or vitamin preparations are also given. Thus, in a study of infant feeding practices in Kenya, Malaysia and Mexico, exclusive breast-feeding was not common in any country even during the very earliest months. Among breast-fed infants , the percentages who were breast-fed exclusively in the first 3 months of life ranged from 0% to 34% (Table II). The highest prevalence of exclusive breast-feeding was seen among poor urban mothers in Mexico during the first month (Dimond et al., 1987).

Supplemented Breast-feeding

Traditional Practices

In traditional societies, the first supplement offered to young infants is often a gruel prepared from the local staple (a cereal or starchy tuber, root or fruit) and water (Table I). Initially the gruels are specially prepared for the infant who is then gradually introduced to the adult diet according to physiological maturity. In pastoral societies, where milk and milk products are staples, these have played a dominant role in the diet of young infants. It has become increasingly recognised that in many cultures supplements have traditionally been introduced at an early age, typically within the first 3 months of life. This is the case among ethnic groups in 5 of the 7 countries surveyed here, the exceptions being India and Mexico, as discussed below.

Malaysia

Among rural Malays, cooked, mashed banana or ground rice cooked with sugar was traditionally fed by hand from the first week of life, since these staples were reputed to have strength-giving properties and breast milk alone was not considered a sufficient food (*e.g.* Firth, 1966). The infants subsequently progressed to the traditional adult diet of rice and sauce with saltfish and occasional fruits (Jelliffe, 1968). With urbanisation, early supplementation with 'starchy' foods persisted; nearly half the Malay mothers in one study had given such supplements by 3 months (Millis, 1958) but one-third of the children received no meat or fish by their first birthday, (since these foods were considered indigestible and fish was believed to cause worms) and fresh vegetables were rarely given due to their 'cooling' properties. More than half the infants, however, received fruit in their second semester.

Kenya

Traditionally, among the Luo, supplementation began as early as 2-3 weeks when the mother's milk was deemed insufficient and generally between 1-3 months when breast milk and gruel played almost equal parts in the diet. After 6 months, gruel formed the major component of the diet, usually made from sorghum and millet flours with a little sour milk added when possible. Gruel was considered especially important in the period up to when the child began to walk, since it was believed to strengthen bones. Frequent tastes of adult food would be provided in the second semester (Odhalo, 1961). Among the Akamba of Machakos in rural Kenya, traditional practices persist although the first supplement offered at 1 to 2 months is cow's milk. The milk is usually boiled and either used freshly or left to ferment and fed when sour. Around the third month, a maize-flour gruel, *uji*, is introduced, to which milk (and more recently sugar) may be added (Steenbergen *et al.*, 1983). Once again there is a perception among Kenyan mothers that breast milk alone is not a sufficient food (Esterik *et al.*, 1986). In the second semester a thicker gruel, *ugali*, is traditionally given together with vegetable stew. After 2 years of age, the local staple dish *isyo* is fed, consisting of a mixture of maize and beans cooked in water for 2 to 5 hours. Most dishes are prepared in large quantities to last over 2 days. While maize is the main ingredient of *uji*, the composition varies to some extent with geographical region. In a nationwide study, the second most popular porridge was maize mixed with millet, followed by millet alone. Others consisted of cassava, alone or with cereals or bananas (Republic of Kenya, undated). An association was observed between the prevalence of malnutrition and porridge composition, with the worst malnutrition occurring in regions where cassava or bananas were the main constituents.

Nigeria

In Nigeria, early supplementation is also practised; the feeding of *agbo* (herb tea) from birth has already been mentioned, and maize 'pap' might be given from as early as 2 months in the east. In a study in an Igbo village, infants in their first semester were given up to half a cup of pap three times a day by spoon or poured from a dish or shell. By 6 to 9 months, mashed or pre-chewed yam was given 1 to 3 times a day, gradually replacing the maize, and by 10 to 12 months the infants received soup or palm oil with the yam. In southern Nigeria yam assumes the dominant role played by rice in Asian cultures, while other food items are considered mere flavourings and therefore not essential components of the infant's diet (Hauck *et al.*, 1963). Animal foods were not given for fear that the child might develop a taste for such luxuries and resort to stealing. In the west, supplementation with maize pap traditionally began later than in the east or south, mainly after 6 months; this was followed by yam, cassava or steamed beancake (Jelliffe, 1953). In the north, supplementation traditionally began later still, a sorghum gruel being introduced from between 5 and 9 months (Osuhor, 1980).

Zaire

Anthropological reports from Zaire describe very early supplementation (in the first few days or weeks) with herbal decoctions, mashed banana or cassava pap, again in the belief that breast milk alone was insufficient. Traditional practices persist in Zaire and recent studies show a varied pattern of supplementation. In the woodland savannah region of Kasai, a gruel of cassava paste or mashed beans was provided at 3 months and, by 5 months, cassava , rice or beans and some fish or meat were given once or twice a week. By 1 year, the children received an adult diet (Vis *et al.*, 1974). In another report from the same region, supplementation from as early as 4 to 5 weeks was noted, and ascribed to the mother's need to prepare the infant to being left at home while she returned to work in the fields. The main supplement, *bidia* (a gruel prepared from cassava and maize flours), was dipped in a sauce of cassava leaves cooked in palm oil with a small piece of fish or meat (Brown *et al.*, 1980). Similarly, in eastern Zaire in the high plateau area of the Great Lakes region, infants received a sorghum-flour and banana-juice gruel from the first or second month and later were also given fish and cow's milk. In the equatorial forest zone, however, supplementation began only from the fourth to seventh month, with foods such as cassava, palm oil, fish and fruits (Vis *et al.*, 1974).

Caribbean

In the Caribbean, traditional infant feeding patterns were distorted by the trauma of slavery which destroyed family structure and resulted in a predominance, persisting today, of households headed by women. Constrained by enforced work, mothers gave supplements at an early age. 'Bread tea', wheatflour or arrowroot pap were fed under unhygienic conditions and an association with diarrhoeal disease was noted in many early medical reports (Marchione, 1980).

In later years, oatmeal or cornmeal porridge, milk (where cows were kept), fruit juices and 'bush teas' were commonly reported first supplements. Older infants were given additional mashed Irish potato, green banana or soft rice (King *et al.*, 1987c). The age at which supplements were first introduced ranged from 2 to 10 months, often related to the mother's breast-feeding performance and the perceived need of the child (Herskovits *et al.*, 1947).

India

In contrast, traditional infant feeding practices in India are characterised by delayed supplementation until 6 months of age, or even later. No special infant foods are prepared; consequently, gruels which are traditional elsewhere are rarely given to Indian infants (WHO, 1981; Wijga *et al.*, 1983). Animal milk is the most common first supplement. Foods from the adult diet such as dhal (lentils), rice and vegetables are given from 1 year or when the child begins to walk.

Mexico

Studies from rural Mexico prior to the 1960s also indicate later supplementation; in one study, 91% of infants were 'exclusively' breast-fed up to 6 months of age and were observed to become progressively malnourished. However, the use of herb teas, initially as pre-lacteal feeds, probably continued throughout infancy and was noted as the most frequently-used supplement at 6 months in another more recent study (Sanjur *et al.*, 1970). Traditional supplements, in order of frequency of use, included cow's or goat's milk, fruit (mainly banana, orange, apple, pawpaw), *caldo de frijol* (red beans cooked and mashed into a watery soup) and *tortilla* (flat cornbread). *Atole*, a watery gruel prepared from maize flour, did not predominate overall in the first semester, but was the most common of all the supplements that were used at all in the first month. As a highly esteemed food, it might be given in preference to breast milk (Fink, 1985).

Summary of Traditional Practices

From the brief review above, it is clear that early supplementation, sometimes in the first few weeks of life, was common in several African societies, Malaysia and the Caribbean. There appear to be two main reasons for very early supplementation in traditional societies. Commonly there is a cultural perception of the nourishing or 'superfood' properties of the local staple while breast milk alone is considered an inadequate food; this may be associated with a perceived inadequacy of breast milk as frequently claimed by mothers. Secondly, in many societies the woman's agricultural or other work commitment meant that the infant might be left with a caretaker for several hours at a time, and thus some alternative provision was necessary. In the next section we consider how these traditional practices have been modified in recent years.

Recent Changes in Supplementation Patterns and Practices

An important factor which has affected supplementation practices undoubtedly relates to the commercial availability and promotion of processed milks and commercial baby foods, notably cereals. In consequence, a move away from the use of traditional gruels and towards these commercial products has taken place in many countries. In those cultures where early supplementation was traditionally practised, this has persisted into modern times but the nature of the supplements has often changed. In those cultures where later supplementation was the norm, a trend towards earlier introduction of supplements has been observed.

Table III.The percentage of breast-fed infants in 3 social groups who received supplementary milk and/or other foods in early infancy								
Social Group	Age Group							
	0-1 Months			1-2 Months			2-3 Months		
	Kenya	Mexico	Malaysia	Kenya	Mexico	Malaysia	Kenya	Mexico	Malaysia
Urban Elite	55	76	60	87	91	86	92	100	80
Urban Poor	34	53	75	75	71	90	74	71	93
Rural	20	57	70	44	42	73	65	70	85
(Data taken from Dimond et al., 1987)								

Malaysia

In rural areas of Malaysia, from the 1950s and 1960s, commercial products such as cornflour and wheatflour have been used for preparing gruels when they could be afforded. Tinned milk, mainly SCM, has also become increasingly popular (King et al., 1987b). Similar changes were observed in urban areas from an even earlier date; processed milks had been available and were being actively promoted in the press by the turn of the century. Initially, advertisements were aimed at expatriates but from the 1950s Malay mothers were increasingly targeted (Manderson, 1982). A nationwide study in the late 1970s showed the persistence of early supplementation; over 80% of mothers from all social groups gave supplements (milk and/or other food by 2 to 3 months (Table III) (Dimond et al., 1987). Non-milk foods still predominated as first supplements among both rural and urban mothers. Commercial cereals were given in preference to unbranded cereals up to 6 months of age, but thereafter unbranded cereals increasingly replaced them. Other milks were used widely, particularly by urban mothers. In recent years, IF has now largely replaced SCM but poorer mothers tend to confine its use to the first semester (Haaga, 1984).

Kenya

In rural areas of Kenya, cow's milk is to some extent being replaced by commercially pasteurised milk bought in paper containers and given, as before, either fresh or sour (the latter occuring spontaneously when packets are stored at ambient temperatures for 1 to 2 days). Milk may be fed by cup or bottle. Early supplementation persists in the rural areas. For example, among the Akamba in the mid-1970s, 14% of mothers gave supplements in the first month, this figure rising to 84% over 2 to 6 months (Steenbergen et al., 1983). In a few districts in one nationwide study, however, between one-

and two-fifths of infants remained unsupplemented at 6 months (Republic of Kenya, 1984).

In urban areas, early supplementation is also the norm; of nearly 1000 mothers with children under 18 months, in the Infant Feeding Practices study in Nairobi, almost half had given supplements by 1 to 2 months. At 3 to 4 months, only 11% of infants were still 'exclusively' breast-fed while 65% were given a combination of breast milk and other foods which included other milk (cow's milk or IF). At the time of the interview, 38% of all the children were receiving breast milk with some other milk (Latham *et al.*, 1986). Nationwide, at least 65% of mothers were giving supplements by 2 to 3 months (Table III) (Dimond *et al.*, 1987).

A 24-hour recall in the Nairobi study showed that the use of other milks rose sharply in the first few months and then levelled off. Over half the infants had received IF at some time (including 44% of those 2-4 months old) while cow's milk was generally given later and was continued into childhood. Similarly, the use of commercial cereals peaked at 4 to 6 months (21%), falling to very low levels beyond 10 months, to be replaced by the traditional gruels, *uji* and then *ugali*. Glucose-water was also given extensively in the early months (21% under 2 months). Fruits and vegetables, with the exception of bananas and (Irish) potatoes, played only a minor role in the young child's diet (Latham *et al.*, 1986). A high rate of usage of commercial products (milk or cereal) was noted in the Kenyan Second Nutrition Survey; 30% of rural and 72% of urban infants had received commercial infant preparations at some time (Republic of Kenya, undated).

Nigeria

In Nigeria, changes in infant feeding practices were first observed in the 1950s, in the use of processed milk (by 13% of infants in one urban study (Jelliffe, 1953)). Most mothers abandoned processed milk after a short time, however, due to its cost and an observed association with diarrhoea, probably as a result of dilution with contaminated water (feeding bottles were rarely used at this time). By the 1970s, however, the use of commercial milks and cereals had increased in urban areas, especially among educated mothers. These supplements were introduced early, often from the first month, and were frequently discontinued after the first semester (except by elite mothers) to be replaced by traditional supplements (Cherian, 1981; WHO, 1981). The use of bottles to feed both processed milks and maize or sorghum pap, either separately or together, is noted in several reports as well as the mothers' perception that both breast milk and processed milks were necessary for their infants' health and strength (*e.g.* Di Domenico *et al.*, 1979; Igun, 1982). The use of processed milk, particularly IF, increased still further in the early 1980s, although lower income mothers tended to confine its use to the first 6 months (Orwell *et al.*, 1984). In urban areas, over 60% of infants received IF at 3 months, declining to 40% at 12 months. Traditional cereals were given to 36% and 69% of infants at 6 and 12 months respectively, while commercial cereals were given to only 19% and 26% of infants at these ages. In rural areas, 45%, 31% and 24% of infants received IF at 3, 6, and 12 months respectively, while 12%, 47% and 76% received traditional cereals and 12% to 13% were given commercial cereals in the first year. Thus IF has come to replace traditional cereals as the first supplement even in rural areas. This trend, however, may now have been halted or reversed by the reduced availability of imported foods as a result of the world recession.

Zaire

Of all the 7 countries surveyed here, Zaire has witnessed the least change in traditional infant feeding practices. In the WHO study, in the late 1970s, almost half the rural mothers gave supplements by 3 months compared to just over one-third of elite and poor urban mothers. Cereals were the predominant first supplement in all groups. Among the elite group, less than half the infants received milk or milk-based supplements in the first 12 months and even fewer in the second year, while among other groups milk was hardly ever used. Processed milks are sold in foodstores in both urban and rural areas, and IF and commercial cereals are available in urban areas but are expensive and infrequently used. In a study in the capital, Kinshasa, use of bottlefeeds (usually containing a milk product, water and sugar) rose to a peak of 35% at 2 to 3 months, falling substantially after 6 months of age (Franklin *et al.*, 1983). In another Kinshasa study, by contrast, first supplementation, with a cassava or maize gruel, was reported to begin later, mainly from 4 to 6 months. In this report, only about 20% of mothers gave processed milks from 3 to 6 months of age, declining to about half that number at 9 to 12 months. One-third of these mothers gave IF and the rest gave DMP (Gussler *et al.*, 1983).

Caribbean

Early supplementation has also persisted in the Caribbean, with an increasing use of bottles to feed a variety of foods such as milk and/or cereal, bush teas or fruit juice. While SCM had been popular earlier in the century, from the 1940s onwards a shift towards DMP and later IF has taken place, together with increasing use of wheatflour in place of arrowroot, although in Jamaica cornmeal remains popular. By the 1960s and 1970s, IF was being introduced very early, often as the first supplement after pre-lacteal feeds of bush teas or glucose-water. At 1 month, 20%-40% of rural and 70%-90% of urban Jamaican mothers gave IF and by 3 months throughout the region 75%-90% of mothers gave it (King *et al.*, 1987a). Use of processed milks persists throughout the first year and into the second, unlike countries such as Malaysia, Nigeria and Kenya where their use ends early, often before breast-feeding stops. Cereal gruels are the first non-milk foods and are given usually from 3 months of age (*e.g.* Gussler *et al.*, 1983). Although commercial cereals may be given at this young age, they are gradually replaced by cornmeal (*e.g.* Landman *et al.*, 1976), a trend observed in other countries. 'Tonic foods' such as malted milk drinks, orange juice and multi-vitamins, are also popular and given early . From 4 to 6 months, Irish potato, plantain/banana and gradually other fruits and vegetables are introduced (King *et al.*, 1987a).

India

In the late 1970s, nationwide, 19% and 12% of urban poor and rural Indian mothers respectively gave regular supplements at 6 to 7 months compared to 66% and 79% of urban middle- and high-income mothers respectively. At 12 to 13 months nearly all the higher-income mothers gave regular supplements but only 54% and 62% of urban poor and rural mothers did so (WHO, 1981). This trend to earlier supplementation is noted even among rural mothers in other reports (*e.g.* Unni *et al.*, 1986). In Gujarat, more than half the infants were on 'solid' foods by 9 months, especially in poorer families, even though the mothers felt these should not be given before the child could walk; they felt constrained, though, by a perceived lack of breast milk and the inability to pay for the preferred supplement, namely animal milk (Wijga *et al.*, 1983). Elsewhere, however, the late introduction of supplements continues, frequent-ly beyond 1 year of age in rural areas (*e.g.* Agarwal, 1982; Rao, 1987). Animal milk continues to be the preferred first supplement, its use remaining high in higher-income groups throughout the first 18 months, but declining among poorer mothers over this period. Cereals are given infrequently in the first semester but almost universally in the second year (WHO, 1981). Locally -manufactured biscuits are commonly given by low-income mothers in Madras and Bombay but not in Calcutta where a well-established dairy favours the use of animal milk (Nutrition Foundation of India, undated). The use of commercial milk and cereals, which is also associated with earlier supplementation, is increasing. This trend was initially seen among the urban elite but is now spreading to poor urban and rural women. About half of the supplemented infants receive commercial milk in Madras and Calcutta but only half as many receive it in Bombay. Across the 3 centres 49%-60% of infants first received commercial cereals at 3 months.

Mexico

Between the 1950s and the 1970s, a trend away from 'exclusive' breast-feeding and towards supplementation with other milks was observed in rural Mexico (*e.g.* Dewey, 1983). Also, in isolated rural communities, commercial carbonated drinks, *refrescos*, are commonly given as early as 2-3 weeks , since they are believed to be cleaner than traditional preparations; poverty limits the amounts that may be given (Fink, 1985).

In a study in the late 1970s, approximately one-third of poor urban mothers breast-fed exclusively in the first month (Table II) while the majority of elite urban mothers were giving supplements of other milks at this age (Dimond *et al.*, 1987). Half the rural mothers were using other milks as supplements by the third month. Among all urban mothers, other milks totally replaced breast milk at earlier ages. Most mothers giving other milk chose IF in the first semester but its use declined markedly in the second semester. Cereals and other foods were given by at least two-fifths of low income mothers by 2 to 3 months, and by over four-fifths of elite mothers at that age. Nearly half the elite Mexican mothers gave commercial cereals by 3 months and continued their use into the second semester, but in contrast to other countries, low-income mothers (both urban and rural) gave commercial cereals predominantly in the second semester and continued their use into the second year. A more traditional form of cereal is *tortilla* soaked in soup, often given at the family dinner table to pacify the infant (Fink, 1985).

Summary of Contemporary Supplementation Patterns

The trends discussed above are summarised in Table IV. While mothers recognise the value of breast milk , many also consider that processed milks, especially IF, are good for their infants (*e.g.* Population Council, 1984). The term 'superfood' has been coined for these commercial products including glucose and tonics of various kinds, which are viewed as having special properties, almost medicinal, and they may be given additional status by being used in hospitals and clinics (Esterik *et al.*, 1986; Meldrum, 1984).

Sevrage

In all the 7 countries surveyed, the traditional practice was for lactation to be prolonged, usually for at least 1 to 2 years and often longer. The first changes occurred in the Caribbean where early sevrage was enforced during slavery and a period of around 9 months' breast-feeding was later recom-

Table IV. Traditional and contemporary patterns of supplementation			
Country	**Timing of Supplementation**	**Nature of Main Supplement**	
		1st Semester	**2nd Semester**
Malaysia			
Traditional	Early	Banana/rice gruel	Gruel contd (A)
Contemporary	Early	IF, commercial cereal (B)	Traditional gruel (A) (C)
Kenya			
Traditional	Early	Cow's milk/maize gruel	Thicker gruel (A)
Contemporary	Early	Processed milk incl. IF; some commercial cereal (B)	Traditional gruel (A)
Nigeria			
Traditional	Medium-late	Maize or sorghum gruel	Gruel contd (A)
Contemporary	Early	IF (declining?) (B)	Traditional gruel (C)
Zaire			
Traditional	Early-medium	Starchy staple gruel	Gruel contd (A)
Contemporary	Early-medium	Mainly traditional gruel limited IF in urban areas	Traditional gruel (A)
Caribbean			
Traditional	Early-late	Cereal/starchy gruel	Cruel contd (A)
Contemporary	Early	IF, commercial cereal	Traditional gruel processed milk (A) (D)
India			
Traditional	Late	Animal milk	Animal milk
Contemporary	Late, rural Early-medium, urban	IF, animal milk commercial cereal (B)	Animal milk (A)
Mexico			
Traditional	Late	Animal milk, soup-soaked cornbread, maize gruel	Gruel contd. (A)
Contemporary	Early	IF	Commercial cereals

Timing defined as commonly given: early <3 months, medium 3-6 months, late >6 months.
Supplementation defined as excluding pre-lacteal and early feeding of infusions and teas.
(A) Including gradual progression to an adult-type diet.
(B) Predominantly in urban areas, to a lesser extent in rural areas.
(C) Elite mothers continue use of IF and commercial cereals.
(D) Reversal of decline towards prolonged breast-feeding by elite mothers.

mended by health workers (Kerr, 1952). Initiation remains almost universal but duration has declined in the past 2 decades with the result that less than 20% of mothers still breast-fed at 6 months in Barbados in 1981 (Ramsey, 1983). Other Caribbean studies, however, indicate a rate of breast-feeding among urban mothers of about 50% at this age and a possible resurgence in breast-feeding has been noted following promotional campaigns in Jamaica (King *et al.*, 1987a).

In the other 6 countries, until the early twentieth century, prolonged breast-feeding continued. In Malaysia, since the 1950s, the duration of breast-feeding has declined substantially in urban areas but initiation has been little affected. Contemporary data indicate that while at least half of rural Malay infants are breast-fed for 6 months, fewer than one-third of urban infants are breast-fed for this period (King *et al.*, 1987b). In Mexican studies in the 1950s and 1960s, at least half the urban mothers breast-fed for more than a year, but by the late 1970s, less than one-fifth were breast-feeding beyond 6 months (Cardenas *et al.*, 1981). A similar trend towards shorter duration of lactation was also noted in rural areas (Dewey, 1983). Continued universal initiation was confirmed in a nationwide study, but less than 10% of elite urban mothers were continuing beyond 6 months and only one-quarter were breast-feeding for 3 months (Dimond *et al.*, 1987). Approximately half of poor urban and rural mothers breast-fed for up to 6 months and only between one-quarter and two-fifths continued up to 12 months.

In both rural and urban Kenya, universal initiation is still found; in rural areas, breast-feeding for over 1 year is the norm, while in Nairobi, 85% and 50% of mothers still breast-feed at 6 and 15 months respectively (Latham *et al.*, 1986). In Nigeria, initiation remains almost universal, and prolonged lactation continues up to 1 year nationally and even longer in rural areas (*e.g.* Orwell *et al.*, 1984). Among urban middle and high income mothers, however, duration has declined; in the WHO study, only one-third of elite mothers at 6 months and only two-thirds of middle income mothers at 9 months were still breast-feeding their infants (WHO, 1981). In Zaire and India, by contrast, most mothers, both urban and rural, still breast-feed for at least 12 months (*e.g.* Franklin *et al.*, 1983; Gussler *et al.*, 1983; Nutrition Foundation of India, undated), although in one study in India half the urban elite mothers had stopped by 1 year (WHO, 1981).

'Abrupt Sevrage'

Abrupt sevrage, whether or not the children are separated from their mothers, is considered one expression of the 'benign neglect' of toddlers (children 13-48 months old) *i.e.* practices which are unintentionally harmful (Cassidy, 1980). The sudden withholding of breast milk is a cause of considerable psychological distress for the infant which may result in loss of appetite and malnutrition. Various methods are used including smearing the nipples with a bitter-tasting substance, sending the child away, and punishment for crying. However harsh these methods may appear to be, the mother often faces serious constraints to continued breast-feeding such as another pregnancy, during which lactation might be forbidden by social norms. Alternatively, she may be guided by a clear set of principles, as described for two rural communities in Mexico (Millard *et al.*, 1985). The term 'principles' is chosen deliberately to denote rational decisions rather than 'beliefs' which implies blindly following a set of rules. According to the mothers, once a baby has teeth it is old enough to eat other foods and so breast-feeding should cease; since dental eruption occurs over a 2-year period, this allows some lee-way in deciding when to stop. However, prolonging breast-feeding is considered to make the child boorish and ill-mannered; again there is flexibility and no precise age could be offered. The mothers also consider that a mixed diet of breast milk and other food will cause sickness and so breast-feeding should not be gradually phased out. Although sevrage is abrupt the child has already become accustomed to other foods by being offered 'titbits' regularly during the course of food preparation or family meals.Thus mothers here take an active role in deciding how and when to apply these principles, based on their perception of their own lactation performance, the child's maturity and past experience.

Determinants of Contemporary Infant Feeding Patterns and Practices

While a number of interacting factors may influence infant feeding patterns and practices, the most important determinants appear to be: maternal employment; health sector activities; commercial availability and promotion of processed milks and cereals; urbanisation and modernisation; and poverty and poor maternal nutrition, as well as a perceived insufficiency of breast milk.

Maternal Employment

In Malaysia and the Caribbean, the trend towards the use of processed milks as breast milk supplements and substitutes began early in the twentieth century and can be attributed to the widespread employment of women on plantations. Processed milks were more convenient than the traditional gruels which were time-consuming to prepare. Even today, women comprise 40% of the workforce in Malaysia, and in the Caribbean 30% of households are still headed by women (King *et al.*, 1987a). In Mexico, women's paid employment is associated with a shorter duration of lactation, and in one study one-third of working mothers had not breast-fed at all (Cardenas *et al.*, 1981).

In Nigeria, traditional women's work varies by region; in the east the Igbos are farmers, the Yorubas in the west are traders while the northern Hausas are largely restricted to the home and its environs by purdah. In each region, their traditional roles are apparently compatible with uninterrupted breast-feeding since the infant accompanies the mother to work, or alternatively the work-pattern is adjusted to allow mother and infant to be together during the first semester (Sudarkasa, 1973). Nigerian women entered the modern employment sector later than women in Malaysia and the Caribbean, so the associated decline in the duration of breast-feeding and the increased use of commercial infant foods occurred later in Nigeria and to a lesser degree. In Kenya, entry into the modern sector has similarly reduced the total duration of breast-feeding, as well as the duration of exclusive breast-feeding, but has not affected its initiation (Population Council, 1984). Maternal employment is an insufficient explanation for the observed high rate of IF use in Kenya (Elliott et al., 1985) since only 11% of nearly 1000 urban Kenyan women surveyed worked outside the home and only 5% could neither visit nor take their infant with them.

In Zaire, in contrast, some female farm workers do not take their infants with them to the fields. This situation is more common in areas where maternal nutritional status is poor and may be due to an inability to fulfil the burdensome duties and competing nutritional demands of both farming and unrestricted lactation (Brown et al., 1980; Vis et al., 1981).

On balance, maternal employment outside the home (or a deeply entrenched tradition of female employment) appears to be an important factor in determining infant feeding practices in many but not all societies. Partial breast-feeding, using processed milks and commercial cereals as substitutes, is the preferred option for the majority of working mothers for whom exclusive breast-feeding is not feasible under present economic and social conditions. The trend towards earlier sevrage may reflect a failing milk supply, either from diminished nipple stimulation as a result of substitution, or from the pressures of a harsh and onerous life which may adversely affect the let-down reflex. Alternatively, a mother may consider that the economic cost of her time, relative to other household members who may substitute for her by bottle-feeding, is too high to spend on breast-feeding (Butz,1977; Popkin et al. 1983; Population Council, 1984).

Health Sector Activities

Medical orthodoxies regarding infant feeding practices have undergone several major changes since the mid-nineteenth century. In particular, with the advent of processed milks, perceived expertise regarding infant feeding and with it the advisory role shifted away from female midwives and towards male doctors. The regimented era of feeding, including complex formulations, scheduled feeds, test weighing etc. began early in the twentieth century in industrialised countries (Apple, 1980; Fisher, 1985) and soon reached out into the colonies. Whether health workers were convinced of the virtues of such practices or were concerned to correct contemporary unhygienic methods of breast milk supplementation and substitution, in Malaysia, by the 1920s, popular annual Baby Shows were held at which health workers demonstrated the preparation of bottle-feeds of processed milk (King *et al.*, 1987b).

By the 1950s in many parts of the world, processed milks (usually DMP) were being distributed from clinics on a large scale, thereby adding a seal of approval to their use. These programmes were initiated at a time when there was a world surplus of dried skimmed milk; they created a demand which later could be met only by expensive imports (Human Lactation Centre, 1979). By the 1960s and throughout the 1970s, maternity units frequently served as venues for distributing free IF samples to newly-delivered mothers. Health workers, however, were growing more aware of the risks associated with such practices, particularly as they gave credence to an apparent sanctioning of processed milk feeds. Health professionals were also more cognizant of other detrimental hospital practices such as giving pre-lacteal and supplementary feeds and separating mothers and newborn infants (*e.g.* Gueri *et al.*, 1977). Consequently, from the mid-1970s, distribution activities were being curtailed and breast-feeding promotional campaigns of varying scope were being inaugurated, although with little formal evaluation taking place (King *et al.*, 1987a). Also the need for health workers to act as role models has been recognised. Most legal maternal entitlements for working mothers are, however, still not conducive to prolonged lactation and thus it can be difficult for health workers to act as role models. Short durations of breast-feeding have been reported in several studies of health personnel (Sinniah *et al.*, 1980; Bamisaiye *et al.*, 1983).

Commercial Promotion of Processed Milks for Infant Feeding

Advertising of processed milks for infant feeding was vigorously directed towards indigenous mothers in Malaysia and the Caribbean in the 1950s (Greiner *et al.*, 1982; Manderson, 1982). Similar activities occurred later in, for example, Nigeria and included regular radio advertisements, visits to clinics by commercial nurses, free milk for doctors' families, pamphlets, posters, calendars *etc.* (Wennen-van der May, 1969). Throughout the 1960s and 1970s such active promotion of infant foods *via* health institutions and the mass media continued in many developing countries. In Nigeria by the late 1970s, there were over 40 brands of milk and milk-based products and 11 brands of feeding bottles on the market, and an estimated 1% of total sales volume was given free, mainly to private health institutions (WHO, 1981).

Advertising may influence behaviour patterns. For example in the Caribbean, mothers with greater exposure to infant food advertising introduced processed milk and stopped breast-feeding earlier than other mothers (Greiner *et al.*, 1982). In Zaire, by contrast, there has been little commercial promotion of infant foods. This may be related to Zaire's very low GNP, which places it amongst the poorest nations of the world and consequently reduces its commercial attractiveness to international companies (King *et al.*, 1987a). Since 1981 when the WHO Code of Marketing of Breastmilk Substitutes was passed by the Assembly of the World Health Organization, Kenya and India have ratified the Code and other countries including Nigeria, Malaysia and some Caribbean countries have passed their own versions of the Code. These have prohibited the advertising of IF in the mass media and direct contact of company personnel with mothers. There are various criticisms of these Codes, however, as well as increasing reports of abuse.

Urbanisation and Modernisation

Increased educational and work opportunities for women in urban areas have been partly responsible for the observed earlier introduction of supplements. Also, as discussed above, with the increased availability of processed milks and commercial cereals, mothers have had access to convenient, although expensive, supplements. These have become all the more attractive with the decline in the extended family and traditional childcare arrangements. In some countries (*e.g.* Nigeria and Zaire) an increase in monogamous marriages in urban areas, coupled with retention of the traditional taboo on sexual intercourse during lactation, has resulted in a shortening of the breast-feeding period and consequent earlier supplementation and substitution (Dow, 1977).

The use of commercial products may reflect a desire to be modern and a perception of breast-feeding as 'primitive' or immodest (Igun, 1982; Narayan *et al.*, 1987; Population Council, 1984). Similarly, since in all the countries studied the elite have led in the use of commercial supplements, there may be a desire for reasons of social prestige, to emulate them. As the elite are usually also more highly eduacated, this emulation may also reflect a belief that IF and bottle-feeding are as good as, if not better than, traditional feeding methods and many mothers expressed the view that both bottle and breast are important for their baby's health (Di Domenico *et al.*, 1979; Population Council, 1984).

Poverty and Maternal Ill-health

Poverty-induced stress, appalling living conditions and maternal ill-health, poor nutritional status and overwork have been implicated as likely causes of lactation failure for many years (*e.g.* Williams, 1938). More recently, poor obstetric outcome and low initiation of breast-feeding among urban slum dwellers have been attributed to low age of marriage, high parity, ill-health and poverty (Leigh *et al.*, 1983). In rural Zaire, reduced milk output is associated with poor maternal nutritional status, with resultant early introduction of traditional supplements (Vis *et al.*, 1981; WHO, 1985). The most common reason for introducing other milks given by mothers in many countries is a perceived lack of breast milk and/or the child not being satisfied with breast-feeds alone (Fink, 1985; King *et al.*, 1987; Population Council, 1984). The maternal poverty-ill-health-overwork syndrome is one that merits consideration in programmes aimed at promoting breast-feeding.

PROBLEMS ASSOCIATED WITH TRADITIONAL INFANT FOODS

In preceding sections we have shown that the first supplement traditionally introduced in many parts of the world is a gruel prepared from a cereal or starchy root, tuber or fruit (usually the local staple) and commonly mixed only with water. The impact of such gruels on the young child's nutritional status is too broad a subject to cover in any comprehensive manner here; consequently, we will focus on two major factors, namely the problems of low nutrient concentration and dietary bulk, and the risks of bacterial contamination and infection.

Low Nutrient Concentration of Traditional Gruels: the Problem of Dietary Bulk and Viscosity.

The Nutrient Content of Traditional Gruels

Many authors have commented on the low energy density and nutrient concentration of cereal or starchy-staple gruels as traditionally prepared and fed to young children. Thin gruels are preferred because they are easier to swallow. Traditionally large amounts of water are added to achieve a thin consistency, thus diluting the nutrients present. In Gambia,the negative correlation between the energy and water contents of local dishes was found to be so highly significant as to permit estimation of the energy content from measurements of water content alone (Hudson *et al.* 1980). In Uganda, the food intake of a group of pre-school children was investigated using 24-hour recall and duplicate diet analysis techniques (Rutishauser, 1974). The most striking feature noted by the author was the low intake of energy, even when appetite was good. This was partly due to the low energy concentration of the diet and to the limited number of meals eaten per day. Protein intake was also low, but this was a direct result of the low energy intake, since the protein:energy ratio of the diet was adequate. Other factors found to be significantly associated with low energy intakes included poor appetite in children over 6 months of age, which showed a seasonal peak that was closely related to the high rates of infection in the rainy season, and the cessation of breast-feeding, since breast milk continued to make a major contribution to energy intakes even in the second year of life. The low energy density and nutrient concentration of traditional gruels has also been noted in relation to Nigerian maize pap, (1.2 MJ (290 kcals) per kg) (Naismith, 1973). In Gambia, the local millet gruel has a similar energy concentration (1.4MJ per kg), half that of the mothers' breast milk (Rowland et al., 1978).

Dietary Bulk

The main constituents of traditional gruels are carbohydrates and these, especially starch, are major contributors to their bulkiness. This is because as starch granules are heated in water, at a certain temperature irreversible swelling occurs (gelatinisation). This causes the mixture to thicken. On cooling a gel forms, making the mixture even more viscous. The viscosity can be reduced by cooking with large amounts of water but this dilutes the nutrients. Diets with a low concentration of energy and nutrients are said to be 'bulky' because large volumes would have to be consumed to meet nutritional require- ments. Due to a small stomach capacity, it is particularly difficult for young children to meet their nutritional needs from gruels. Various studies have examined the upper limits of intake that young children can achieve; for 1 to 3 year olds, a total daily intake of 700 to 900 g. of solid and liquid foods was a common finding (Ljungqvist et al., 1981). Hospitalised children in Uganda fed a traditional diet 5 times daily were able to achieve only a minor increase in energy intake over those eating 3 meals a day at home (Rutishauser , 1974). Using results from Nigeria and current WHO recommended intakes, a 2- to 3- year old would need to consume approximately 4.5 kg of pap daily to meet energy requirements (Naismith, 1973). Several possible solutions to the prob- lem of low dietary intakes from traditional gruels have been proposed, includ- ing 1) increasing the amount of food consumed at each meal, 2) increasing the number of meals per day and 3) increasing the energy concentration of each meal (Ljungqvist et al., 1981). The foregoing discussion, however, suggests that neither of the first two recommendations would have much effect on energy intake unless the composition of the traditional gruel is modified. Furthermore, if the gruel is merely made thicker by reducing the water content, it becomes more viscous and less easy for young children to swallow, and the amount consumed is consequently reduced.

Viscosity

Viscosity is a measure of the internal friction of a liquid or semi-solid and determines its ease of pouring, stirring and being swallowed. As noted previously, when starchy gruels cool after cooking they become more viscous. A recent study examined various factors influencing the viscosity of traditional food mixtures used as supplements for young children including: the type of starch and protein in the food; the presence of fat; and the effects of different processing techniques (Hellstrom et al., 1981). Starch from different staple foods and different sizes of starch granule from the same staple were found to produce varying viscosity effects in a blended weaning product; it may therefore be possible to develop varieties of staples with favourable viscosity properties relating, for example, to the size of the starch granule or the amylose/amylopectin ratio. Certain proteins, e.g. those from soybean, were found to increase viscosity whereas the presence of fat, by reducing the swelling of the starch granules, led to a decrease in viscosity. Consequently, gruels may be made with less water if they contain fat without increasing their viscosity. In addition, fats greatly increase the energy density of the gruel, although they introduce the risk of rancidity if the dry ingredients have to be stored for long periods.

The application of processing techniques such as pre-cooking, extrusion and enzyme (amylase) treatment of starch can effectively reduce dietary bulk by reducing the swelling of the starch granules. Extrusion cooking is a relatively new technology which is most suited to cereals or cereal-legume mixes. The raw materials are passed through a rotating screw in a fixed barrel at controlled temperatures; this compression and heating results in a product with an expanded, puffed characteristic (Jansen et al., 1980). The final viscosity of the extruded food will depend on various factors such as the extrusion temperature, moisture content and the amylose/amylopectin ratio. Studies on wheat, maize and sorghum have shown a much lower viscosity in gruels prepared from extruded materials than unextruded grains, though when various flours are blended prior to extrusion, viscosity may be affected by interactions between the constituents. For example, an extruded mixture of maize and soybean flours had a higher viscosity than the unextruded mixture of raw materials (Hellstrom et al., 1981).

A traditional processing method, malting, has been shown to have a significant effect on viscosity and hence bulk (Brandtzaeg et al., 1981). Malting is the controlled germination and subsequent drying of seeds. During this process, enzymatic reactions result in important nutritional changes such as an increase in the content of some vitamins and essential amino acids, and a decrease in trypsin inhibitors and phytic acid. Also, changes occur in starch composition due to localised amylase activity. Consequently, the concentration of the gruel can be increased 3- to 4- fold while the volume and viscosity remain the same. In India, sprouted dried red millet (*ragi*) has traditionally been fed to young children; however, with increasing pressures on women's time, this practice has declined. A study of the effects of malting showed a major decrease in viscosity with increasing germination time in thick *ragi* and sorghum gruels. Various other treatments also led to a decrease in viscosity: mixing the malted flour with cold water and slowly heating, rather than placing it directly in boiling water; retaining the husk; and first toasting the dried product. The use of malted grain for preparing gruels results in a liquid slurry rather than the bulky, sticky gruel formed by cooking the unmalted flour. The authors conclude that malting has good potential for increasing the concentration of energy and other nutrients in gruels made from cereals and some cereal-legume mixes and has the added advantage of a technology that can be applied at both village and industrial level.

Recent work in India has shown that only a small amount of malted flour added to the cooked, thick gruel results in thinning, since adding it after cooking prevents the amylase activity being destroyed by heat. This method is time-saving as less malting is required. In Tanzania, 'power flour' is produced in a similar way (*i.e.* using maize flour which has been hydrolysed by the addition of germinated cereal) and has been associated with increased intakes of gruel in children (Tomkins *et al.*, 1987).

Fermentation is a traditional food processing technique used widely throughout the world. It involves the breakdown of carbohydrates and related compounds by microbial enzymes and results in reduced viscosity, due perhaps to the presence of lactic or acetic acids and/or to increased amylase activity as in malting. Fermentation also improves the digestibility of proteins and other nutrients in cereals and this property, together with the preferred texture and taste and increased nutrient concentration, confer added value to fermented gruels during sickness and loss of appetite. We have shown that increasing the amount of food and even the frequency of meals will not necessarily result in a sufficiently improved energy intake in young children because of the bulkiness of the traditional diet. Similarly, a more concentrated gruel will be highly viscous and consequently unpalatable. More promising approaches are:

extrusion cooking for industrially processed foods, but with due regard to the interaction effects of certain combinations of cereals and legumes on viscosity.

malting which has been shown to favourably influence viscosity and taste in some cereal flours and can be used at village level.

addition of fat or other energy-rich foods such as nuts, seeds, oil-rich legumes. There is a need for more research on the nutritional effects and keeping properties of these methods for different foods and food combinations, as well as on other processes, such as fermentation, which may also decrease bulk and hence provide a more nutrient-dense diet for young children.

The Contamination of Traditional Dishes Fed to Young Children

The setting in which traditional gruels are prepared is usually hazardous; water supplies may be of poor quality, intermittent and/or distant, kitchen facilities primitive and the mother's education and consequent awareness of hygiene minimal. The gruel will commonly be prepared once a day and left to stand for use when required, due to the time-consuming and tedious method of preparation and the many other calls on the mother's time. There is now a wealth of evidence showing that traditional gruels may be heavily contaminated by bacteria both at the time of preparation and increasingly with storage at ambient temperatures.

A thorough investigation of this problem was carried out in Gambia. Samples of a traditional millet gruel were tested, at different intervals after preparation, for the presence of common pathogens. The flour itself, prepared by pounding the dampened grain, was found to be contaminated, as was the water in which it was cooked. Since prolonged boiling would increase viscosity, the perfunctory simmering of the mixture enabled a considerable proportion of organisms to survive (up to 10^4 total count per g). This increased to almost 10^8 per g over an 8 hour storage period. Among the potentially pathogenic organisms isolated were E. coli, B. cereus, S. aureus and C. welchii. Although the feeding bowls were scrupulously cleaned by scrubbing with palm leaves and rinsing in fresh water, high counts were also obtained from these empty bowls (Rowland et al., 1978). A comparison was made of rates of contamination between the millet gruel and commercial milks prepared in the traditional setting; freshly made up with boiled water, these contained a similar total viable count to the freshly prepared gruel (10^2-10^3 per g), reflecting the contamination of the container. With unboiled water, counts of 10^4-10^7 per g were found, depending on the degree of pollution of the well water which was greatest in the wet season. On storing both milks and gruel for 8 hours, levels of *E. coli* and *B. cereus* were little higher in the milk than in the traditional gruel, regardless of whether the milk was made up with boiled or unboiled water. However, contamination with *S. aureus* was greater, except in the 'biologically acidified' milk, while *C. welchii* was essentially absent from both milks (Rowland *et al.*, 1978; Barrell *et al.*, 1980). Therefore prepared and fed in the customary way, traditional gruels were at least as hazardous as commercial milk preparations.

Further studies were done in Gambia on seasonal changes in contamination rates. A variety of local millet and rice dishes, some containing groundnut sauce, dry fish, sour milk, palm oil etc. were tested. A higher proportion of wet season foods were found to contain unacceptable levels of potential pathogens, using international reference standards, compared to the dry season throughout an 8 hour sampling period.; the proportion increased from 35% to 98% in the wet season compared to from 7% to 71% in the dry season. At all sampling times, *E. coli* was present at unacceptable levels in a higher proportion of foods that had been boiled rather than steamed. Although no direct association was shown, the authors note that the wet season is also the period of highest incidence of diarrhoeal disease (Barrell)*et al.*, 1979).

Similarly, in a rural area of Kenya, a high contamination rate was found in foods given to children; 44% were unsafe with respect to *Enterobacteriaceae* (which include *E. coli*, *Salmonella*, and *Shigella*) and 12% with respect to *S. aureus*. Colonisation again increased with storage time, but in contrast to the Gambian studies, drinking water drawn from rivers and open wells was surprisingly uncontaminated (van Steenbergen *et al.*, 1983). In India, samples of children's meals, mainly rice, dhal (lentils) and vegetables, were unacceptably contaminated with *E. coli* and *S. aureus*. This was the case in 60% of samples from low-income groups compared to only 15% from high-income families. Similarly, milk samples were significantly more contaminated among the low-income group who did not attempt to sterilise the feeding utensils and whose water supply was often contaminated. Hand-feeding was common and hand-washings prior to a feed showed a similarly high level of contamination in both income groups (Mathur *et al.*, 1983). Other studies have found high contamination rates in maize paps in Nigeria (Elegbe *et al.*, 1984) and in the contents of bottles (milk and/or cornmeal or oatmeal) in the Caribbean (Hibbert *et al.*, 1981).

From the above it is clear that the risks of contamination *via* traditional weaning foods are considerable, increase with storage at room temperature and, where water supplies are unsafe, with the rainy season. Various implications for prevention emerge (see Table V). Handwashing is clearly one simple and effective method of reducing the risks of contamination; however it

Table V. Potential interventions to reduce the risks of contamination of traditional gruels

			Aetiological Factor				
	Dirty Hands	Poor Water Supply	Contaminated Raw Food		Contaminated Stored Food		
Preventive Measures	hand washing	provision of good supply	improve storage	cook well	re-heat thoroughly, difficult if thick mixture	cook several times a day	ferment food
Resources Required	water, soap	high level of investment	capital investment	fuel, time	fuel	time, fuel	time
Means of Implementation	health education	govt/internat programme	health educ/ community development	health educ.	health educ.	health educ.	health educ/ community development

presupposes adequate supplies of water. Food preparation techniques may also be modified *e.g.* cooking at a temperature high enough to kill pathogens and shorter periods of storage. These assume adequate fuel supplies and time to prepare smaller portions of food, constraints which could be overcome by the provision of low cost nutritious infant foods that are easy to prepare.

CONCLUSION

It is important to recognise that certain misconceptions have prevailed concerning infant feeding practices in developing countries. One is the notion of prolonged 'exclusive' breast-feeding. We have shown that in many cultures other substances besides breast milk have traditionally been offered in the first few weeks of life, a practice which persists today. A second is the idea that 'abrupt weaning' means mothers withdrawing the breast suddenly with little preparation for the new dietary regime; however the evidence suggests that infants have already been well accustomed to other foods. Mothers around the world are influenced by various combinations of factors in their choice of infant feeding method or 'style'. A major determinant is clearly the economic pressures on their time; others include various messages and advice (commercial advertisements, contact with health workers), social trends and influences. Underlying all these are the mothers' own perceptions of their children's needs and maturity and of their own lactation performance.

From the available evidence, early supplementation would appear to be satisfactory in nutritional terms; in both Kenya and India, supplemented infants grew as well as those who were exclusively breast-fed (Sathian *et al.*, 1983; Kusin *et al.*, 1985). Indeed, prolonged unsupplemented lactation will result in inadequate growth as noted in many reports (*e.g.* Chavez *et al.*, 1977; Underwood *et al.*, 1982). The main concern lies in the nutritional quality of the supplement, risks of contamination and the effect of its purchase on the household budget. To date, most low income mothers have faced the choice of preparing a time-consuming but cheap traditional gruel (generally of low energy density and often contaminated with potentially pathogenic organisms) or of purchasing expensive commercial products which are convenient to prepare and nutritious, but equally likely, under the usual conditions of preparation, to be contaminated and constituting a major drain on the family's resources.

Strategies aimed at improving the diets of young children must first realistically address the constraints (economic, social, environmental and time) under which the majority of Third World mothers live (Anyanwu *et al.*, 1985). Measures will vary according to the socio-cultural situation. In urban areas, the production of low cost infant foods from local ingredients using

Table VI. Potential measures to improve infant feeding practices in diffferent situations

Infant Feeding Practice		Country Examples	Identified Needs	Appropriate Measures
Breast-feeding	Supplementation			
High initiation Long duration	early	Nigeria Kenya Zaire	good supplements later supplementation (after 3 months)	education/food processing education and better maternity leave provision (urban areas)
High initiation Short duration	early	Mexico Caribbean Malaysia	good supplements later sevrage later supplementation (after 3 months)	education/food processing education and better maternity provision, creches, support networks
High initiation Long duration	late	India	good supplements earlier supplementation	education/food processing education

techniques such as extrusion or malting is a promising approach which has already been applied in some countries (*e.g.* Tanzania). A second is the production of more nutritious snacks based on those already popular, such as the wheatflour biscuits and chin-chin of India and Nigeria respectively. Breast-feeding working mothers must be supported, both by realistic maternity leave entitlements (the present 6 weeks' leave postpartum is clearly inadequate) and by providing creches and/or time to breast-feed during the day. In rural areas, measures would more appropriately be directed towards mothers and home preparation, such as encouraging the malting of grain, addition of fat-rich foods to traditional gruels etc.

In both situations, carefully articulated education messages relating to maternal and child nutritional requirements, hygiene etc. are essential,using a mode of delivery appropriate to the lifestyle of the target population. Programmes should involve maximum community participation. It is now well recognised that when people are directly involved in identifying and devising solutions to their problems then development programmes are more likely to succeed than where outside agents move in to impose an externally devised programme (*e.g.* Praun, 1982). Appropriate measures for improving infant feeding practices in the 7 countries surveyed in this chapter are suggested in Table VI.

Two other factors are crucial to the success of programmes such as those outlined above: one is the political will to mount programmes cutting across ministerial boundaries (health, education, agriculture, community development) and aiming to empower the powerless to improve their own life situation. The second is the role of health workers; we have shown that the health sector played a major part in the popularisation of bottle-feeds and processed milks in infant feeding. We argue that they can have an equally important impact on redirecting infant feeding (King *et al.*, 1987a). Realistically, this will not be the advocacy of 4 to 6 months' unsupplemented breast-feeding, which was a response to the perception in the 1970s of a crisis in breast-feeding worldwide. We now know that Third World mothers have not abandoned breast-feeding wholesale, indeed the vast majority still initiate lactation but for increasingly shorter periods of time. What these mothers need is every possible support in their harsh daily routine to enable them to continue supplemented breast-feeding for as long as possible, together with cheap, convenient and nourishing supplements.

REFERENCES

Agarwal, D. K., Agarwal, K. N., Tewari, I. C., Singh, R., and Yaday, K. N. S.: Breast-feeding practices in urban slum and rural areas of Varanasi. *J. Trop. Pediat.*, 28:89-92 (1982).

Akenzua, G. I., Akpovi, S. U., and Ogbeide, O.: Maternal and child care in rural areas: the role of traditional birth attendants in Bendel State of Nigeria. *J. Trop. Pediat.*, 27:210-214 (1981).

Anyanwu, R. C., and Enwonwu, C. O.: The impact of urbanisation and socioeconomic status on infant feeding practices in Lagos, Nigeria. *Fd. Nutr. Bull.*, 7:33-37 (1985).

Apple, R. D.: 'To be used only under the direction of a physician': commercial infant feeding and medical practice. 1870-1940, *Bull. Hist. Med.*, 54:402-417 (1980).

Bamisaiye, A., and Oyediran, M. A.: Breast-feeding among female employees at a major health institution in Lagos, Nigeria. *Soc. Sci. Med.*, 17:1867-1871 (1983).

Barrell, R. A. E., and Rowland, M. G. M.: Infant foods as a potential source of diarrhoeal illness in rural West Africa. *Trans. Roy. Soc. Trop. Med. Hygn.*, 73:85-90 (1979).

Barrell, R. A. E., and Rowland, M. G. M.: Commercial milk products and indigenous weaning foods in a rural West African environment: a bacteriological perspective. *J. Hygn.*, 84:191-202 (1980).

Bhandari, S., Tak, S. K., and Goyal, S.: Breast-feeding versus top feeding: impact on growth, morbidity and mortality in neonatal period. *Ind. J. Nutr. Dietet.*, 20:255-258 (1983).

Brandtzaeg, B., Malleshi, N. G., Svanberg, U., Desikachar, H. S. B., and Mellander, O.: Dietary bulk as a limiting factor for nutrient intake - with special reference to the feeding of pre-school children III Studies of malted flour from ragi, sorghum and green gram. *J. Trop. Pediat.*, 27:184-189 (1981).

Brown, R. C., Brown, J. E., and Teeter, R. A.: Evaluation of a nutrition center program in rural Africa. *J. Trop. Pediat.*, 26:37-41 (1980).

Butz, W. P.: *Economic Aspects of Breastfeeding.* The Rand Paper Series. P-5801, The Rand Corporation, Santa Monica, California, 1977.

Cardenas, A. M., Gonzalez, L. M. P., Garcia de Alba, J. E., San Roman, R. T., and Becerra, A. D.: Some epidemiological aspects of maternal breast-feeding in a population entitled to social welfare services in Mexico. *Bull. Pan. Am. Organ.*, 15:139-147 (1981).

Cassidy, C. M.: Benign neglect and toddler malnutrition. In: *Social and Biological Predictors of Nutritional Status, Physical Growth, and Neurological Development* (L. S. Greene and F. E. Johnston Eds.) New York, Academic Press, 1980.

Chavez, A., Martinez, C., Opheuis, A. O., and Basta, S.: Nutrition and development of children from poor rural areas. VI. Effects of mild malnutrition on body morphology during early growth. *Nutr. Rep. Int.*, 15:407-419 (1977).

Cherian, A.: Attitudes and practices of infant feeding in Zaria, Nigeria. *Ecol. Food. Nutr.*, 11:75-80 1981.

Dewey, K. G.: Nutrition survey in Tabasco, Mexico: patterns of infant feeding. *Am. J. Clin. Nutr.*, 38:133-138 (1983).

Di Domenico, C. M., and Asuni, J. B.: Breastfeeding practices among urban women in Ibadan, Nigeria. In: *Breastfeeding and Food Policy in a Hungry World* (D. Rapheal, Ed.) New York, Academic Press, pp 51-57, 1979.

Dimond, H. J., and Ashworth, A.: Infant feeding practices in Kenya, Mexico and Malaysia: the rarity of the exclusively breast-fed infant. *J. Hum. Nutr., Appl. Nutr.*, 41A:51-64 (1987).

Dow, T. E., Breast-feeding and abstinence among the Yoruba. *Studies in Family Planning*, 8:208-214 (1977).

Elegbe, I. A., and Ojofeitimi, E. O.: Early initiation of weaning foods and proliferation of bacteria in Nigerian infants. *Clin. Pediat.*, 23:261-264 (1984).

Elliott, T. C., Agunda, K. O., Kigonda, J. G., Kinoti, S. N., and Latham, M. C.: Breastfeeding versus infant formula: the Kenyan case. *Food Pol.*, 10:7-10 (1985).

van Esterik, P., and Elliott, T.: Infant feeding style in urban Kenya. *Ecol. Fd. Nutr.*, 18:183-195 (1986).

Fildes, V.: Neonatal feeding practices and infant mortality during the eighteenth century. *J. Biosoc. Sci.*, 12:313 (1980).

Fink, A. E.: Nutrition, lactation and fertility in two Mexican rural communities. *Soc. Sci. Med.*, 20:1295-1305 (1985).

Firth, R.: *Housekeeping Among Malay Peasants*, LSE Monograph on Social Anthropology No. 7, University of London. The Athlone Press, 1966.

Fisher, C.: How did we go wrong with breast-feeding? *Midwifery*, 1:48-51 (1985).

Franklin, R. R., Bertrand, W. E., Mock, N. B., Nkamany, K., and McCaw, A.: Feeding patterns of infants and young children in Kinshasa, Zaire. *J. Trop. Pediat.*, 29:255-259 (1983).

Greiner, T., and Latham, M. C.: The influence of infant food advertising on infant feeding practices in St. Vincent. *Int. J. Hlth. Serv.*, 12:53-73 (1982).

Gueri, M., Jutsum, P., Mohammed, I., and McDowell, M. F.: Breast-feeding campaigns and hospital practices as factors affecting age of weaning. *Envir. Child Hlth.*, 23:267 (1977).

Gussler, J. D., and Mock, N. B.: A comparative description of infant feeding practices in Zaire, the Philippines and St. Kitts-Nevis. *Ecol. Fd. Nutr.*, 13:75-85 (1983).

Haaga, J. G.: *Infant feeding and nutrition policy in Malaysia*, The Rand Paper Series, P-6995-RGI, The Rand Corporation, Santa Monica, California (1984).

Hauck, H. M., and Tabrah, F.: Infant feeding and growth in Awo Omamma, Nigeria. *J. Am. Dietet. Assoc.*, 43:327-330 (1963).

Hellstrom, A., Hermansson, A., Karlsson, A., Ljungqvist, B. Mellander, O., and Svanberg, U.: Dietary bulk as a limiting factor for nutrient intake - with special reference to the feeding of pre-school children II. Consistency as related to dietary bulk - a model study. *J. Trop. Pediat.*, 27:127-135 (1981).

Herskovits, M. J., and Herskovits, F. S.: *Trinidad Village*. New York, Alfred A. Knopf (1947).

Hibbert J. M., and Golden, M. H. N.: What is the weanling's dilemma? *J. Trop. Pediat.*, 27:255-258 (1981).

Hudson, G. J., John P. M. V.,and Paul, A. A., Variation in the composition of Gambian Foods: the importance of water in relation to energy and protein content. *Ecol. Food Nutr.*, 10:9-17 (1980).

Human Lactation Centre, Milk in foreign aid and the developing dairy industries in the Third World. In: *Breast-feeding and Food Policy in a Hungry World* (D. Raphael, ed.) New York, Academic Press,pp 99-104 (1979).

Igun, U. A., Child-feeding habits in a situation of social change: the case of Maiduguri, Nigeria. *Soc. Sci. Med.*, 16:769-781 (1982).

Jansen, R., and Harper, J. M.: Application of low-cost extrusion cooking to weaning foods in feeding programmes Part 1, *Food and Nutrition*, 6:2-9 (1980).

Jelliffe, D. B.: Infant feeding among the Yoruba of Ibadan. *W. Afr. Med. J.*, 7:114-122 (1953).

Jelliffe, D. B.: *Infant Nutrition in the Tropics and Sub-tropics*. WHO Monograph Series No. 29, Geneva, World Health Organisation (1968).

Karnawat, B. S., Sirgh, R. N., Gupta, B. D. and Chaudbury, S. P.: Knowledge and Attitude of Hospital Employees Regarding Infant Feeding Practices. *India Pediatrics* 24:929-948 (1987).

Kerr, M.: *Personality and Conflict in Jamaica*. Liverpool University Press (1952).

King, J., and Ashworth, A.: Historical review of the changing pattern of infant feeding in developing countries: the case of Malaysia, the Caribbean, Nigeria and Zaire. *Soc. Sci. Med.*, 25:1307-1320 (1987a).

King, J., and Ashworth, A.: *Changes in Infant Feeding Practices in Malaysia*, Occasional Paper No. 7, Department of Human Nutrition, London School of Hygiene and Tropical Medicine, London (1987b).

King, J., and Ashworth, A.: *Changes in Infant Feeding Practices in the Caribbean*, Occasional Paper No. 8, Department of Human Nutrition, L.S.H.T.M., London (1987c).

King, J., and Ashworth, A.: *Changes in Infant Feeding Practices in Nigeria*, Occasional Paper No. 9, Department of Human Nutrition, L.S.H.T.M., London (1987d).

King, J. and, Ashworth, A.: *Changes in Infant Feeding Practices in Zaire*, Occasional Paper No. 10, Department of Human Nutrition, L.S.H.T.M., London (1987e).

Kushwaha, K. P., Mathur, G. P., and Prakash, O.: Infant feeding practices of peri-urban areas of Gorakhpur, *Indian Pediatrics*, 24:899-901 (1987).

Kusin, J. A., Kardjati, S., and van Steenbergen, W.: Traditional infant feeding practices: right or wrong? *Soc. Sci. Med.*, 21:283-286 (1985).

Landman, J. P., and Shaw-Lyon, V.: Breast-feeding in decline in Kingston, Jamaica. *W. Ind. Med. J.*, 25:43-45 (1976).

Latham, M. C., Elliott, T. C., Winikoff, B., Kekovole, J., and van Esterik, P.: Infant feeding in urban Kenya: a pattern of early triple nipple feeding. *J. Trop. Pediat.*, 32:276-280 (1986).

Leigh, B., Ebrahim, G. J., Lovell, H., and Yusof, K.: The urban poor and obstetric outcome. *J. Trop. Pediat.*, 29:265-267 (1983).

Ljungqvist, B., and Mellander, O.: Dietary bulk as a limiting factor for nutrient intake in pre-school children I. A problem description, *J. Trop. Pediat.* 27:68-73 (1981).

Manderson, L.: Bottle-feeding and ideology in colonial Malaya: the production of change. *Int. J. Hlth Serv.*, 12:597-616 (1982).

Marchione, T. J.: A history of breast-feeding practices in the English-speaking Caribbean in the twentieth century. *Food and Nutr. Bull.*, 2:9-18 (1980).

Martines, J. C., Ashworth, A. and Kirkwood, B. Breastfeeding among the urban poor in southern Brazil : reasons for termination in the first 6 months of life. *Bull. Wld. Hlth. Org.* 67, 151-161 (1989).

Mathur, R., and Reddy, V.: Bacterial contamination of infant foods. *Ind. J. Med. Res.*, 77:342-346 (1983).

Meldrum, B.: Traditional child-rearing practices of the Ojo market women of Ibadan. In: *Nigerian Children: Developmental Perspectives* (H. V. Curran Ed.) London, Routledge and Kegan Paul, pp. 174-196, (1984).

Millard, A. V., and Graham, M. A.: Principles that guide weaning in rural Mexico. *Ecol. Food Nutr.*, 16:171-188 (1985).

Millis, J.: Infant feeding among Malays. *Med. J. Malaya*, 13:145-152 (1958).

Naismith, D. J.: Kwashiorkor in western Nigeria: a study of traditional weaning foods, with particular reference to energy and linoleic acid, *Brit. J. Nutr.*, 30:567-575 (1973).

Narayanan, I., Saxena, M., Tarafdar, S., Scindi, A., Murthy, N. S., and Singh, S., Adolescent girls' perspectives on breast-feeding - pointers for health education. *Indian Pediatrics*, 24:927-932 (1987).

Nutrition Foundation of India: *Infant feeding practices with special reference to the use of commercial infant foods*. Scientific Report 4 (undated).

Odhalo, J.: *A Report on the Luo Culture and Health*. Paper presented to the UNICEF Seminar on Health Education. Makere College, Kampala, 13-18 November (1961).

Omolulu, A.: Breast-feeding practice and breast milk intake in rural Nigeria. *Hum. Nutr. Appl. Nutr.*, 36A:445-451 (1982).

Orwell, S., Clayton, D., and Dugdale, A. E.: Infant feeding in Nigeria. *Ecol. Food Nutr.*, 15:129-141 (1984).

Osuhor, P. C.: Weaning practice among the Hausas. *J. Hum. Nutr.*, 34:273-280 (1980).

Popkin, B. M., Bilsborrow, R. E., Akin, J. S., and Yamamoto, M. E.: Breast-feeding determinants in low-income countries. *Med. Anthropol.*, 7:1-31 (1983).

Population Council, *The Determinants of Infant Feeding Practices: Preliminary Results of a Four-Country Study*. Research Consortium for the Infant Feeding Study, Working Paper No. 19, New York, The Population Council (1984).

Praun, A.: Nutrition education: development or alienation? *Hum. Nutr. Appl. Nutr.*, 36A:28-34 (1982).

Ramsey, F. C.: An analysis of breast-feeding findings in the Barbados National Health and Nutrition Surveys of 1969 and 1981, with special reference to the International Code of Marketing of Breast-Milk Substitutes, *Cajanus*, 16:14-18 (1983).

Rao, M.: Ecological factors and nutritional status of nursery school children in rural Dharwad, India. *Ecol. Food Nutr.*, 19:323-332 (1987).

Republic of Kenya. *Report of the child nutrition survey 1978-79.* Central Bureau of Statistics, Nairobi, Kenya (undated).

Republic of Kenya, *Situation analysis of children and women in Kenya, Section 4 : the wellbeing of children.* Central Bureau of Statistics, Nairobi, Kenya (1984).

Rowland, M. G. M., Barrell, R. A. E., and Whitehead, R. G.: Bacterial contamination in traditional Gambian weaning foods. *Lancet.*, 1:136-138 (1978).

Rutishauser, I. H. E.: Factors affecting the intake of energy and protein by Ugandan preschool children. *Ecol. Food Nutr.*, 3:213-222 (1974).

Sanjur, D. M., Cravioto, J., Rosales, L. et al.: Infant feeding and weaning practices in a rural pre-industrial setting. *Acta Paediatr. Scand.*, 200: (Suppl.) (1970).

Sathian, U., Joseph, A., and Waterlow, J. C.: Exclusive breast-feeding versus supplementation: a prospective study in a rural south Indian community. *Ann. Trop. Paediatr.*, 3:157-161 (1983).

Sinniah, D., Chon, F. M., and Arokiasamy, J.: Infant feeding practices among nursing personnel in Malaysia. *Acta Paed. Scand.*, 69:525-529 (1980).

van Steenbergen, W. M., Kusin, J. A., de Lacko, C. E., and Jansen, A. A. J.: Lactation performance of mothers with contrasting nutritional status in rural Kenya. *Acta Paediatr. Scand.*, 72:805-810 (1983).

Sudarkasa, N.: *Where Women Work: a Study of Yoruba women in the Market Place and in the Home.* Anthropological Papers No. 53, University of Michigan, Ann Arbor (1973).

Tomkins, A., Alnwick, D., and Haggerty, P.: *Household Level Food Technologies for Improving Young Child Feeding in Eastern and Southern Africa.* Paper prepared for UNICEF multidisciplinary workshop, Nairobi, October (1987).

Underwood, B. A., and Hofvander, Y. Appropriate timing for complementary feeding of the breast-fed infant. *Acta Paed. Scand.*, 294 Suppl. (1982).

Unni, J. C., and Richard, J.: Infant feeding in urban south Indian families. *Indian Pediatrics*, 23:41-45 (1986).

Vimala, V., and Ratnaprabha, C.: Infant feeding practices among tribal communities of Andhra Pradesh. *Indian Pediatrics*, 24:907-920 (1987).

Vis, L. H., and Hennart, P.: L'allaitement maternel en Afrique centrale. *Les Carnets de l'enfance (Assignment Children)*, 25:87-107 (1974).

Vis, L. H., Hennart, P., and Ruchababisha, M.: *Some issues in breast-feeding in deprived rural areas.* Assignment Children, 55/56:183-200 (1981).

Wennen van der May, C. A. M.: The decline of breast-feeding in Nigeria. *Trop. Geog. Med.*, 21:93-96 (1969).

WHO, *Contemporary Patterns of Breast-feeding.* Report of the WHO Collaborative Study on Breast-feeding, Geneva, World Health Organisation, 1981.

WHO, *The Quantity and Quality of Breast-milk.* Geneva, World Health Organisation, 1985.

Wickes, I. G.: A history of infant feeding Part II. The 17th and 18th centuries, *Archs. Dis. Childh.*, 28:232-240 (1953).

Wijga, A., Vyas, U., Vyas, A., Sharma, V., Pandya, N., and Nabarro, D.: Feeding, illness and nutritional status of young children in rural Gujarat. *Hum. Nutr. Clin. Nutr.*, 37C:255-269 (1983).

Williams, C. D., Common diseases of children as seen in the General Hospital, Singapore. *J. Malaya Brch Brit. Med. Ass.*, 2:113-124 (1938).

7

Social and Psychological
Factors in Breast-feeding

Manuel Carballo

Social & Behavioral Research
Global Programme on AIDS
W.H.O.
Geneva, Switzerland

Gretel H. Pelto

Department of Nutritional Science
University of Connecticut
3624 Horse Barn Road
Storrs, Connecticut 06269

INTRODUCTION

During the past two decades of intensive research on lactation, substantial attention has been devoted to the investigation of the social, cultural and psychological factors involved in breast-feeding. Studies have ranged from the collection of survey data on large population groups to ethnographic research with small samples; sociological, psychological, and anthropological theories and research techniques have all been brought to bear on questions concerning the incidence and prevalence of breast-feeding in the modern world. Historians have provided data on infant feeding practices of the past. Investigators representing a number of disciplines and many nations have created a large body of new knowledge about the socio-cultural and psychological factors that influence breast-feeding. They have also provided impressive evidence that breast-feeding is a very complex behavior, which does not yield easily to simple generalizations about its determinants.

The purpose of this chapter in to highlight some of the significant dimensions that emerge repeatedly in social science research on lactation. However, it is not general review of all relevant social and psychological factors related to breast-feeding, and there are many issues not addressed. We focus particularly on factors that influence the *decision-making* of mothers to breast-feed or continue breast-feeding, and on the factors that constrain or support her decisions. In addition to beliefs, attitudes and psychological characteristics of mothers, we focus also on the influence of work roles and social support. We do not deal here, however, with the larger socio-political context within which breast-feeding behavior occurs, nor have we attended to the substantial body of literature on the role of the medical system in influencing breast-feeding, although these are obviously of great significance for understanding the full picture.

THE SELECTION OF FEEDING MODE VERSUS DURATION OF BREAST-FEEDING

The prevalence of breast-feeding in any given environment is a function of two distinct processes: (1) the decision by mothers about whether to breast-feed or bottle-feed their babies ("feeding mode"), and (2) the duration of breast-feeding among those mothers who elect initially to breast-feed. A substantial portion of the newly born are immediately removed from the pool of breast-fed infants because they are bottle-fed from birth.

A number of social and psychological features have been identified as factors that influence the initial decision-making process on feeding mode. Having made the decision to breast-feed, additional factors come into play in determining the length of time that infants receive breast milk. Duration, however, is not a simple matter that can be reduced merely to whether or not the infant receives breast milk. In the first few months of life when exclusive breast-feeding is the biomedically-recommended practice, there is substantial intra- and inter-societal variation in the extent to which infants receive other fluids (including artificial milks) and solids.

Even in traditional societies, exclusive breast-feeding generally appears to be the exception rather than the rule. As the infant matures, other foods need to be added in order to maintain adequate nutrition. Cross culturally, the variation in the percent of total intake from breast milk at any given age varies extremely widely. In some societies the duration of breast-feeding is commonly extended beyond two years, but the later contribution of breast milk to the child's diet is relatively minimal because extensive supplementation with other foods begins at an early age. In other societies the average duration may be much shorter but the proportion of the diet contributed by breast milk is large during the period the infant is breast-fed.

There is often substantial overlap in the factors that influence the initial decision about feeding mode and those that influence duration. For example, lack of confidence in the ability to breast-feed may lead one woman to decide to bottle-feed from birth, while the same situation leads a woman who selected breast-feeding to conclude that her milk isn't "sufficient" to satisfy her infant and to make an early shift to the bottle. Similarly, a woman may select bottle-feeding as the feeding mode because she plans to return to paid employment outside the home; while another woman initially breast-feeds, but shifts to the bottle at 3-4 weeks postpartum because she returns to her job. Another maintains breast-feeding for many months but practices "mixed feeding" (breast and bottle) when she returns to work. The discussion below explores the social and psychological factors influencing breast-feeding from the perspective of both selection of feeding mode and duration.

WAGE LABOR AND BREAST-FEEDING

Historically, changes in infant feeding behavior have coincided with the emergence of new technologies, changing patterns of male and female work, and increasing regimentation of time. It has often been asserted that the changing economic role of women in modern society is a primary cause of the rapid decline of breast-feeding since World War II. This argument is based on the supposition that babies are being bottle-fed because their mothers are engaged in wage labor, and are therefore away from home for long hours at a time.

The economic factors that may influence reproductively active women to seek employment and utilize substitute caretakers for their infants include the following possibilities:

(1) In both developed and developing countries, increased opportunities for paid employment have attracted women to seek work outside the home;

(2) Economic necessity, fueled by rapid inflation in basic commodities, has forced women into wage work to help support their families;

(3) The nearly geometric rise in single parent, female-headed households means that many women have become the sole economic support for their children and themselves, and must therefore return to work as rapidly as possible following childbirth, particularly in societies where social welfare services are poorly developed;

(4) The rising desire for manufactured goods, particularly those that are associated with modern, urban lifestyles, has influenced women to work even when the additional income is not critical for household survival;

(5) Labor policies in many sectors of the economy, particularly those requiring substantial skill and training, often do not permit women to take extended maternity leave, and women must therefore return to their jobs shortly after childbirth or lose their positions, their seniority or their benefits.

THE EVIDENCE FOR THE "EMPLOYMENT HYPOTHESIS"

The evidence concerning the importance of women's employment as a primary factor in the decline in breast-feeding is equivocal, and suggests that much of the discussion has been over-simplified. The relevant data for addressing this question come from many sources: - large scale national surveys, community-based studies and in-depth studies with small samples. Synthesizing the results of empirical investigations into a coherent interpretation is complicated by large differences in the methods of data collection and analysis. Moreover, the data are often amenable to more than one interpretation, depending on the perspective of the analysers.

On the one hand, a number of investigators have suggested that wage labor plays a relatively small part in determining infant feeding patterns. For example, from their review of survey data from a number of countries on reasons for terminating breast-feeding, Winikoff and Baer (1980) determined that employment is seldom given by women as a reason for weaning their infants. Van Esterik and Greiner (1981) reviewed 81 studies from both industrialized and developing countries all of which included some mention of the role of employment on infant feeding decisions. They concluded that employment is not the major reason for selection of bottle-feeding or the termination of breast-feeding for the majority of women.

On the other hand, there is evidence that in some populations infant feeding practices of at least a subset of women are strongly influenced by the matter of employment. Data from 4,000 women in Sri Lanka interviewed in connection with the World Fertility Survey showed that the selection of bottle-feeding at birth was associated with maternal work away from home (Akin et al., 1981). This finding remained statistically significant even when a number of other socio-demographic characteristics were taken into consideration. A similar picture emerged in a 1980 survey of 850 women in Taiwan. This survey revealed that wage work away from home, as opposed to work for income at home, predicted the selection of bottle-feeding - again with statistical control for potentially confounding variables (Milman, 1981). In Bangkok 210 women were interviewed concerning their feeding practices; 54 mothers reported that they selected bottle-feeding at birth, and, of these, 28 percent said that their reason for choosing bottle-feeding was "work away from home" (Tamchareon et al., 1980).

In addition to these findings concerning the initial selection of feeding mode, there are also data that reflect the influence of employment on duration of breast-feeding and level of supplementation. Foreman (1984) carried out an extensive review of the literature on this subject, reporting the results of her analysis on a region by region basis. In south Asia (India and Bangladesh) return to work was associated with an earlier introduction of supplementary foods but not with the termination of breast-feeding. In East Asia and the Pacific Islands, maternal work away from home was related to both duration of breast-feeding and degree of supplementation. In the Caribbean, maternal work, or intention to return to work, was associated with the introduction of supplementary bottle-feeding and the cessation of breast-feeding. In studies in Africa, both work in general and distance to work have been shown to relate to duration and supplementation practices. Data from the World Fertility Survey in four countries in Latin America revealed that "work categorized by type and place was not associated with length of breast-feeding after controlling for maternal age, parity, education, place of residence and husband's occupation."

Foreman suggests that further research is needed to clarify the effects of maternal work on choice of feeding mode and duration of breast-feeding. She points out that much of the research to date has used oversimplified definitions of "work," and investigators often fail to examine inter-relationships with other confounding variables.

Under the direction of researchers at the Population Council and Cornell University, a large scale study of social determinants of breast-feeding was carried out in Thailand, Indonesia, Colombia, and Kenya. The study used survey techniques and ethnographic research methods to examine a series of questions, including the role of maternal employment in infant feeding (Winikoff *et al.*, 1983; Winikoff *et al.*, 1988; Winikoff & Lautaran, 1989). The results are generally similar to the composite picture that emerges from the reviews described above. Reviewing the data, Van Esterik (1989) suggests: "The four-country study demonstrates that work outside the home is not the primary determinant of duration of breast-feeding, although it is strongly implicated in the early initiation of bottle-feeding. Conditions at work and distance from work are extremely important also."

Through multi-variate analyses, Winikoff and Laukaren (1989) showed that in all four countries, a significant intervening variable in the association between employment and bottle-feeding is early introduction of the bottle, which is associated with early weaning in both employed and unemployed women. They conclude that "...it is clear that work has a strong effect, in most cases, of pushing women towards bottle-feeding." However, since "early supplementation and weaning are much more common than is working outside the home," it is obvious that other influences must be operating to affect the duration of breast-feeding.

Employment in wage labor is clearly not the strongest factor that accounts for declines in breast-feeding in the twentieth century. However, the evidence suggests that it is a determinant in some segments of the population, particularly for poor women in urban communities. The conditions of employment also have important influences on infant feeding practices. For example, Popkin and Solon (1976) found that among Cebuano women in the Philippines, women breast-feed if they work close to their homes, but they begin mixed feeding if they work in a different barrio.

WOMEN'S WORK ROLES AND BREAST-FEEDING PATTERNS

Studies of employment and breast-feeding practices point to the larger issue: the relationships of infant feeding to women's work roles. A number of investigators have presented arguments concerning the need to consider the management of infant feeding in the context of women's multiple economic and domestic roles (Van Esterik, 1989; Pelto, 1981; Nerlove, 1974; Popkin, 1978 and Popkin). Whether the competing demands on women's time come in the form of paid labor activities, agricultural and animal care responsibilities, domestic chores (including the provisioning of water and fuel), or combinations of these, infant feeding must nearly always be carried out as part of a complex of women's multiple roles.

The widespread availability of infant feeding bottles and breast milk substitutes provides new opportunities for mothers to solve time management problems that were previously handled in other ways. Until the last few decades only a minority of mainly privileged women could elect not to breast-feed. But the early introduction of foods to supplement breast-feeding has often been a strategy that women in many societies use to extend the period between breast-feeds.

Nerlove (1974) examined the relationship of women's work loads to infant feeding practices in traditional societies. Using ethnographic data from 83 traditional cultures, she demonstrated a strong tendency for infants to receive supplementary foods before one month of age in societies in which there is high female participation in food production. When women have less responsibility for production, supplements to breast milk tend to be given later. Nerlove concludes that "...child care responsibilities may be adjusted to accommodate the mothers' subsistence activities"

Recently, Levine (1988) carried out a study of infant feeding in a remote area of Nepal where nearly all women breast-feed their children for a prolonged period of time. She compared the age of introduction of supplementary feeding in two farming communities that differed in average size of landholding and female labor participation. In the village where households had smaller plots, and women did more of the farm labor, foods were introduced at an earlier age than in the community in which households could afford to hire extra labor. Typically, women who were away from their infants for extended periods of time fed them in the morning before leaving for work, returned to feed them at mid-day (when possible) and fed them immediately upon returning in the evening. Infants also slept with their mothers and suckled freely at night.

Levine (1988) comments on the implications of her study for infant feeding patterns in urban areas. "The patterns I have described for Humla, where supplementary cereal foods commonly are introduced within the first few months, where breast-feeding is prolonged for at least two years and often more, where there is a mix of frequent and indulgent nursing when the mother is present and supplementary foods when she must work, still may be found among traditional groups...The existence of such long-standing, traditional patterns of early supplementation to facilitate mother's work may lend a certain perspective on the use of bottle-feeding by urban working mothers in less developed countries today." She goes on to note a potentially important difference between earlier supplementation with paps in traditional societies and use of bottles. "The difference is that bottle-feeding seems likelier to replace, than to supplement, breast milk, and thus carries greater risks."

To summarize this discussion, we conclude that maternal work roles, including wage labor, are a major influence on breast-feeding. When competing demands for mothers' time take precedence over breast-feeding, the results may appear in several forms: the selection of bottle-feeding at the time of birth; the early introduction of breast milk substitutes given by bottle, with or without cessation of breast-feeding, and/or the introduction of supplemental foods, initially in highly liquid form and followed later by semi-solid foods. Breast-feeding is not *intrinsically* incompatible with women's employment, as evidenced by the substantial upturn in rates of breast-feeding in some industrialized countries with high rates of women's employment (Hofvander & Sjolin, 1979). There is, however, also substantial evidence to suggest that breast-feeding must be highly valued and protected when the multiple pressures from other economic and domestic roles can lead to premature weaning or other inappropriate infant feeding practices. The institutionalization of new work patterns and employment conditions that promote successful feeding routines requires legislative procedures that are unlikely to emerge in the near future.

THE ROLE OF MATERNAL BELIEFS AND ATTITUDES

In the past two decades considerable efforts has been expended to promote breast-feeding through health education campaigns. These activities are based on the proposition that breast-feeding behavior is strongly influenced by maternal beliefs and attitudes, particularly concerning what is best or healthiest for infants. The now well-known slogan, "breast is best," epitomizes the educational focus on infant health.

Interviews with women in many parts of the world provide evidence in support of the proposition put forth by Marshall and Marshall (1979) that "a mother frequently base(s) her decision [on infant feeding mode] on considerations of optimal health for her child and herself -- the perceived adequacy of her milk supply, medical problems experienced by her child or herself or her opinion on the relative merits of breast milk and commercial formulas."

The concern about doing what is best for infant and maternal health can lead to the selection of either breast *or* bottle-feeding, depending on people's beliefs and perceptions. Recently Weller & Dungy (1986) conducted a study of beliefs about infant feeding among Hispanic and Anglo mothers in southern California. They found some differences in attitudes between women who selected breast-feeding and those bottle-fed. Breast-feeders, for example, were more likely to mention "protecting babies from illness," while bottle-feeders were likely to include "no embarrassment" as a reason for selecting bottle-feeding. A major finding of the study, however, was that "similar characteristics are preferred by both breast and bottle-feeders." Differences in perceptions about the two feeding modes permit women to select breast-feeding because "baby will grow up healthier," or to select bottle-feeding because "it provides complete nutrition when the mother is not eating right."

The authors interpret the results as suggesting that "Mother's beliefs about their lifestyles and health behaviors may be the most important factors in determining which method to use. Although research shows breast-feeding to be superior, a mother who believes she does not eat well or that she may not be able to provide the nutrients, *etc.* that an infant needs, would certainly be more likely to bottle-feed...assuming that bottle-feeders and breast-feeders are equally concerned or cautious in their choice of a method, bottle-feeders may be less sure of their physical ability to do so."

THE PROBLEM OF "INSUFFICIENT MILK"

A primary expression of maternal fears concerning the ability to meet infant's needs is the often reported problem of "insufficient milk." In surveys from both developed and developing countries "inadequacy of the milk supply," is very commonly given as the reason for beginning supplementation or for ceasing breast-feeding (Gussler & Briesemeister, 1980). The interpretation of these results has been a subject of considerable debate.

Some observers have suggested mothers give this as a convenient excuse or socially acceptable response as a cover up for other motives. For example, these authors reported that on the island of St. Kitts, where there is a high rate of initial breast-feeding and a rapid shift to bottles, "several nurses expressed the opinion that 'insufficient milk' is an excuse for mothers on the island to switch to bottle-feeding 'too early'." On the other hand, some researchers have suggested that there is often a true insufficiency in many cases, which is caused by poor maternal diet or nutritional status (Wichelow, 1979).

There are very few data on which to base an assessment of the relationship of perceived milk insufficiency to milk value; it is thus not possible to determine the frequency with which insufficiency relative to infant needs actually exists. It is unlikely, however, that this occurs in the majority of cases in which insufficiency is perceived to be a problem. The explanation for the wide-spread perception of insufficiency on the part of mothers is probably best sought in the realm of maternal interpretation of infant behavior and growth, and the role of maternal insecurity and anxiety (Allen & Pelto, 1985).

There has been little examination of the process by which women decide that their milk is inadequate in either quality or quantity. In some - probably a small minority of cases in industrialized countries - this conclusion may be based on medical advice that the baby is "not growing well." The appropriateness of this judgment depends on the growth reference values the health care practitioner is using to assess development, since breast-fed infants grow more slowly than bottle-fed infants after the first few months of life (Whitehead & Paul, 1984).

In the great majority of cases, however, it is the infants' behavior, not their growth, that is the basis on which mothers (and their advisors) determine that the baby is "not satisfied" or not "doing well" on breast milk. Crying, restlessness, changes in sleep patterns, and sucking rapidly at the breast are among the characteristics that indicate breast milk problems to mothers. Before the advent of bottle-feeding as a nearly universal option, these behaviors may have been given a different interpretation in many cases.

On-demand feeding, which is generally characteristic of feeding patterns in traditional societies may, in part, reflect a feeling on the part of mothers that infants are not adequately satisfied with any single feed and that the restlessness which, in modern societies might lead to complementary feeding has been responded to by additional breast-feeding.

On-demand feeding may also reflect a physiological reality that the quantity of milk available to the infant on any given feed is low and has to be supplemented by frequent, but short, suckling episodes. Frequent feeding, by definition, requires proximity to the infant and the time devoted to putting the infant to the breast. The work patterns imposed on mothers in highly regimented industries typical of modern society do not easily lend themselves to this responsiveness.

Duthie (1983) examined the matter of maternal interpretation of infant crying in her study in Scotland of factors influencing the duration of breast-feeding. She visited mothers on a weekly basis following the birth of their infants and interviewed them about a number of issues, including infant behavior. The majority of women in her study reported problems of fussing, crying and restlessness. Women who shortly thereafter went on to terminate breast-feeding had a strong tendency to blame problems with their milk as the cause of the baby's discomfort, whereas the women who had alternative explanations (*e.g.* "stomach ache," "natural development," "wants attention") were more likely to continue to breast-feed. One young mother expressed her frustration and disappointment in the misinterpretation that led her to premature weaning to the bottle: "I thought he was fussing because I didn't have enough milk so I gave him the bottle. But it was colic, and he didn't stop crying after I changed. It was a mistake."

Martin (1978) examined reasons for early weaning among women in England and Scotland and found that mothers tended to assume that any crying by their babies was the result of hunger and thus a reflection of their inadequate milk supply. Kocturk (1986) conducted a prospective study of 24 mothers in Istanbul, Turkey. There, also, it appears that "the crying infant was the most important cue leading the mother to believe her milk was insufficient." In addition to fears about inadequate quantity, mothers' concerns about the quality of their milk led to early supplementation. The author notes that there was no evidence in this study to suggest that "the milk insufficiency syndrome is a rationalization for reasons which otherwise might be frowned on by society," and concludes that "over-anxiety and preoccupation in being a 'better' mother seemed to contribute to anxiety over the milk yield and introduction of complements more than anything else. Findings of this study tend to support the view that urban environments contain elements which impart a sense of insecurity in the mother on her ability to satisfy the needs of her infant."

Expressions of anxiety and lack of confidence about their ability to breast-feed occur commonly when women are interviewed prenatally to obtain information on their choice of feeding mode. In the Scottish study, women who expressed doubt about their likelihood of success at breast-feeding also tended to purchase bottles "just in case" they were needed. Both of these factors proved to be predictive of an early shift to bottle-feeding (Duthie, 1983). While it may be argued that such behaviors are indicative of ambivalence or lack of commitment to breast-feeding, there is also a physiological effect of anxiety on the "let down reflex," which can have subsequent effects on breast-feeding (Newton & Newton, 1967; Jelliffe & Jelliffe, 1978).

SOCIAL LEARNING, SOCIAL SUPPORT AND BREAST-FEEDING

Anxiety about insufficient milk may be correlated with inadequate preparation and social support for breast-feeding among young, primiparous women. In the absence of advice that might be forthcoming from older, more experienced women, young mothers increasingly have to interpret fussiness or crying in infants according to adult expressions of hunger. They also have to struggle with other problems, such as sore nipples and breast engorgement, which can usually be easily resolved, in fact, by advice on effective management.

Margaret Mead, one of the first social scientists to draw attention to the importance of a supportive environment (Mead & Newton, 1967), argued that new mothers not only need psychological support, they also require teaching and guidance from women with experience and expertise. In most traditional societies, *doulas* help women through the early postnatal period (Raphael, 1976). The *doula* is almost always an older woman; sometimes, but not necessarily, a relative of the new mother. Their role is to initiate the new, primiparous mother into the intricacies of breast-feeding, to help her through the first days of learning a new behavior, and support her until lactation is firmly established.

With urban migration and other social changes associated with modernization, the support and instruction provided by the *doula* has often been lost or seriously attenuated. In industrialized countries, the growth of childbirth preparation classes and breast-feeding support groups represent new developments to replace this traditional role. With respect to preparation for breast-feeding, data suggest that where careful, sensitive and systematic preparation and support for breast-feeding has been available to women in urban, industrialized societies, the incidence and prevalence of breast-feeding has been enhanced.

Preparation for breast-feeding in modern society, however, increasingly depends upon the capacity and willingness of health care workers and systems to include it in prenatal and maternity care. To date, educational programs to promote breast-feeding have primarily emanated from breast-feeding mothers groups that have drawn upon the experiences of middle class families. The content of the educational and promotional programs and the manner in which they have been communicated has implicitly restricted messages to educated, middle class women. There have been few examples of educational or promotional programs implemented by and through health and social service systems designed to reach a wider population. Moreover, in the few cases where such programs have evolved, there has been little consideration of the social conditions in which working class mothers function, and the range of occupational, economic, time and cultural factors that might constrain the capacity of these mothers to incorporate breast-feeding into their life conditions.

In addition to preparation for breast-feeding and assistance in problem solving during the period in which lactation is established, social support for breast-feeding from family members and friends is a significant factor in both selection of feeding mode and duration of breast-feeding. For example, a study of 255 women in rural Missouri found that the most important influence on women's decisions about feeding mode was the attitude of the husband, and almost all women chose the method the husband preferred (LeFevre *et al.*,

1987). Among low-income women in New York City, the feeding method preference of the baby's father significantly influenced both the incidence and duration of breast-feeding (Bevan *et al.*, 1984).

Barnowski and colleagues (1983) examined the role of sources of support in a multi-ethnic population in Texas. Using sophisticated statistical methodology to control for confounding factors, they discovered that the influence of various sources of support differs by ethnic group. Among Anglo-American women, "the male partner is clearly the single most important source of spouse support in promoting breast-feeding." For Black American mothers the attitude of the "best friend" is the only significant predictor of feeding mode, whereas it is the mother herself who is the significant individual for Mexican American women. Bryant (1982) has reported a very similar picture from her multi-ethnic study in Miami, Florida. Taken as a whole, these and other similar studies provide ample evidence that the attitudes of family members and friends represent a significant sector for influence on breast-feeding.

THE MARKETING OF BREAST MILK SUBSTITUTES

The marketing of breast milk substitutes has increasingly constituted one of the principal sources of information on infant feeding for both health practitioners and the public at large. In the absence of systematic education and information on infant nutritional needs, the value of breast-feeding, together with the importance of frequent mother-infant contact, industry messages concerning the nutritional value of breast milk substitutes, their effectiveness and their "scientifically-researched composition" have become pivotal sources of advice. The WHO study of infant feeding (1981) indicated that even in small, rural communities, large proportions of mothers had been exposed to information on such substitutes and the majority of them could identify these substitutes by brand name. While no clear correlation could or should be made between this indicator and decisions to breast-feed or maintain breast-feeding, it is important to note how pervasive such information had become in the 1970s and how little "competing" information on the value of breast-feeding has been available to mothers and the health sector. Since that time the situation has changed substantially, but the wide-spread availability of breast milk substitutes and the marketing of these commodities must be seen as a continuing source of influence on breast-feeding.

PROMOTING BREAST FEEDING AS A AN INTEGRAL COMPONENT OF CARE GIVING

Among modern, educated mothers, the decision to breast-feed is likely to be associated with a greater awareness of, and commitment to, principles of child care that involve physical and psychological stimulation, a sensitivity to the emotional needs of the young in infant, and a willingness to dedicate time to the infant. Studies of growth and development in infants have consistently indicated that an important variable in positive development and physical growth is the psycho-social stimulation of the infant, expressed in such ways as picking up, cuddling, talking to, eye contact, exposure to toys and visual movement, and so on. By the same token, assessments of inadequate growth and development should take into account the role played by the reduction of these experiences, which, in turn, may reflect the limited time available to mothers and the pressures of competing demands and responsibilities.

Changing patterns of infant feeding in modern, industrialized societies suggest a relatively clear association between education, socioeconomic background, employment status and decisions to breast-feed. In industrialized societies, breast-feeding today is more common among the well educated than it is among women who have not completed secondary education. A further correlation is that between educational status and exposure to information about infant and young child needs, including education about the importance of frequent stimulation and physical contact with the infant. Thus, infants of better educated and higher income mothers may be benefitting more from the physical and psycho-social advantages of child care practices that include a complex of supportive, growth-promoting behaviors.

Programmatic activities aimed at the promotion of breast-feeding are increasingly undertaken in an atmosphere of awareness about the multiple factors that influence feeding practices. In addition to considering these factors and seeking ways to modify the constraints to breast-feeding, it is also important to promote breast-feeding as an integral part of child care. To achieve this, greater attention must be given to an examination of the factors that constrain or facilitate effective and sensitive care giving.

REFERENCES

Akin, J., Belsborrow, R., Guilkey, D., *et al.* The Determinants of Breast-Feeding in Sri Lanka. *Demography*, 18:287-307 (1981).

Allen, L. H., and Pelto, G. H. Research on Determinants of Breast-Feeding Duration: Suggestions for Biocultural Studies. *Med. Anthro.*, 9:97-105 (1985).

Baranowski, T., Bee, D. E., Rassen, D. K., Richardson, C. J., Brown, J. P., Guenther, N., and Nader, P. R. Social Support, Social Influence, Ethnicity and the Breast-Feeding Decision. *Soc. Sci. and Med.*, 17:1599-1611 (1983).

Bevan, M. L., Mosley, D., Lobach, K. S., and Solimano, G. R. Factors Influencing Breast-Feeding in an Urban WIC Program. *J. Amer. Diet. Assoc.*, 84:563-567 (1984).

Bryant, C. A. The Impact of Kin, Friend, and Neighbor Networks on Infant Feeding Practices. *Soc. Sci. and Med.*, 16:1757-1765 (1982).

Duthie, A. M. *Biological and Sociocultural Predictors of the Extent and Duration of Breast-Feeding.* Ph.D. Dissertation. University of Connecticut (1983).

Foreman, M. R. Review of Research on the Factors Associated with Choice and Duration of Infant Feeding in Less-Developed Countries. *Pediatrics*, 74:(4, part 2) 667-694 (1984).

Gussler, J. D., and Briesemeister, L. H. The Insufficient Milk Syndrome: A Biocultural Explanation. *Med. Anthro.*, 4:1-24 (1980).

Hofvander, Y., and Sjolin, S. Breast-Feeding Trends and Recent Information Activities in Sweden. *Acta Pediat. Scand.*, 275:16-27 (1979).

Jelliffe, D. B., and Jelliffe, E. F. P. *Human Milk in the Modern World.* Oxford: Oxford University Press (1978).

Kocturk, T. O. Events Leading to the Decision to Introduce Complementary Feeding to the Breast Among a Group of Mothers in Istanbul. *Scand. J. Prim. Health Care*, 4:231-237 (1986).

LeFevre, M., Kruse, J., and Zweig, S. Selection of Infant Feeding Method: A Population-Based Study in a Rural Area. *J. Fam. Prac.*, 24:487-491 (1987).

Levine, N. E. Women's work and infant feeding: a case from rural Nepal. *Ethnology*, 27(3):231-252 (1988).

Marshall, L. B., and Marshall, M. Breasts, Bottles and Babies: Historical Changes in Infant Feeding Practices in a Micronesian Village. *Ecol. Food and Nutr.*, 8:241-249 (1979).

Martin, J. Infant Feeding 1975: *Attitudes and Practice in England and Wales.* London: Office of Population Censuses and Surveys, Social Survey Division, Her Majesty's Stationery Office (1978).

Mead, M., and Newton, N. Cultural Patterning of Perinatal Behavior. In: *Childbearing - Its Social and Psychological Aspects.* (S. A. Richardson and A. F. Guttmacher, Eds.) New York: Williams and Williams (1967).

Milman, S. Breast-Feeding in Taiwan: *Trend and Differentials, 1966-1980.* Paper presented at the Annual Meeting of the Population Association of America. March 26-28, 1981.

Nerlove, S. Women's workload and Infant Feeding Practices: A Relationship with Demographic Implications. *Ethnology*, 13:207-214 (1974).

Newton, N. R., and Newton, M. Psychologic Aspects of Lactation. *New Engl. J. Med.*, 277:1170-1188 (1967).

Pelto, G. H. Perspectives on Infant Feeding: Decision-Making and Ecology. *Food and Nutr. Bull.*, 3 (3):16-29 (1981).

Popkin, B. M., and Solon, F. S. Income, Time, the Working Mother and Child Nutriture. *J. of Trop. Ped.*, 22:156-166 (1976).

Popkin, B. M. Economic Determinants of Breast-Feeding Behavior. In: *Nutrition and Human Reproduction.* (W. H. Mosley, Ed.) New York: Plenum Publishing Co. (1978).

Popkin, B. M. Time Allocation of the Mother and child nutrition. *Ecology of Food and Nutrition*, 9:1-14.

Raphael, D. *The Tender Gift.* New York: Schocken Books (1976).

Temchareon, P., Temchareon, P., Sirivunaboot, P. Relationship between Mother's Attitudes Toward Breast-Feeding and Types of Feeding Practices. *J. Med. Assoc. Thailand*, 63:548-552 (1980).

Van Esterik, P., and Greiner, T. Breast-Feeding and Women's Work: Constraints and Opportunities. *Studies in Family Planning*, 12 (4):182-195 (1981).

Van Esterik, P. *Beyond the Breast-Bottle Controversy.* New Brunswick, N. J.: Rutgers University Press (1989).

Weller, S. C., and Dungy, C. I. Personal Preferences and Ethnic Variations Among Anglo and Hispanic Breast and Bottle Feeders. *Soc. Sci. and Med.*, 23:539-548 (1986).

Whichelow, M. Breast-Feeding - Keeping Up the Milk Supply. *Health Visitor*, 52:217-220 (1979).

Whitehead, R. G., and Paul, A. A. Growth Charts and Assessment of Infant Feeding Practices in the Western World and Developing Countries. *Early Human Development*, 9:187-207 (1984).

Winikoff, B., and Baer, E. The Obstetrician's Opportunity: Translating 'Breast is Best' from Theory to Practice. *Am. J. Obstetrics and Gynecology*, 138 1:105-117 (1980).

Winikoff, B., Latham, M., and Solimano, G. *The Infant Feeding Study: Semarang, Nairobi, Bogota and Bangkok Site Reports*. New York: Population Council (1983).

Winikoff, B., Castle, M., and Laukaran, V. *Infant Feeding in Four Societies*. Westport, CT.: Greenwood Press (1988).

Winikoff, B., and Lautaran, V. H. Breast-Feeding and Bottle-Feeding Controversies in the Developing World: Evidence from a Study in Four Countries. *Soc. Sci. and Med.*, 29:859-868 (1989).

World Health Organization. *Contemporary Patterns of Breast-Feeding: Report of the WHO Study on Breast-Feeding*. Geneva: WHO (1981).

8

Weaning: Why, When and What?

Angel Ballabriga

Childrens Hospital
Vall d'Hebrón
Autonomous University
Barcelona, Spain

DEFINITION

Weaning is an ambiguous term. Sometimes it signifies different things in different countries, sometimes different things in the same country according to who defines it. It could be said that it is a process that starts when any nutrient other than breast milk or formula is introduced into the diet of the baby and starts with the introduction of semi-solids or solids and continues up to the time when the purely sucking period has finished. The term "to wean" would be that of accustoming or familiarizing the child with the family diet and during this period of weaning children pass from dominant milk feeding to a diet in which they receive solids. Weaning from the breast is the process of retiring the breast, which can be abrupt or gradual. In the former, it may be called complete weaning because the breast has been completely retired. When we speak of complementary feeding we refer to something that can be given following, or in addition to lactation and which does not interfere with the process of sucking. In some cases it can be a breast milk substitute, which in some countries is called supplementary feeding. On the other hand mixed feeding would be the addition of semi-solid or solid supplements or paps in a regular daily fashion and in significant quantities.

Weaning foods are considered those that are used during the transitional period which is started with complementing breast-feeding, or formula with semi-solids or solids, and which finishes when the child receives a completely tablefood diet. Complementary feeding does not act as a substitute for the breast as it does not condition lessening of the frequency of sucking. The process of weaning is a long one during which the contribution of calories comes from other nutrients that are not breast milk or formula; this process has great geographical and cultural variations. In some societies it is extended over years. The word *beikost* has been used to refer to any type of food that is neither breast milk nor formula and is employed during the period of weaning.

PREVALENCE OF BREAST MILK AND HISTORICAL BACKGROUND

Retrospective data studied by Hirschman and Butler (1981) show that between 1911 and 1915, 30% of infants were breast-fed at nine months in the USA, whilst in the period 1946-50 only 1% were.

In the decade of the forties, approximately 65% of newborn infants in the USA were breast-fed after delivery in hospital (Bain, 1948). In 1972 (Martinez, 1974) only 28% of North American babies were being breast-fed at one week of age. Andrew *et al.* (1978) in a survey of feeding practices, reported that 32% of infants were breast-fed during the first month of life, and in a study by Crawford *et al.* (1978) they showed that at six months, 27% of infants surveyed were breast-fed. A review of the USA literature between 1955 and 1980 showed the newborn infant breast-fed at one week of age had the following percentages 29.2% in 1955, 24.9% in 1970, 33.4% in 1975 and 54% in 1980 (Martinez *et al.*, 1981). In Sweden, around 60% of all infants were breast-fed at six months of age in 1940, while in 1970 this was only 6% (Persson and Samuelson, 1984). Studying the trends in breast-feeding, Martinez and Nalezienski (1981) pointed out that between 5 and 6 months of age the incidence of breast-feeding rose from 5.5% in 1971 to 23% in 1979. Two national surveys carried out in France in 1972 and 1976 (Roumeau-Rouguette, 1980) on representative samples of births showed an increase in the frequency of breast-feeding in the neonatal period from 36.6% to 45.5%. In 1977 reports of various child health centres in Sweden (Hofvander and Sjölin, 1979) showed that at six months an average of 20-25% of infants were breast-fed and in another study in Uppsala in 1978 the rate of breast-feeding at 6 months was 36% (Hofvander and Petros-Barvazian, 1978). A survey in Barcelona in a very large maternity hospital in 1985, gave initial percentages of breast-feeding of around 75%. This figure decreased to 40% at one month of age (Ballabriga and Schmidt, 1987). A European survey called attention to the notable differences existing between different countries, reaching maximum figures at 12 months of age of 80% in Turkey, and of 20% in Finland, although due to different reasons. This trend back to breast-feeding is observed very clearly in many countries in the second half of the decade of the seventies, related to a change in maternal attitude as well as recommendations of various authorities (*e.g.* Protein Advisory Group of the United Nations System, 1972; ESPGAN Committee on Nutrition, 1982).

Traditionally, infants with very lengthy breast-feeding did not receive solids until the end of the first year of life. Some reports, such as those of Hamburger (1923), Jundell (1924) and Glazier (1933), who administered supplements of solid food, were the exception to the rule. From the moment when the trend of a decline in breast-feeding occurred with a substitution by different infant formulas, a concurrent tendency arose of the early introduction of mixed feeding. As a result of this trend there are the reports of Steward (1943), with introduction of solids between 4 and 8 weeks of life, and that of Sackett (1956) with the introduction of beikost right from the early days. The survey of Butler and Wolman (1954) showed that 66% of infants received solids before 8 weeks of age. Fomon (1974) noted that in a 1970 market research it was found that 30% of the energy intake at 3 months was given in the form of beikost, and Shukla *et al.* (1972) demonstrated that 93% of infants in the USA were taking solid foods at 13 weeks. The study of Oates (1973) showed that the introduction of beikost between 3-4 weeks was a normal practice. In the seventies, between 80-95% of British babies received non-milk solids by three months (DHSS, 1983). With the improvement of the downward trend of breast-feeding and an increase in its frequency and duration, a new tendency was begun towards the late administration of solid foods, and 1975, according to Whitehead *et al.* (1986), 18% of babies received non-milk foods at 4 weeks whilst in 1980 this figure had been reduced to 4%.

COMPLEMENTARY FEEDING

If we consider the weaning period as starting with the introduction of some food other than breast milk, or infant formula, and finishing with definite stopping of breast-feeding or of formula, complementary feeding means the introduction of any nutrient complement made with the objective of maintaining breast-feeding for as long as possible, and given as additional supply to compensate for individual needs. The idea is not weaning from the breast but to start a complementation generally in about three months of age, because the mother considers that there is an inadequate milk flow or not enough weight gain. Particularly in developed countries, in which frequency of sucking is less, the start of complementary feeding very often represents the first step of weaning in a relatively short space of time. The experience in developing countries shows that if the frequency of sucking is maintained or even increased, there is no decrease of breast milk output due to the initiation of an additional complement. For us, this complement is not a substitute. In a study in an urban community in India (Ghosh *et al.*, 1976) with 802 mothers of children exclusively breast-fed at 3 months, showed that 48% receive some complements, particularly in the form of buffalo milk or infant formula; 57% of these mothers stopped breast-feeding by 12 months and 20% stopped by 24 months. Solids were introduced in this study between 13 and 18 months. In infants fed with formula, the introduction of regular complements really represents the start of a semi-solid mixed diet and progressive substitution of infant formula for weaning foods. In any case, the complement should not interfere with the sucking frequency, it should be given after a breast-feed and be offered with a cup or spoon, never with a bottle.

The WHO Collaborative Breast-Feeding Study (1981), included 9 countries, and showed that the percentage of breast-fed babies receiving regular complementary food varies widely, ranging from 86% in rural areas of Nigeria to only 12% in rural areas of India. Underwood and Hofvender (1982) consider that the appropriate timing for complementary feeding of the breast-fed infant should not be before 4 months.

WEANING: WHY?

The most important reason for the introduction of beikost in the infant diet is nutritional. The infant fed by the breast, or with infant formula, reaches a point at which his energy requirements are not being met. Protein requirements in the second semester of life can be met by a quantity of milk that is well tolerated by the infant but the energy supply obtained from the mother's milk output can be too low to meet the energy requirements. Individual mother's variations of milk output also prompt the need for additional energy with very variable limits. Individual variations in daily milk output can be almost three-fold. As Waterlow and Thomson (1979) point out, breast milk in some infants just meets the energetic needs at 3 months of age. It is impossible to reach the large volume of breast milk required for long-term breast-fed infants not receiving daily supplements with the passing of time. FAO/WHO (1973) have estimated the energy requirements of infants as 120kcal/kg/d at 2 months and 110kcal/kg/d at 6 months. Whitehead *et al.* (1981) showed that energy intake in infants was about 15% lower than those recommended and established it as 104kcal/kg/d at 2 months and 87/kcal/kg/d at 6 months instead of the 110kcal/kg/d recommended by FAO/WHO. Critical analysis of the data used by the FAO/WHO/UNU Committee (1985), summarized by Bëhar (1986), give the following energy intake established during the first year of life: 0-2months = 118-114kcal/kg/d; 6-7m. = 91kcal/kg/d; 8-9m. = 90kcal/kg/d; 10-11m. = 93kcal/kg/d; 12m. = 102kcal/kg/d. In fact the difference between the 1971 data and the latter, especially between 3 and 9 months is important, and just at a period in which the process of weaning begins. It also supposes that breast milk alone can cover the needs of the great majority of infants between 4 and 6 months (Ahn and Maclean, 1980). As in the first months of life, fat stores increase rapidly so that, according to individual needs, energy requirements during weaning can be covered, in part, by energy stored as fat. The energy requirements at 6 months can vary with relation to the degree of activity. It has been suggested that infants living in developing countries have energy and protein requirements that may be different from those of infants in developed countries (Seward and Sedula, 1984). Energy efficiency changes during weaning because during the first months of life a very important part of energy is provided by fat, and stored with low energy cost. During the weaning period energy supply is obtained mainly from carbohydrates which in part will be transformed to fat with a very important loss of energy. Infants can adapt themselves to low energy intakes during weaning by reducing activity (Poskitt, 1987).

The greater need for food can be perceived by the mother, who appreciates the sensation of hunger, and this implies an increase in the frequency of sucking in order to try to obtain a greater milk volume and the progressive step towards a mixed diet.

An interesting question is that of knowing the reasons why mothers start weaning, sometimes very early. In many cases of trying to keep up exclusive lactation until 5-6 months is unrealistic, and in fact it is the mother herself who interprets the needs of her baby. From there, for example, stems the fact that in different countries, pertaining to similar cultural areas, there are notable differences regarding the time of introduction of beikost. In the Hindley *et al.* (1965) study median age for weaning was 0.92 months in Brussels and 4.5 months in the Stockholm samples. Mothers of a high social class effect longer lactation than those of a lower social class (Klackenberg and Klackenberg-Larsson, 1968). Sjölin *et al.* (1977) found that problems of mother-infant interaction, a perception of insufficient milk and work outside the home, played a role in short breast-feeding periods. For 243 mothers who stopped breast-feeding before the end of two weeks, the reasons given were: insufficient milk (48%), painful breast (16%) and rejection of breast by the infant (11%): Martin (1978) gives others. In our study of 218 mothers who stopped breast-feeding before three months, the reasons given were: insufficient milk (50.5%), no weight gain (21.7%) and tiredness and local pain and discomfort (20.4%), (Ballabriga and Schmidt, 1987). It is always difficult to affirm when exclusive breast-feeding is inadequate, but it seems that breast milk outputs of 800, 930 and 1020ml daily at 2,4 and 6 months can assure the fiftieth percentile for normal patterns of development (Whitehead, 1985).

WEANING: WHEN?

The onset of the weaning period implies that a degree of gastrointestinal tolerance and a capacity for the intestinal absorption of the new nutrients to be offered to the infant has been reached, both from a qualitative and quantitative point of view. It also supposes the development of mechanical factors, such as suction of the food, coordination of deglution and the beginning of mastication. The ability to chew includes an innate component and others that are acquired by means of a learning process which develops with the existence of a good integration of neurological functions. Illingworth and Lister (1964) consider that there surely exists a critical period of development during which mastication must be learned; this period would extend from 5 months to the end of the first year of life. In the neonatal period there is an extrusion reflex when something is introduced into the anterior part of the mouth. Later, between 6-8 months, there are biting movements. In those cases where this learning has not been gained, such as in infants who have received an enteral tube or parenteral feeding for a long time, or who have been fed by gastrostomy, enormous difficulties can be encountered in trying to initiate the normal oral route due to lack of habit. Between 4-6 months the extrusion reflex disappears and the infant is capable of transporting semi-solid food towards the posterior part of the mouth and then to swallow it. The infant is also able to maintain neuromuscular control of head and neck, facilitating feeding, and is able to reflect the sensation of hunger or satiation, with acceptance or refusal of food offered. In parallel fashion, during these first months, a maturative process of the gastrointestinal tract, with integration between gastric, intestinal and biliary secretions, motor intestinal activity and local immune response has taken place (Milla, 1986). Many of these changes are induced by the presence of nutrients in the intestinal lumen, the activity of gut hormones and the development of the local immune system regulation mainly by the production of secretory IgA.

A complete study of the developmental structures and function of the gastrointestinal tract has been reported by Schmitz and McNeish (1987). In industrialised countries the time to begin the weaning period with the introduction of mixed feeding is influenced by standards of life, traditions, habits, individual needs and the type of food employed up to that moment, breast-feeding or infant formula. The age for the introduction of semi-solids and solids has changed in the last 15 years from early weaning to a general recommendation of later weaning. ESPGAN (1982) has recommended this age as not being before three months and not later than six months. The Committee on Nutrition, the American Academy of Pediatrics (1980), points out that there are no nutritional advantages for the introduction of beikost before 4-6 months. These recommendations are valid both for infants receiving breast milk and for those receiving infant formula. If the infant is breast-fed, weaning must be slow in order to continue providing the protective factors present in breast milk, such as IgA antibodies, lysozine and lactoferrin for as long as possible (Goldman et al., 1983). In Europe, in a study with data from 20 countries, the trend observed in the greater number of countries was the introduction of beikost at 4-5 months. Only in two was the introduction as early as 2-3 months and, exceptionally, after 6 months in one country (Ballabriga and Schmidt, 1987). In affluent societies, generally, the infant does not suck the breast so often and the milk output decreases between 3-4 months, the mother having the sensation of "insufficient milk" and starting weaning with the use of some infant formulas and thereon to mixed feeding. Socioeconomical and emotional factors, of course, participate in the weaning decision and likewise there are differences between rural and urban factors and social class where the age of introduction of beikost usually correlates inversely with the duration of maternal lactation (Klackenberg & Klackenberg-Larsson, 1968; Sjolin *et al.*, 1977). The sensation of hunger between 4 and 6 months can also depend to a certain degree on the increase of energy requirements due to the greater activity of the infant. The introduction of beikost at earlier ages supposes a forced situation when overcoming the extrusion reflex is necessary. In developed countries the inconveniences and problems of weaning are not so important, given that the danger of infection is much less, the quality of water is good and the weaning foods are "safe" and of good nutritional value. It should be born in mind that one of the reasons in this situation for not proceeding to early weaning, is the immunological response that can occur with foreign proteins. If the infant is taking a homemade milk formula, the time for weaning can be somewhat advanced so that the infant can receive complements of vitamin C, linoleic acid, iron and other minerals by means of the beikost.

In developing countries, with generally poor sanitation, the indication of a long breast milk feeding period and late weaning is clear. The question is, what length of time will the mother's milk output be sufficient, as unique food, to cover the needs for growth? Under the most favourable circumstances, breast-feeding can be maintained exclusively for 4-6 months, or with the addition of some complement. It is rare that, between the second and fourth month, the mother's milk output, even with large individual variations, is sufficient, and a faltering in infant growth appears (Waterlow *et al.*, 1980; Chandra, 1981). Large variations in milk output have been observed, related to yearly seasons, with decreased values during the wet season (Prentice, 1980). The administration of some complement allows prolongation of lactation. From 10 to 50% of mothers in rural areas, continuing to breast-feed, gave complements (WHO, 1981). If the infant is breast-fed for too long a time, with an insufficient energy intake, slight malnutrition presents and the alternative is to wean in unfavourable conditions. Beikost is frequently the origin of weanling diarrhoea due to the use of contaminated weaning foods (Woodruff *et al.*, 1983) or to the bad quality of water used in their preparation. In these cases, there is really a "weanling dilemma" (Rowland, 1980). The choice is that the infant receives a low calorie intake which leads to malnutrition, or receives weaning foods that lead to infection and secondarily to malnutrition. The need of multimixes, using local sources at low cost is imperative but, on the other hand, failure to thrive is accentuated in poorer environments, as is the case in underdeveloped areas. Efficient measures presuppose the necessity of improving the mother's breast milk output and the quality of weaning foods, together with nutritional education for their employment.

WEANING: WHAT?

The question of what type of foods should be given during the weaning period depends on different aspects of geographical factors, cultural habits, development of appetite, availability of nutrients, local customs and the level of socioeconomical-cultural development of the family. All nutrients must be free of substances with adverse pharmacological content, aflatoxins, pesticide residuals and hormones. In the introduction of weaning foods there may have diverse affects, not only with regard to timing, that is to say, early or late weaning, but also to which sort of foods should be given from the start. In almost all countries fruit juices are introduced very soon. The data of Stolley *et al.* (1981) show that at 6-9 weeks, 92% of German infants receive fruit juice, and 32% vegetable juice, and that at 10-11 weeks these percentages reach 100 and 42% respectively. Fruit juice should not be administered by bottle so as not to create the habit of sweetened liquids intake because infants already with teeth may contract "nursing bottle caries." Large quantities of fruit juice needs to be avoided as loss of appetite is caused. Our European survey showed that cereals were introduced between 4 and 7 months in 12 of the 16 countries surveyed. Some countries showed a preference for their introduction as first weaning food. The breast-fed infant should receive weaning foods that contain a little more protein and if the infant is not breast-fed, but receives a follow up formula, mixed feeding that has a greater energy density is preferable. Infants not receiving routine milk formulas during the first months but, instead, homemade milk preparations, particularly in rural areas and almost always for economical reasons, require an early diversification of the diet when weaning from the bottle is begun. Fruit juice for a greater supply of Vitamin C, cereals for the supply of linoleic acid and meat which assures a supply of heme iron are needed. The solids administered must have a nutritional value which is not less than that of milk and should preferably be fortified with iron, as is the case of cereals. Acceptance of the food offered with a spoon is generally good from 3-4 months. It should be born in mind that fresh vegetables and fruit have a high potassium content. The calories contained in beikost should cover half of the energy requirements between 6 and 9 months, and around two thirds between 9 and 12 months.

In developed countries, in which the quality of foods is well guaranteed and the possibility of infection much less, the infant develops well and enjoys good health in spite of the existing differences in feeding practices, although the long term consequences, if any, are not known. Up to 5-6 months, infants receiving only breast milk and supplements of vitamin D, iron and fluor (Committee on Nutrition, 1980) can develop well without other complements.

The infant should often be introduced to new foods, with different tastes and textures, food preference being mediated by social aspects and cross cultural variations for taste. British and Swiss babies show a preference for yogurt though this is not the case in the United States. In Switzerland the use of homemade formulas has recently declined and the preference for cereals with milk has been substituted by yogurt, thus a tendency to reduce carbohydrate intake (Toenz & Schwaninger, 1978).

The kidney solute load increases with the consumption of meat and eggs due to salt content, on the other hand, though there is less renal charge with the consumption of desserts, puddings and fruit.

Although desiccated beef has been administered between 1 and 3 weeks of age (Sanford and Campbell, 1941) a general trend is to offer meat preparations around 5 months of age. Strained meat supposes a high concentration of proteins and little water. Eggs are recommended between 5-7 months of age.

In developing countries, solid weaning foods are usually of great bulk and with a low energy density. The consumption of large volumes satiate the infant and the risk is run of reducing the amount of milk intake with a lessening of the frequency of sucking and a decline in breast milk output (see Chapter 6). Homemade preparations that are modifications of the family diet are recommended. Through health education balanced diets may be achieved, with, for example, multimixed vegetables in which there is a good distribution of aminoacids. The use of cereals and vegetables with high fibre content and retention of great quantities of water during cooking greatly increases volume and because of the high content in phytates absorption of minerals may be diminished. It is clearly important to avoid monotony of diet. Foods should be consumed quickly after preparation, thus avoiding storage. In a study in Kenya (Van Steenbergen et al., 1983), bacterial counts increased after 3 hours of storage. In a rural area of Bangladesh, 41% of foods and 50% of samples of water were contaminated by E. coli (Black et al., 1982).

The quality of water is one of the most important factors in the prevention of gastroenteritis associated with weaning food administration. Fresh or steamed bananas and papaya can be a good source of energy. It must be recommended insistently that the infant receive 4 meals a day and a family habit of only two be avoided. The main object is to obtain a pattern of normal development without trying to alter the cultural patterns of weaning by the use of local weaning foods. Dietary education should modify the inconvenient local habits. In the weaning diet of Hong Kong children, fish and meat is largely used in cooking congee, which has low energy value, but around 20% of mothers remove meat particles before serving their infants (Li et al., 1985). The fortification of staple weaning foods adapted to different developing countries is an important problem, bearing in mind that the weaning period can carry on for up to 18-24 months (Ransome-Kuti, 1983). The use of enriched precooked instant weaning foods from local sources is highly recommendable, but always encounters the usual problem of cost.

WHOLE COW'S MILK AND FOLLOW UP FORMULAS AS COMPONENTS OF THE WEANLING'S DIET

After 4-6 months of life, when mixed feeding is begun, milk is still an important contribution to the diet, both for the supply of proteins and of calcium. If the infant is breast-fed, the mother should continue lactation for as long as possible, using weaning foods in a diversified diet to cover needs. If the infant has been weaned from the breast or has been fed with a starting infant formula (ESPGAN, 1987) then the choice of a suitable milk is an important decision. The use of whole cow's milk as a contribution of milk to the weaning period has been a subject of contention.

WHOLE COW'S MILK

Data from normal infants aged between 112 and 196 days that received whole cow's milk and had never done so before, showed an increased number of guaiac positive stools until 140 days of life when compared with infants receiving infant formula or heated cow's milk. After 140 days, the results were the same. Iron and ascorbic acid supplements were given to infants receiving whole cow's milk. The study showed (Foman et al., 1983) no untoward effects when whole cow's milk was given after 140 days, but did not allow an opinion on the possibility of development of iron deficiency. The Committee on Nutrition of the American Academy of Pediatrics (1983) reported the opinion that after 6 months whole cow's milk can be administered if adequate mixed feedings are given. This opinion has been strongly criticised by Oski (1985). In a study of infants aged 6-9 months receiving whole cow's milk, it was shown that 31.3% were iron deficient (Sadowitz and Oski, 1983). This iron insufficiency is related to the poor iron content of the milk and to the gastrointestinal bleeding produced. The association between occult enteric blood loss and whole cow's milk administration is a long and well established fact (e.g.: Wilson et al., 1974; Rasch et al., 1960; Ayon and Clarkson, 1971). Bovine milk content is 0.6mg of iron/l and the bioavailability of this iron ranged from 5-10% (Dalman, 1980). From this, one can deduce that either the cow's milk must be fortified with iron, or supplements of iron must be given. The total solute load of the diet is another important question. The solute load of non-modified whole cow's milk is high and to this is added the solute load of other components of the diet, such as meat or eggs, which means that the total renal charge will depend on the balance of the diet in general. Another question to be borne in mind is the low content of vitamin C and essential fatty acids in whole cow's milk. The study of Van Woelderen and Goedhart (1987) on the daily nutrient intake of American and Dutch infants fed cow's milk as the milk component of a diversified diet, reviewing 4 reports in the literature, shows that the total daily sodium intake was higher when compared with infants fed infant formula as milk component during the weaning process, or compared with recommendations for infants aged 6-12 months (F.R.G., 1979; USRDA, 1980; ESPGAN, 1981). We believe that we can adhere to the conclusion quoted by Kretchmer (1985) "that whole cow's milk, especially if given alone, may carry unacceptable risks for the infant." In Europe our survey (Ballabriga and Schmidt) showed that in 13 countries fresh cow's milk is given between 4 and 8 months, although not frequently, and in 6 it is used after this age. The actual trend is towards the use of follow-up formulas as the milk component of the diet of the weanling infant in significant number of European countries.

Cow's milk with low fat content is not suitable for infants (Committee on Nutrition, 1976). The energy density is so low that a large volume would be necessary to cover energy needs. With the use of skimmed or semi-skimmed milks, body energy stores also decrease (Fomon *et al.*, 1977) and biochemical essential fatty acid deficiency appears (Ballabriga and Martinez, 1976).

FOLLOW-UP FORMULA

As follow-up formulas, we address those that form part of the milk component from the period of 4-6 months onwards, differing from the starting formulas used until 4-5 months (ESPGAN 1981). During the second semester, the needs for growth impose an increase in the energy intake, maintenance of protein intake, of essential fatty acids and increased needs of calcium and iron. The follow-up formula must be destined to cover the minimal requirements of essential nutrients during the weaning period. 500ml daily of follow-up formula should meet approximately half the energy requirements and the rest be covered by beikost. This type of formula is generally, but not necessarily, cow milk-based. In its composition, a proportion of 3-5.5g proteins/100kcal, 3-6g of fat/100kcal and 8-12g of carbohydrates/100kcal have been recommended (ESPGAN 1981). Given that at the age at which it is employed, the enzymatic systems responsible for the metabolism of aminoacids are well developed, but it does not deal with a whey enriched formula, which differentiates it from starting formulas. The recommended intake of proteins in the second semester of life has been established as 2g of proteins/kg/day (Food and Nutrition Board, 1974) and the minimal protein requirement as 1.5g/k/day. The intake of proteins is divided between those received from the milk supply and those coming from other non-milk solids, mainly cereals, meat, fish and eggs. The quantity of proteins recommended in the formula of 3-5.5g/100kcal or 2-3.7g/100ml, has been criticised (Raiha, 1985; Axelsson, 1987) as being too high on the basis of theoretical calculations of requirements for growth and maintenance, and from the point of view of anthropometrical measurements when they are compared with breast-fed infants. It would seem that the upper limit of 3.7g/100ml is too high, and if the other components of proteins that come from beikost are borne in mind, the total protein given is in excess of needs. The reevaluation of protein intake during the second semester is in need of consideration. The recommended sodium content of follow-up formulas has been of the order of 1-3.7mEq/100kcal. Between 6 months and 1 year, the capacity to adapt to higher intakes of sodium increases but there is a more pronounced tendency to retain sodium than water (Aperia et al., 1987). This is aggravated if the diet contains high quantities of salt, as is the general case when the use of tablefoods is started.

Regarding fat, it has been said that the total intake should not be over 35% of the total energy supply (Royal College of Physicians, 1976). The Netherland recommendations of this age were 45% (Dutch recommendations, 1983) and in the German Federal Republic between 35-50% for the first year. The total fat intake will depend both on the milk supply and on the fat content of the beikost. A high content is usually combined by the fat and oil in table foods. In our opinion, figures up to 35% seem correct. Fat absorption at this time is well developed and reaches 85% because the bile salt synthesis capacity is fully developed and the critical micellar concentration in the intestine is 4mM (Polley, 1976). The linoleic acid content in the follow up formula is on the order of 300mg/100kcal, that is, higher than that of whole cow's milk, and is obtained by substituting part of the animal fat by vegetable fat rich in essential fatty acids. Cereals are an important supply of EFA (0.5-1.0g of EFA per 100g of cereal). One of the most important reasons for the use of follow-up formulas is that it acts as a vehicle for the intake of iron and calcium. There is no reason for iron supplementation in starting formulas used during the first four months of life, but a fundamental element of the follow-up formula rests in its fortification with iron. A total content ranging from 0.7-1.4mg/100ml or 1.0-2.0mg/100kcal is recommended and the total iron intake recommended at this age is 10-15mg/day, mainly given as supplemental iron in milk and cereals.

Calcium requirements from 6 months to 1 year of age range between 500-600mg daily (Committee on Nutrition, 1978), and the major part of this intake is met by follow-up formula, of which the estimated minimal calcium concentration is 60mg/100ml or 90mg/100kcal. A concentration of around 800 mg/l would be preferable, and in this way the consumption of 500ml of follow-up formula daily represents the greater part of total calcium requirement, the rest being covered by solids. This signifies a greater quantity of calcium than that included in the starting formulas. It is not advisable to add any sort of thickener to follow-up formulas as some of them contain starch or maltosedextrine. Once prepared, they should be kept at 0-4° for not more than 24 hours, in order to avoid contamination.

CEREALS AND STARCH

Many infants receive cereals as their first solid food and these contribute to energy intake, given their high content of carbohydrates and, sometimes, that of added sugar. "Milk cereal" formulas imply that some milk is in the product, while others are to be used only with water and do not contain milk. "Complete" milk cereals contain fruit or vegetables. ESPGAN recommendations (1981) suggest a protein content of 1-3g/100kcal except for the milk containing cereals and so called protein enriched products. Cereals containing milk or described as enriched with proteins and to be prepared with water, should contain no less than 3.75g/100kcal of protein of a nutritional quality containing a minimum of 70% of casein or an equivalent level in relation to a higher biological value as determined by protein efficiency ratio; that is to say, the protein level in a milk cereal should be linked to the nutritional value of the protein. It is recommended that all or part of sucrose be exchanged by partially enzymatically hydrolyzed flour, and by this method polysaccharides may be cut down to shorter and sweeter units.

Cereal foods derived from soya should be supplemented with methionine because in soya there is a deficiency of sulphur containing aminoacids. A mixture of different cereals can produce a balanced distribution of different aminoacids.

Cereals are relatively rich in essential fatty acids (0.5-1g/100g cereal). The EFA intake of infants fed artificially with non-adapted formulas is low. Early introduction may be useful in these infants, but a daily supply of 500ml of milk is necessary to cover the daily protein and calcium requirements. Fortification of cereals with iron has been strongly recommended. One reason to introduce beikost is the prevention of iron deficiency. Ferrous salts are usually added to infant formulas and their bioavailability is relatively high. However, ferrous salts cause organoleptic problems in cereals, and other preparations, such as elemental iron, have therefore been used (*e.g.*:hydrogen-reduced, carbon monoxide-reduced, electrolytic or carbonyl iron). Other forms of iron in cereals are ferric pyrophosphate, ferric orthophosphate, and ferric oxide saccharated. Hydrogen-reduced elemental iron is probably the most available and the least expensive source of iron (Hurrell, 1984). Iron enriched milk formulas give the recommended amount of iron (Committee on Nutrition, 1976).

Although the total content of iron in breast milk is similar to unfortified cow's milk formulas (Murthy and Rhea, 1971), the iron in breast milk has a high bioavailability (McMillan *et al.*, 1976; Saarinen *et al.*, 1977) which allows the establishment of an iron adequacy in breast-fed infants until 4-6 months, but this high bioavailability of iron from breast milk can be decreased with the introduction of solid foods (Cook *et al.*, 1972; Oski and Landaw, 1980). For this reason, supplementary iron is necessary after 4-6 months in infants on prolonged breast-feeding (Saarinen, 1978; Siimes *et al.*, 1984), given that a decrease in the concentration of iron in breast milk is observed during lactation (Siimes *et al.*, 1979) and maternal iron supplementation during breast-feeding has no effect on breast milk iron content. It has been suggested that solid food be given separately from a breast-feeding (Dallman, 1986). For all these reasons, iron fortification of cereals is useful but it is not an absolutely definitive method for coverage of all the iron requirements because the bioavailability of iron coming from fortified cereals depends on the source of iron, and also, the satisfactory bioavailability of elemental iron powders is questioned (Foman, 1987). The question of maintaining a good iron intake to prevent iron deficiency is very important because a relation has been established between iron deficiency and mental development scores (*e.g.*: Lozoff *et al.*, 1982; Walter *et al.*, 1983; Oski *et al.*, 1983).

Up to the fourth month of life, amylase activity in duodenal fluid is very low or absent (Auricchio *et al.*, 1955; Zoppi *et al.*, 1972), for pancreatic amylase fragments the molecules of starch which results in the production of small polysaccharides, especially maltose and maltotriose. On the other hand, at one month of age there is intestinal glucoamylase hence disaccharides are ready for digestion and the absorption of starches (Lebenthal and Lee, 1980). Normally, starches are hydrolyzed by the action of x-amylase and the later action of maltase and isomaltase in order to be absorbed. In infants, an alternative pathway is the action of glucoamylase that directly hydrolizes starch to glucose. In use of native starches coming from wheat, corn, tapioca, potatoes and rice given to infants during the first months of life, results show that when given as flour cooked for 10 minutes there is 98% absorption (De Vizia *et al.*, 1975). Modified food starches (MFS) have been largely used,

added to strained and "junior" foods or soya milk, and act as a good stabilizer
and for changing the consistency and texture of the food; its concentration in
the food ranges from 5-6.5%. Starches are principally amylopectin and
amylose. It has been considered whether the residuals of chemical products
employed in the industrial modification of MFS could cause toxic effects; but,
The National Academy of Science points out that there is no toxicological
basis to exclude MFS in the diet of infants (Filer, 1971). The possibility has
also been raised that MFS can chelate minerals, thus interfering with their
absorption (Hood and Oshea, 1977). In many products MFS give from 10 to
30% of the total energy, and *in vivo* and *in vitro* digestibility studies of corn
syrup sugars show that each of the sugars was well hydrolyzed (Lebenthal *et
al.*, 1983).

SALT

Arterial hypertension has been observed in experimental animals after an
increase in the consumption of salt (Maneely and Dahl, 1961; Dahl *et al.*,
1970). Correlation has also be found between the prevalence of hypertension
and the intake of salt in different cultures (Dahl, 1972). Dahl and Love (1957)
also suggested that dietary salt intake in infants and children could be one of
many factors contributing to the development of hypertension. Evidence
to-date is incomplete. For example, the study of Whitten and Steward (1980)
shows no difference in the blood pressure of infants with two different diets
containing a mean daily intake of 323mg or 1570mg sodium respectively,
given for five months form 3 months of age. The infants were followed at 4
and 8 months of age and later at 8 years. Extracellular fluid volume was
increased in children receiving the higher sodium intake and reduced in the
group with low intake in most of the cases. It should be borne in mind that
with a salt intake in the upper limits and restriction of water intake the risk of
hypernatremia is increased and the extra renal losses of salt can lead to saline
depletion, as occurs in diarrhoea. Glomerular filtration rate is low in the
newborn and reaches two thirds of its normal values at 3 months of age.
During the first semester there are some limitations concerning regulation by
the kidneys of salt, water and acid loads (Rodriguez-Soriano, 1987) and in the
second semester these limitations disappear but there is still a certain degree
of incapability when faced with an overload of salt. During the first months
of life, the intake of salt depends fundamentally on the content of salt in breast
milk or in the formula used (starting formula or follow-up formula). Salt
requirements in infants should be considered alongside the needs for growth
and for the compensation of losses in urine, stools and skin. As a safe intake,
amounts have been established as 115 to 350mg daily up to 6 months of age,

and as 250-750mg from 6 months to 1 year (Food and Nutrition Board, 1980). ESPGAN (1981) recommends a sodium intake of 10mEq/100kcal, that is 2.5mmol/100kcal. Minimal requirements for sodium in infants have been established in the order of 6-8mEq/day (Gamble *et al.*, 1951; Fomon *et al.*, 1970) and the limits of tolerance between 8 and 100mEq/day (Committee on Nutrition, 1974). Infants, in fact show a good tolerance to salt and intakes of 100mEq/day have been reported without complications (Puyau and Hampton, 1966). The daily intake may increase from about 30mEq at 2 or 3 months of age to 60mEq at 12 months, and it is preferable that intake of sodium should be kept below 40mEq/day. The ratio of sodium/potassium in humans is usually greater than 0.5 and fresh whole milk, fruits and fruit juices are the most important sources of potassium in the infant diet (Shank *et al.*, 1982). The major food sources of salt are bread, presalted cereals, milk and milk products, which provide approximately 44% of the total sodium intake; 14% comes from meat, fish and vegetables and 35% from homemade preparations. The study by Yeung and coworkers (1982) on the sodium intake of babies of 1 to 18 months of age, shows that this intake increases rapidly when table foods are introduced. From 8 months onwards it was more than twice as high as the Canadian recommendations (Bureau of Nutritional Sciences, 1975). Salt consumption increases considerably when beikost is introduced. Cultural aspects and the mother's appetite for salt play an important role and mothers should be warned not to add salt when preparing food at home and not to add salt to manufactured products, at least for children under 1 year of age. The study of Kerr *et al.* (1978) concerning 70 samples of homemade products prepared by 36 mothers, showed that the mean amount of added salt was 64% higher than the maximum recommended in infants between 3 and 14 months of age. The addition of salt to fruit preparations or desserts is not recommended. Since 1977 two manufacturers in the United States voluntarily discontinued adding salt in weaning foods (Food and Nutrition Board, 1971). The quantity of salt present in most industrially prepared products, which now do not have added salt, is actually less than the quantity in many homemade products, which can contain up to ten times as much salt. The National Academy of Science recommended that no more than 0.25% salt should be added to any beikost product. The fact is, actually, that industrial products consumed as weaning foods in developed countries are products with low salt content, but a sharp increase in intake is observed after 8-9 months of use due to the use of table foods. At present we consider that although the administration of some nutrients, amongst which is salt, can exercise some degree of influence on blood pressure (Boulton, 1987), in infancy there is no convincing data with regard to long term effects, although neither is there any benefit in administrating quantities higher than those recommended. Contrary to that observed in laboratory animals (Contreras and Korsten, 1983), salt intake during the first 8 months of life in humans does not seem to imprint salt preference in early childhood or later. Young infants do not show a definite preference for salted foods; however, the majority of children show a definite preference for salted products after the age of 2 years (Filer, 1975).

SUGAR

Mothers have a natural tendency to sweeten their babies' foods, both homemade and manufactured products, even when the latter sometimes already contain added sucrose. The addition of sucrose to cereals increases the energy density but the cariogenic action of sugar should also be considered. ESPGAN (1981) suggested a maximum of 5g/100kcal additional sucrose in "complete" cereals. Some manufacturers add corn syrup of fructose; others try to substitute enzymatically hydrolyzed flour for all or part of the sucrose. By this method, polysaccharides are split up into smaller units with a higher sweetening power, allowing the use of more flour instead of sucrose, and at the same time increasing indirectly the proportion of protein of cereal origin in the diet. No proved benefits are obtained with the addition of sucrose. There is some evidence that infants like to consume sweet formulas (Fomon *et al.*, 1983) but it is recommended that mothers be instructed not to add more sugar to fruits and desserts prepared by them. The caloric density in manufactured weaning foods has lessened considerably due to the decrease in sugar content; this decrease in caloric density has been about 34% in preparations containing fruits, and 17% in desserts in 1984 compared with 1972 data (Anderson and Ziegler, 1987). Corn sweeteners have generally been used as a substitute for sucrose. The use of saccharine and cyclamate sweeteners was banned in the late 1960's. The use of aspartame, a dipeptide with a sweetening power 180 to 200 times of sucrose, has been the subject of long debate. The Food and Drug Administration approved its use as a low-calorie food sweetener in 1982. The taste of aspartame and sugar is the same, but aspartame does not promote tooth decay and is metabolized as protein, since it is composed of aspartic acid and phenylalanine. It is particularly useful in cold breakfast cereals and gelatine desserts and in foods that normally contain relatively high levels of sucrose or corn syrup. Aspartame cannot be used in baked products because its components break down at high temperatures (Morris, 1981).

DIETARY FIBRE

The plant material residue remaining after strong acid or base hydrolysis is called "crude fibre." Dietary fibre comprises plant-cell skeletons, which resist digestion and are formed from noncarbohydrate substances such as lignin, and from carbohydrate compounds including cellulose, hemicellulose, pectin, gums, mucilages and alginates. The administration of high levels of dietary fibre has been recommended for adults, because fibre decreases intestinal transit time and lowers blood cholesterol levels. However, it has been suggested that fibre could reduce protein digestibility and energy absorption in young children and could also have undesirable effects on the intestinal mucosa in infants (Jansen, 1980). The Codex Alimentarius Commission (1976) did not establish an upper limit for fibre in infant cereal, but the Protein Advisory Group of the United Nations (1975) suggested an upper limit of 5% crude fibre in supplementary foods. The intake of dietary fibre from weaning foods in developed countries is low and comes from grains, fruits and vegetables with a low fibre content (0.5/100g) such as oats, carrots, white potatoes, tomatoes, apricots and bananas, or with an intermediate fibre content such as found (1.5/100g) in peas, lentils and apples. Brown wholemeal bread and fibre rich breakfast cereals are also a common source of fibre supply. In developing countries, the diet during the weaning period includes much use of cereals and legumes with high fibre content which results in an increased food bulk. Weaning mixtures are based on the principle of multimixes (Jelliffe, 1971) which are a mixture of plant proteins so that a balanced content of aminoacids is established. The result is usually a less energy dense food with high viscosity. The bulk increases with cooking because there is high water retention. Fibre is not a totally non-nutrient substrate because a portion of certain fibres is partially degraded in the gastrointestinal tract by colonic bacteria which produce volatile fatty acids. The content of fibre in different foods modifies alimentary behaviour in relation to the volume of food taken, the energetic density of the same, its palatableness and the sensation of satiety it produces. In developing countries, the diet is characterized by large volume, high dietary fibre content, low energy density and low fat content, which can lead to malnutrition, whilst in the developed world, the diet has less volume, high fat, more refined carbohydrates and high energy density, leading to overnutrition.

The danger in developing countries is that the effect of a diet with high fibre content can result in decreased nitrogen absorption and binding of minerals, including iron, zinc magnesium and copper (Rheinhold, 1971; Rheinhold et al., 1973, 1975; Garcia et al., 1975).

The Committee on Nutrition of the American Academy of Pediatrics (1981), reported that fibre is probably unnecessary for infants of less than 1 year of age.

We believe that in infants of nine months and older, foods with a low and intermediate fibre content can be useful, particularly if there is a tendency to constipation.

COMMERCIAL BABY FOOD PREPARATIONS

The consumption of commercial baby food preparations has increased considerably during the last 20 years, although large variations are observed in different European countries. In some of the most affluent, such as Sweden, per capita consumption has been as high as 600 jars per year, and in others it is as low as 15. These preparations can be classified as dehydrated products, requiring reconstitution with water, and those ready for use. The size of fragments in different preparations varies. Strained preparations for younger children can be swallowed without chewing, others, such as "junior" foods, contain larger fragments. The ESPGAN Committee on Nutrition (1982) recommended the following composition: 70kcal/100g in meat or fish preparations with vegetables, rice, potatoes etc.; not less than 6.5g protein/100kcal in meat or fish preparations without vegetables, rice or potatoes and not less than 4.2g protein/100kcal in meat or fish preparations with vegetables, rice or potatoes. It has been recommended that in preparations with meat or fish that also contain vegetables, 15% of energy should come from proteins. Meat containing baby foods fortified with iron and ascorbic acid have been recommended as appropriate for the prevention of iron deficiency in infants (Haschke et al., 1988). Nutritional advances in industrial preparations have resulted in, among other features, reduction of sodium, sugar and fat, freedom from nitrates and that many of them are fortified with iron and ascorbic acid. Both of these fortifiers have also been added to jarred products containing cereals and fruits. Sodium has been limited to less than 10mEq/100kcal. However, milk remains the most important source of protein between 6 and 12 months of age and should not be less than 500ml daily. The choice of industrial preparations or homemade strained foods in the different age groups differs in various European countries according to habits, traditions, degree of industrialization and socioeconomical conditions. In Sweden only 11% of families cook infant beikost at home (Kohler et al., 1977) and jars are predominantly bought and used. Industrial preparations should have a minimum density of 60kcal/100g and products of less should be avoided.

DISTURBANCES THAT CAN APPEAR IN WEANLING INFANTS

These can either be immediate or appear after some time. The principal objective should be to maintain a well balanced diet from the point of view of energy intake and balance between the different nutrients in order to avoid resultant deficiencies or intolerances. The maintenance of a sufficient energy intake will avoid malnutrition, which is a danger is developing countries due to low density weaning foods; overnutrition in developed countries can also be avoided. Protein deficiency can be avoided by maintaining a good milk intake during the second semester. Early weaning, with the introduction of foreign proteins may lead to food allergy. Appropriate fat intake (not too little and not to much) avoids either unspecific chronic diarrhoea after a short fat intake (Cohen et al., 1979), or intolerance due to fat excess since the fat absorption mechanism is not completely developed (Rey, 1982). Adequate intake of vitamin D and fluoride prevents rickets and caries, and iron supplements in cow or soya milks and iron enriched beikost prevent iron deficiency with or without resultant anemia. Restrictions in the intake of salt and sugar and in the early introduction of gluten can prevent subsequent negative nutritional consequences.

Zinc requirements are covered by foods of animal origin, such as meat, poultry, fish and eggs. Zinc from vegetables and cereals are poorly absorbed because of the high content of fitates and fibre that can modify bioavailability. Mild nutritional zinc deficiency has been reported in some areas as a cause of failure to thrive (Hambridge, 1986), and iron fortification has been incriminated as a dietary factor that can adversely affect zinc absorption (Solomons and Jacobs, 1981).

It is possible that the early introduction of gluten-containing cereals increases the risk of celiac disease in predisposed infants, particularly when formula fed. For this reason, it has been suggested that it could be advisable to postpone the introduction of gluten until the age of 6 months (ESPGAN, 1982).

Clearly, absence of nitrates, contaminants, residual pesticides and aflatoxins lead to high tolerance of weaning foods. Danger of infection is closely related to water quality and good hygienic conditions during food preparation and storage, and every effort needs to be made to avoid the risk of gastroenteritis when new foods are introduced (Surjono et al., 1980; Barrel and Rowland, 1980).

FLUORIDE

During the weaning period the development of future teeth is very important and non-cariogenic foods should be employed. Fluoride is considered as an essential nutrient (Food & Nutrition Board, 1968), and it plays a key role in the prevention of caries. Fluoride concentration in breast milk is low and a 0.25mg/day fluoride supplement has been recommended for breast-fed infants, with an increase in dosage after two years (Fomon *et al.*, 1979). A revised dosage schedule concerning fluoride recommended between 2 weeks and 2 years is a dosage of 0.25mg/day if the concentration of fluoride in drinking water is less than 0.3ppm and no supplement should be given above this concentration (Committee on Nutrition, 1979). In the weanling infant, fluoride drops can cover these needs. In formula fed infants the need for fluoride supplementation will depend on whether the drinking water of the community is fluoridated or not. The concentration of fluoride in infant foods has been considered low but commercially prepared baby foods can show a great variability in fluoride content, depending too on the content of fluoride in the water of the area where the food has been processed (Wiatrowski, 1975). Fluorosis can occur with a fluoride intake ranging between 0.1-0.3mg/kg/day (Forsman, 1977). Sugar also plays a very important role in the aetiology of caries, this is one of the main reasons for the recommendation to reduce sugar in baby foods, and not adding sugar to fruit juice, together with the restriction of sweet drinks to prevent the "nursing bottle syndrome" (Jelliffe, 1977). This syndrome can occur, although very rarely, in breast-fed infants (Brams and Maloney, 1983). A survey of British mothers showed that between 8-11 months, 77% of infants receive sugar during meals and separate candy "sweets" during the day on 4.3 occasions (King, 1978). This reflects maternal habits and even small amounts of sugar can be extremely cariogenic when consumed between meals (Konig, 1986).

MONOSODIUM L-GLUTAMATE

Glutamic acid is present in most nutrients, either free or bound to peptides and proteins. The average intake of glutamic acid depends, of course, on the type of food. The concentration of glutamate in human milk is 10 times higher than in rodent milk and about five times that of cow's milk.

The addition of monosodium glutamate to infant foods has been widely debated. Early observations indicated that monosodium L-glutamate could produce defects in the retina, and could modify the structure of neurons of the nucleus arcuatus in the hypothalamus in newborn animals (Olney, 1969). Subsequent studies could not attribute any neurotoxic effect to monosodium glutamate given in different doses with food or drinking water to different animal species at various ages and under different experimental conditions (Garattini, 1979). No adverse reactions could be demonstrated in children (Filer *et al.*, 1979; Salmona *et al.*, 1980; Tung and Tung, 1979), and there is evidence that term and premature infants metabolize glutamate in the same way as adults. Glutamate is easily metabolized by the human infant without adverse effects when added to meals, even at high levels (150mg/kg). It was therefore concluded that glutamate was a safe food additive. However, the addition of glutamate to infant food products does not present any specific advantage, and since some transient side effects such as the "Chinese restaurant syndrome" may be attributed to glutamate, manufacturers have not incorporated glutamate in infant and "junior" foods since the end of 1969, and the National Academy of Science had recommended that it should not be added to infant food preparations (Food & Nutrition Board, 1970).

NITRATES AND NITRITES

Since the early description by Comly (1945) of methemoglobinemia in young infants caused by the administration of water containing high amounts of nitrates, the relationship between nitrate levels in different vegetables and methemoglobinemia has been well established. The high content of nitrates was due to the use of nonorganic fertilizers. The relationship between intestinal flora and methemoglobinemia has also been studied. When water with a high content of nitrates was used for diluting dried milk preparations, *Bacillus subtilis* contained as spores in the dried milk reduced nitrates to nitrites (Knotek and Schmidt, 1964). Coliform bacterias of the upper small intestine in infants with diarrhoea are able also to reduce nitrates to nitrites (Cornblath and Harmann, 1948). Some vegetables such as spinach, beets and carrots easily accumulate nitrates from fertilizers. Strained foods containing beets and spinach should be used preferably after 6 months of age, and under no circumstances before 3 months. Special attention should be given to fresh and frozen spinach. In any case, these vegetables need to be consumed rapidly after preparation, or after opening a jar. Carrot water for diluting baby formulas, carrot soup for treatment of gastroenteritis, and carrot juice for normal infants have been used for many years in Europe. When their nitrate content is high, these preparations, either manufactured or homemade, can produce methemoglobinemia. In our experience, this more often the case with homemade preparations than with manufactured products. The reduction of nitrates to nitrites in homemade products may be attributed to coliform bacteria in the gut or to bacterial contamination due to lack of hygiene or to too long conservation of the preparation. We observed 57 cases of

methemoglobinemia in infants less than 1 year of age; 15.7% were of unknown origin, 12.2% were due to drinking well water, 5.2% to ingestion of
aniline, 42.1% to drugs, and 24.5% to homemade carrot soup. The legal upper
limit of nitrates - 250mg/kg - has been questioned, since this amount in carrot
preparations is probably unsafe during the first months of life (Stolley *et al.*,
1978). French regulations do not allow more than 50m/kg for infants less than
3 months of age expressed as NO_3.

FOOD ALLERGY

The incidence of food allergy increases with the early introduction of
cow's milk or beikost (Wood, 1986) and this is probably due to the immaturity
of the immune system of the intestine during the first months of life, and to
the absorption of protein antigens at a time when there is a functional immaturity of absorption. However, it is possible that an early introduction of
foods produces less allergic effects than has been supposed while some data
suggest that prolonged breast-feeding up to 6 months and a delay in the
introduction of cow's milk and solid foods lessens the risk of the appearance
of allergic manifestations in babies from atopic families (Saavinen *et al.*,
1979; Foucard, 1985; Jarrett, 1977). Studies in experimental animals have
demonstrated that sufficiently large quantities of antigens capable of activat-
ing the IgE immunoregulating mechanisms are usually absorbed through the
intestinal mucosa, producing an inhibition rather than a stimulation of the IgE
response. The practical human application of this fact is that demonstrated by
Björksten and Saarinen (1978), that lesser quantities of cow's milk protein
favour the production of milk specific IgE and these authors suggest that
greater quantities of antigen can inhibit the response (Firer *et al.*, 1981;
Hatterig *et al.*, 1985). This question has not in fact, yet been completely
clarified.

Infants from atopic families, should be breast-fed for 6 months, if this is
not possible they need to receive a hypoallergenic infant formula together
with exclusion of the most common allergenic foods during the weaning
period. There may be important geographical differences with regard to food
allergy. In our series in Spain, the most common allergens in children presenting with symptoms of food allergy during the first year of life are eggs (33.3%
of cases), cow's milk (30.7%), dried fruit (10.2%), peaches (10.2%), oranges
(7.6%), soya (5.1%), oats (2.5%) and fish (2.5%). Other common allergenic
foods observed have been wheat, tomato, chocolate, nuts, peanuts and honey.
Eggs are probably one of the most potent sensitising agents in the Western
world, egg-white can even produce transitory responses of IgE antibodies of
a higher frequency than with other foods in healthy children. Sometimes a

clinical reaction may not be due to milk constituents themselves but to foreign substances contained in the milk or in the weaning foods - for instance, food additives acting by immunological or non-immunological mechanisms (FAO/OMS, 1974). Antigenic similarity between goat and cow milk proteins has been demonstrated (Superstein, 1960) and heat denaturation of milk does not exclude potential allergenicity (Bahna and Heiner, 1980). Water soluble soy protein formulas have a good nutritional value, but it must be noted that soy protein can also cause clinical allergic manifestations in infants immediately after prolonged administration. Soy protein can be as antigenic as cow milk protein (Saarinen and Kajosaari, 1980; Eastham et al., 1978) and be associated with cow milk allergy Powell, 1976; Whitington and Gibson, 1977) or with monosaccharide intolerance (Goel et al., 1978). If a correct diagnosis of milk allergy has been established, a milk free diet must be administered early and maintained during 6-18 months. Some sensitive children can present clinical reactions to antigens contained in breast milk as a consequence of the cow's milk received by the mother. In these cases, infantile colic disappeared immediately when the mother was put on a diet free from cow milk proteins (Jakobsson and Lindberg, 1978). Wheat antigens in human breast milk have also been identified (Hemings and Kulangava, 1978). On the other hand, it has been suggested that human milk can also contain tolerogenic factors when faced with allergy (Ferguson and Strobel, 1987). Cord blood containing IgE antibodies to a food presupposes that the baby will present allergenic reaction to this food sooner or later. It has been discussed whether weaning in allergic families should be established early or late, with a progressive introduction of small quantities of possible allergens. It would appear wise to delay the beginning of weaning until 6 months of age maintaining breast-feeding, while the mother reduces her consumption of cow's milk and eggs. At the start of weaning a new food is regularly offered of two or three small spoonfuls each week. In this way, easier detection of an offending food is obtained in the case of adverse reactions.

OBESITY

Not too much is known about the long term consequences of the different practices of infant feeding. With relation to obesity a correlation has been established between obesity at 12 months of age and its occurrence later in life (Johnston and Marck, 1978). It has been suggested that overfeeding contributes to later obesity. An Australian study of 394 healthy children (Hitchcock et al., 1985) showed that between 3 and 6 months weight gain was greater in infants fed artificially from birth, or breast-fed only for a short time, than those that had been exclusively breast-fed during 6 months, greater weight gain continued in the former group. The prevalence of obesity in British babies in the decade of the 70's was attributed to overfeeding and early weaning, but scrutiny of the different papers published as to whether early weaning predisposes to obesity showed contradictory results. Whilst some authors (Shukla *et al.*, 1972; Taitz, 1971) were of the opinion that there was a correlation, others (Davies *et al.*, 1977; de Swiet *et al.*, 1977; Thoragood *et al.*, 1979; Wilkinson and Davies, 1978) did not observe it. These same contradictions exist concerning whether breast-feeding itself protects against obesity.

Experimental studies in animals suggest that food intake and appetite are related to early feeding (Oscai and McGarr, 1978). It must though be accepted that a large component of the causation of obesity is genetically determined (Hahn, 1987). This, together with a genetic predisposition to deposit fat easily, other non-nutritional environmental factors can also play a role, such as degree of activity, social class, family structure and, perhaps, quality of food rather than energy quantity (Poskitt, 1986). It must be accepted that introducing solids before four months of age can induce different eating habits and contribute to overfeeding. On the other hand, on many occasions the early introduction of solids does not substitute for the calories of the formula, they are an additive calorie supply. Early weaned formula fed infants rapidly develop medium to high skin fold measurements when compared to other groups not weaned early, but afterwards the differences decrease and they are equal at 5 months of age (Ferris, 1979).

In an attempt to prevent obesity in infants, Piscano *et al.* (1978) recommended an adapted "prudent" diet started at 3 months of age, which not only limited excess of sugar and salt but also employed skimmed milk. The idea was to obtain a diet modifying the taste preference of the infants in order to influence eating habits without interfering with normal growth, but with the prevention of early obesity. The risk of depletion of energy body stores though, results in reduction of milk fat (Fomon *et al.*, 1979) and dietary fat should not be restricted at this age when weaning foods may be introduced (Committee on Nutrition, 1983). Perhaps a balanced diet should be the goal with, in particular a good balance in essential fatty acids.

As overfeeding in great part relates to the amount of energy intake, it is necessary to bear in mind the different caloric densities of different industrial foods, and labels clearly should show the caloric content of the product.

CHOLESTERINE AND ATHEROSCLEROSIS

It is very different to establish a true relationship between dietary practices in infancy and resultant future artherosclerotic disease. Human milk is a
cholesterine containing food containing more than cow's milk and than formulas derived from it. Obesity in children is associated with increased serum
cholesterol levels, and children of parents with high cholesterine values have
greater possibilities of having mean cholesterine levels high than those of the
general population. Familial influences on childrens' total serum cholesterol
levels become increasingly important after the end of the first years of life
(Boulton, 1980). Serum cholesterol screening should be effected only in
children of more than two years old that are at risk because of their family
history (Committee on Nutrition, 1983). Postmortem examination of
youngsters who died in the Korean and Vietnam wars (Emos *et al.*, 1953)
showed a high incidence of atherosclerosis, but diet-atherosclerosis is only
one aspect of the multifactorial etiology of this condition that also involves
genetic factors. Infants with high levels of blood lipids, who have a tendency
to maintain these values, should be longitudinally followed and any excess in
their supplementary feeding should be avoided. In the normal infant a high
cholesterol diet during infancy does not seem to have any adverse consequences in adulthood (Hahn, 1987). Recent recommendations do not advise any
change in normal diets for infants and children of less than two years with
regard to the prevention of adult atherosclerosis (LaRosa & Finberg, 1988).

WEANING IN VEGETARIANS

Due to religious or cultural motivation, there are important groups of
children who follow restrictive dietetic habits that are notably different from
those of the general population, and in these families important problems of
nutrition can be posed in infants of weaning age. Inside these vegetarian
groups different categories are established, which generally speaking are:
lacto-ovo vegetarians, in whose diet meat is excluded but in which consumption of milk and eggs occurs; lacto vegetarians, who exclude meat and eggs
but include milk in their diet; total vegetarians that refuse any food of animal
origin, including milk and eggs. A subgroup of these total vegetarians, the
Vegan, apart from the dietetic restriction, also refuse the use of any material
of animal origin. Amongst other subgroups, semi-vegetarians can be included,
some of which sporadically include fish and chicken in their diet but who
exclude the consumption of red meat, and other small subgroups are included
under the umbrella of food faddism (Robson, 1977), and the ZEN macrobiotic
diet, whose philosophy leads to particular dietary restrictions and habits.

From a nutritional point of view, it is theoretically possible for a total vegetarian diet to be comparable with nutrition, although the achievement of this with a rational intake of different aminoacids and vitamins is extremely difficult. It is much easier to achieve a good nutritional balance with lacto-vegetarian and lacto-ovo vegetarian diets.

Total vegetarian diets, as in the Vegan, lead to a low intake of energy, low fat and protein intakes and difficulty to provide calcium, iron, riboflavin, vitamin D and vitamin B_{12}. Lacto-vegetarians receive a diet with low energy and iron deficiency and lacto-ovo vegetarians generally receive a diet with low energy intake.

All "eliminating diets" are potentially dangerous (David *et al.*, 1984). In moderate restriction form, at weaning the infant has the risk of growth retardation of failure to thrive. In the more exaggerated forms, such as total vegetarians, macrobiotic diets or food faddism, serious risks can occur with the appearance of protein calorie malnutrition, osteoporosis, rickets, zinc deficiency and nutritional anemia (Zmora *et al.*, 1979; Roberts *et al.*, 1979; Shinwell and Gorodischer, 1982). Other diets, such as those made up of barley water, corn syrup and whole milk have conditioned deficiencies in iron, vitamin A and vitamin C, and some infants, such as those fed with Kokoh - a ZEN macrobiotic food mixture -suppose an energy intake of only 40% of the recommended dietary allowances for the United States (Fabius *et al.*, 1981; Robson *et al.*, 1974).

The use of poorly balanced diets at an early age with a predominance of cereals, vegetables and legumes generally lead to a deficient caloric intake and facilitate a deficit in proteins. These diets need a great volume of food in order to reach a certain energetic density, and poor digestibility of some plants decrease the amounts of available aminoacid for intestinal absorption. By means of multimixes of different vegetables, cereals and legumes a balanced aminoacid intake can in fact be achieved.

Values of vitamin B_{12} in serum are usually lower in vegetarians than in non-vegetarians (Armstrong, 1974), but infants in the weaning period that are breast-fed by totally vegetarian mothers can exhibit deficiencies in vitamin B_{12} if they do not receive exogenous supplementation (MacLean and Greham, 1980). The deficit in iron due to the malabsorption of non-heme iron because of the excess of fibre and phytates in the diet, causes anemia, although in part the absorption of iron can be improved by the quantity of vitamin C received with offered fruit (Hanning and Zlotkin, 1985). The high content of dietary fibre decreases the bioavailability of minerals on the whole, and all vegetarian diets contain low quantities of zinc. In Vegan children low serum zinc levels have been reported (Roberts *et al.*, 1979). Calcium deficiency can be present if calcium supplements or fortified soy milk based formula are not given. Rickets among vegetarian children has also been described (Dwyer *et al.*, 1979), because vitamin D_2 is lacking in most of vegetable foods, and many children may get very little sunshine due to cultural reasons or industrial pollution. The low calcium intake and low Vitamin D diet leads to what Finberg (1979) very rightly calls "vegetarian rickets." Dietary abnormalities in infants during the weaning period with intentional withdrawal of milk can induce kwashiorkor that is not associated with poverty (John *et al.*, 1977). Some peculiarities in the diets of immigrant Asian communities that maintain traditional habits also lead to a nutritional deficiency (Jivani, 1978). In vegetarian families, weaning needs to be established in a way that, through professional advice, medical support and nutritional education, diets can be recommended and put into practice that allow maintenance, to a certain point, of traditional eating habits without provoking clinical disturbances. The Health Professional will, however, surely encounter great resistance from the families concerned for the intention to modify their practices (Committee on Nutrition, 1977).

The vegetarian diet should include at least two different classes of vegetable proteins that can complement themselves, such as rice and beans, or corn and beans, with which a better balance between different aminoacids is established. The use of soy based milk fortified with vitamin B_{12} or soy-meat-like-steaks and different legumes such as chick peas and lentils and other foods such as nuts, almonds, bread, cereals, leafy vegetables, fresh and dried fruits, oil seeds and peanut butter, allow the establishment of balanced diets (Vyhmeister *et al.*, 1977).

In the case of lacto-vegetarian and lacto-ovo vegetarian families, the problem is easier as the children can take milk and dairy products and eggs that contain vitamin B_{12} and proteins of excellent quality. Eggs contain sufficient iron but also a factor that interferes with the absorption of non-heme iron.

The British Paediatric Association (1988) has established recommendations for vegetarian weaning, emphasizing, amongst other things, that the infants must receive at least four meals a day; that breast-feeding should be continued, or a cow's milk based formula or soy protein fortified formula given; and fortified margarine with vitamins A and D and fats should be added to weaning cereals to better energy density. Neither whole cow's milk or skimmed milk is recommended.

VITAMIN SUPPLEMENTATION

The recommendations of the Department of Health and Social Security of the United Kingdom point out that all breast-fed infants should receive supplements of vitamin D (DHSS, 1983) although the antirachitic effect of breast milk of well nourished mothers seems adequate for full term infants (Committee on Nutrition, 1980). Reports of rickets in breast-fed infants are not exceptional and are probably due to the combination of a low vitamin D intake and limited exposure to sunlight. Supplementation with 200-400 IU/day of vitamin D has been recommended until a regular exposure to sunlight can be assured (Fomon and Strauss, 1978). Infants fed formulas fortified with vitamin D that follow the recommendations of the Committee do not need such supplements during the first 6 months of life. During the weaning period, milk supplemented with vitamin D should be continued until one year of age. Special attention, during weaning, should be given to those children who due to socio-cultural factors receive specific diets that can be deficient, or who are almost never exposed to sunlight. Factors such as bad housing conditions and increasing urbanization lead to a greater likelihood of rickets (Belton, 1986). Asian and dark skinned children have a poorer vitamin D status than white children, and differences have been found in the regulation of metabolism of vitamin D between black and white children (Bell *et al.*, 1985). Under normal circumstances there is no real indication to use hydroxylated forms of vitamin D3 (Particularly 1,25-OH-D3) and preference should be given to native forms of vitamin D (Orzalesi, 1982). In any case, preparations of vitamin D should always be administered with caution thus avoiding accumulation of the vitamin in the body that can cause toxic effects.

Supplementation with vitamin A does not seem necessary as a general rule and should be reserved for those cases with specific indications. In developing countries, vitamin A status is an important factor for the determination of health (Sommer *et al.*, 1988). The association, for example, is well known between vitamin A deficiency and diarrhoea (WHO, 1988) as well as the protective effect of vitamin A in the evolution of measles (WHO/UNICEF, 1987) and these situations condition special indications for the use of this vitamin. Finally, the diet should needs to contain adequate sources of vitamin C so that supplementation is unnecessary.

REFERENCES

Ahn, C. H., and Maclean, Jr., W. C. Growth of the exclusively breast-fed infant. *Am. J. Clin. Nutr.*, 33:183, (1980).

Anderson, T. A., and Ziegler, E. E. Recent Trends in Weaning in the United States. In: *Weaning: Why, What and When?* Edited by A. Ballabriga, and J. Rey, Raven Press, New York, (1987).

Andrew, E. M., Clancy, K. L., and Katz, M. G. Infant feeding practices of families belonging to a prepaid group practice health care plan. *Pediatrics*, 65:978, (1980).

Anyon, C. P., and Clarkson, K. G. Cow's milk: A cause of iron-deficiency anaemia in infants. *New Zealand Med. J.*, 74:24, (1971).

Aperia, A., Broberger, O., Thodenius, K., and Zetterström, R. Development of renal control of salt and fluid homeostasis during the first year of life. *Acta. Paediatr. Scand.*, 64:393-398, (1975).

Armstrong, B., Davis, R. E., and Nicol, D. J. et al. Hematological vitamin B_{12} and folate studies on Seventh-Day Adventist vegetarians. *Am. J. Clin. Nutr.*, 27:712, (1974).

Auricchio, S., Rubino, A., and Munset, G. Intestinal glycosidase activities in the human embryo, fetus and newborn. *Pediatrics*, 35:944, (1955).

Axelsson, I., Borulf, S., Righard, L., and Räihä, N. Protein and Energy intake during weaning: I. Effects on growth. *Acta. Paediatr. Scand.*, 76:321-327, (1987).

Bahna, S. L., and Heiner, D. C. *Allergies to Milk.* Grune & Stratton New York, (1980).

Bain, K. The incidence of breast-feeding in hospitals in the United States. *Pediatrics*, 2:313, (1948).

Ballabriga, A., and Schmidt. Actual trends of the diversification of infant feeding in industrialized countries in Europe. In: *Weaning: Why, What and When?* Edited by A. Ballabriga, and J. Rey, Raven Press, New York, (1987).

Ballabriga, A., and Martinez, M. Changes in erythrocyte lipid stroma in the premature infant according to dietary fat composition. *Acta. Paediatr. Scand.*, (1976).

Barrel, R. A. E., and Rowland, M. G. M. Commercial milk products and indigenous weaning foods in a rural West African environment: a bacteriological perspective. *J. Hygiene*, 84:191-202, (1980).

Behar, M. Physiological development of the infant and its implications for complementary feeding. *WHO/MCH/NUT/86*. 2:1-20, (1986).

Bell, N. H., Stern, P. H., and Paulson, K. Tight regulation of circulating la,25-dihydroxyvitamin D in black children. *N. Engl. J. Med.*, 313:1418, (1985).

Belton, N. R. Rickets - Not only the "English Disease." *Acta. Paediatr. Scand.*, suppl., 323:68-75, (1986).

Björksten, F., and Saarinen, U. M. IgE antibodies to cow's milk in infants fed breast milk and milk formulae. *Lancet.*, 2:624-625, (1978).

Black, R. E. at al. Contamination of weaning foods and transmission of enterotoxigenic Escherichia coli diarrhoea in children in rural Bangladesh. *Trans. R. Soc. Trop. Med. Hyg.*, 76:259-264, (1982).

Boulton, J. Hypertension as a consequence of early weaning. In: *Weaning, Why, What and When?* Edited by A. Ballabriga, and J. Rey, Raven Press, New York, (1987).

Boulton, T. J. C. Serum cholesterol in early childhood: Familial and nutritional influences and the emergences of tracking. *Acta. Paediatr. Scand.*, 69:441-445, (1980).

Brams, M., and Maloney, J. "Nursing bottle caries" in breast-fed children. *J. Pediatr.*, 103:415-416, (1983).

British Paediatric Association, Nutrition Committee: *Vegetarian Weaning.* London p. 1-13, (1988).

Bureau of Nutritional Sciences, Department of National Health and Welfare: *Dietary standard of Canada*. Ottawa: Information Canada, (1975).

Butler, A. M., and Wolman, I. J. Trends in the early feeding of supplementary foods to infants; an analysis and discussion based on a nationwide survey. *Quart. Rev. Pediat.*, 9:63, (1954).

Chandra, R. K. Breast-feeding, growth and morbidity. *Nutr. Res.*, 1:25-31, (1981).

Codex Alimentarius Commission. Joint FAO/WHO Food Standards Program. Recommended international standards for foods for infants and children. Rome: Secretariat of the joint FAO/WHO food standards programme, *CAC/RS* 72/74, (1976).

Cohen, S. A., Hendricks, K. M., Mathis, R. K., Laramee, S., and Walker, W. A. Chronic nonspecific diarrhea: dietary relationships. *Pediatrics*, 64:402-407, (1979).

Comly, H. H. Cyanosis in infants caused by nitrates in well water. *JAMA*, 129:112, (1945).

Committee on Nutrition, American Academy of Pediatrics. On the feeding of supplemental foods to infants. *Pediatrics*, 65:1178-81, (1980).

Committee on Nutrition, American Academy of Pediatrics: On the Feeding of Supplemental Foods to infants. *Pediatrics*, 65:1178-1181, (1980).

Committee on Nutrition: The use of whole cow's milk in infancy. *Pediatrics*, 72:253-255, (1983).

Committee on Nutrition: Commentary on breast-feeding and infant formulas, including proposed standards for formulas. *Pediatrics*, 57:278-285, (1976).

Committee on Nutrition, A. A. P.: Calcium Requirements in infancy and childhood. *Pediatrics*, 62:826-834, (1978).

Committee on Nutrition, A. A. P.: Iron Supplementation for Infants. *Pediatrics*, 58:765-768, (1976).

Committee on Nutrition. American Academy of Pediatrics: Salt intake and eating patterns of infants and children in relation to blood pressure. *Pediatrics*, 53:115-121, (1974).

Committee on Nutrition, A. A. P.: Plant fiber intake in the pediatric diet. *Pediatrics*, 67:572-5, (1981).

Committee on Nutrition, A. A. P.: Fluoride supplementation: Revised dosage schedule. *Pediatrics*, 63:150-152, (1979).

Committee on Nutrition: Toward a prudent diet for children. *Pediatrics*, 71:78-80, (1983).

Committee on Nutrition American Academy of Pediatrics: Nutritional aspects of vegetarianism, health foods and fad diets. *Pediatrics*, 59:460-464, (1977).

Committee on Nutrition, A. A. P.: Vitamin and mineral supplement needs in normal children in the United States. *Pediatrics*, 66:1015-1021, (1980).

Contreras, R. J., and Korsten, T. Prenatal and early postnatal sodium chloride intake modifies the solution preferences of adult rats. *J. Nutr.*, 113:1051-62, (1983).

Cook, J. D., Layrisse, M., Martinez-Torres, C., Walker, R., Monsen, E., and Finch, C. A. Food iron absorption measured by an extrinsic tag. *J. Clin. Invest.*, 51:805, (1972).

Cornblath, M., and Hartmann, A. F. Methemoglobinemia in young infants. *J. Pediatr.*, 33:421-5, (1948).

Dahl, L. K., Heine, M. A., Leitl, M. A., and Tassinari, L. Hypertension and death from consumption of processed baby foods by rats. *Proc. Sec. Exp. Biol. Med.*, 133:1405, (1970).

Dahl, L. K. Salt and hypertension. *Am. J. Clin. Nutr.*, 25:231, (1972).

Dahl, L. K., and Love, R. A. Ethiological Role of Sodium Chloride intake in essential hypertension in humans. *JAMA*, 164:397-400, (1957).

Dallman, P. R. Iron deficiency and related nutritional anemia, In: *Hematology of Infancy and Childhood*. Nathan, D. G., Oski, F. A. (Eds.) Philadelphia, W. B. Saunders Co., pp. 298-343, (1981).

Dallman, P. R. Iron deficiency in the weanling: A nutritional problem on the way to resolution. *Acta. Paediatr. Scand.*, Suppl. 323:59-67, (1986).

Davies, D. P., Gray, O. P., Elwood, P. C., Hopkinson, C., and Smith, S. Effects of solid foods on growth of bottle-fed infants in first the three months of life. *Br. Med. J.*, 2:7-8, (1977).

David, T. J., Waddington, E., and Stanton R. H. J. Nutritional hazards of elimination diets in children with atopic eczema. *Arch. Dis. Childh.*, 59:323-325, (1984).

de Swiet, M., Fayers, P., and Cooper, L. Effect of feeding habit on weight in infancy. *Lancet*, 1:892-894, (1977).

De Vizia, B., Ciccimarra, F., De Cicco, N., and Auricchio, S. Digestibility of starches in infants and children. *J. Pediatr.*, 86:50-55, (1975).

DHSS. *Present day practice in infant feeding: 1980*. Rep. Health Soc. Subj. No. 20. London. HMSO, (1983).

Dutch recommendations. Nederlandse Voedingsmiddelentabel: Aanbevolen hoeveelheden, 34th ed., (1983).

Dwyer, J. T., Dietz, W. H., Hass, G., and Suskind, R. Risk of nutritional rickets among vegetarian children. *Am. J. Dis. Child.*, 133:134-140, (1979).

Eastham, E. J., Lichauco, T., Grady, M. I., and Walker, W. A. Antigenicity of infant formulas: role of immature intestine on protein permeability. *J. Pediatr.*, 93:561-564, (1978).

Enos, W. F., Homes, R. H., and Beyer, J. Coronary disease among United States soldiers killed in action Korea. *JAMA*, 152:1090, (1953).

ESPGAN Committee on Nutrition: Guidelines on Infant Nutrition. III Recommendations for infant feeding. *Acta. Paediatr. Scand.*, suppl. 302:1-27, (1982).

ESPGAN Committee on Nutrition. Guidelines on Infant Nutrition. I. Recommendations for the composition of an adapted formula. *Acta. Paediatr. Scand.*, suppl. 272:1-20, (1977).

ESPGAN Committee on Nutrition. Guidelines on Infant Nutrition. II. Recommendations for the composition of Follow-up Formula and Beikost. *Acta. Paed. Scand.*, suppl. 287:1-25, (1981).

Fabius, R. J., Merritt, R. J., Fleiss, P. M., and Ashley, J. M. Malnutrition associated with a formula of barley water, corn syrup and whole milk. *Am. J. Dis. Child.*, 135:615-617, (1981).

FAO/WHO, WHO Technical Report Series No. 522, 1973, Geneva, *Energy and protein requirements: report of Joint FAO/WHO Ad. Hoc. Expert Committee*, (1973).

FAO/OMS: *Evaluation de certains additifs alimentaires* (Serie rapports techniques): Geneve, OMS, (1974).

Ferguson, A., and Strobel, S. Potential effects of weaning on intestinal immunity. In: *Weaning: Why, What and When?* A. Ballabriga and J. Rey (Eds.), Raven Press, New York, (1987).

Ferris, A. G., Beal, V. A., Laus, M. J., and Hosmer, D. W. The effect of feeding on fat deposition in early infancy. *Pediatrics*, 64:397-401, (1979).

Filer, Jr.,L. J. Modified food starches for use in infant foods. Summary of report by Subcommittee on Safety and Suitability of MSG and other substances in baby foods, Food Protection Committee, Food and Nutrition Board, National Academy for Sciences-National Research Council. *Nutr. Rev.*, 29:55-9, (1971).

Filer, L. J. *Studi della preferenza del sale nell'infanzia e fanciullezza. Problemi attuali de nutrizione in pediatria.* Le Giornate di Studio Plasmon. San Remo, March (1975).

Filer, Jr., L. J., Baker, G. L., and Stegink, L. D. Metabolism of free glutamate in clinical products fed infants. In: *Advances in biochemistry and physiology: Glutamic Acid*, L. J. Filer, Jr. (Ed.) Raven Press, New York (1979).

Finberg, L. Human choice, vegetable deficiencies and vegetarian rickets. *Am. J. Dis. Child.*, 133:129, (1979).

Firer, M. A., Hosking, C. S., and Hill, D. J. Effect of anitgen load on development of milk antibodies in infants allergic to milk. *Br. Med. J.*, 283:693-696, (1981).

Fomon, S. J. *Infant nutrition.* 2nd ed. Philadelphia: W. B. Saunders, (1974).

Fomon, S. J., Ziegler, E. E., and Nelson, S. E. et al. Cow milk feeding in infancy; Gastrointestinal blood loss and iron nutritional status. *J. Pediatr.*, 98:540, (1981).

Fomon, S. J., Filer, Jr., L. J., Ziegler, E. E., Bergmann, K. E., and Bergmann, R. L. Skim milk in infant feeding. *Acta. Paediatr. Scand.*, 66:17-30, (1977).

Fomon, S. J. Bioavailability of supplemental iron in commercially prepared dry infant cereals. *J. Pediatr.*, 110:660-661, (1987).

Fomon, S. J., Thomas, L. N., and Filer, Jr., L. J. Acceptance of unsalted strained foods by normal infants. *J. Pediatr.*, 76:242-4, (1970).

Fomon S. J., Ziegler, E. E., Nelson, S. E., and Edwards, B. B. Sweetness of diet and food consumption by infants. *Proc. Soc. Exp. Biol. Med.*, 173:190-3, (1983).

Fomon S. J., Filer, Jr., L. J., Anderson, T. A., and Ziegler, E. E. Recommendations for feeding normal infants. *Pediatrics*, 63:52-63, (1979).

Fomon, S. J., and Strauss, R. G. Nutrient deficiencies in breast-fed infants. *N. Eng. J. Med.*, 299:355-356, (1978).

Food and Nutrition Board, National Research Council. *Recommended Dietary Allowances. 8th ed.* Washington D.C.: National Academy of Sciences (1974).

Food and Nutrition Board, National Research Council. *Recommended dietary allowances. 9th ed.* Washington D.C.: National Academy of Sciences (1980).

Food and Nutrition Board, National Academy of Sciences, National Research Council: Salt in infant foods. *Nutr. Rev.*, 29:27-30, (1971).

Food and Nutrition Board, National Research Council: *Recommended Dietary Allowances, 7th ed, revised.* Publication 1694. Washington D.C.: National Academy of Sciences, p.55, (1968).

Food and Nutrition Board, Food Protection Committee: *Safety and suitability of monosodium glutamate for use in baby foods.* Washington D.C.: National Academy of Sciences -National Research Council, pp. 42, (1970).

Forsman, B. Early supply of fluoride and enamel fluoresis. *Scand. J. Dent. Res.*, 85:22, (1977).

Foucard, T. Development of food allergies with special reference to cow's milk allergy. *Pediatrics*, 75 part 2:177-181, (1985).

FRG Recommendations. Deutsche Gesellschaft Für Emaehrung: Empfehlungen für die Nahrstoffzufuhr. Umschau Verlag. Frankfurt/Main, (1979).

Gamble, J. L., Wallace, W. M., Eliel, L., Holliday, M. A., Cushman, M. Appleton, J., Shenberg, A., and Piotti, J. Effects of large loads of electrolytes. *Pediatrics*, 7:305-9, (1951).

Garattini, S. Evaluation of the neurotoxic effects of glutamic acid. In: *Nutrition and the brain (vol. 4).* R. J. Wurtman, and J. J. Wurtman, (Ed.), Raven Press, New York, 79:115, (1979).

Garcia, V., Leon, C., Armas, M. R., Muros, M., Garcia, M., and Gonzalez, R. Deficit dietetico de magnesio en la infancia. *Acta. Pediatr. Esp.*, 42:293-8, (1984).

Ghosh, S., Gidwani, S., and Mittal, S. K. et al. Socio-cultural factors affecting breast-feeding and other infant feeding practices in an urban community. *Indian Pediatr.*, 13:827-832, (1976).

Glazier, M. M. Advantages of strained solids in the early months of infancy. *Pediatr.*, 3:883, (1933).

Goel, K., Lifshitz, F., Kahn, E., and Teichberg, S. Monosaccharide intolerance and soy-protein hypersensiticity in an infant with diarrhea. *J. Pediatr.*, 93:617-619, (1978).

Goldman, A. S., Goldblum, R. M., Garza, C. Nichols, B. L., and O'Brian Smith, E. Immunologic components in human milk during Weaning. *Acta. Paediatr. Scand.*, 72:133-4, (1983).

Hahn, P. Obesity and atherosclerosis as consequences of early weaning. In: *Waning: Why, What and When?* A. Ballabriga and J. Rey (Eds.), Raven Press, New York (1987).

Hamburger, R. Uber milchfreie Aufzucht von Sauglingen. *Jahrb. Kinderh.*, 103:277, (1923).

Hambidge, K. M. Zinc deficiency in the weanling - How important? *Acta. Paediatr. Scand.* supp. 323:52-58, (1986).

Hanning, R. M., and Zlotkin, S. H. Unconventional eating practices and their health implications. *Pediatr. Clin. A. Amer.*, 32:429-445, (1985).

Haschke, F., Pietschnig, B., Vanura, H., Heil, M., Steffan, I., Hobiger, G., Schuster, E., and Camaya, Z. Iron intake and iron nutritional status of infants fed iron-fortified beikost with meat. *Am. J. Clin. Nutr.*, 47:108-12, (1988).

Hattevig, G., Kjellman, B. and Johansson, S. G. O. Quoted by Foucard In: Development of Food allergies with special reference to cow's milk allergy. *Pediatrics*, 75 part 2:177-181, (1985).

Hemmings, W. A., and Kulangara, A. C. Dietary Antigens in Breast Milk. *Lancet*, ii:575, (1978).

Hindley, C. B., Filliozat, A. M., Klackenberg, G., Nicolet-Meister, D., and Sand, E. A. some differences in infant feeding and elimination in five European longitudinal samples. *J. Child. Psychol. Psychiat.*, 6:179, (1965).

Hirschman, C., and Butler, M. Trends and differentials in breast-feeding: An update. *Demography*, 18:39-54, (1981).

Hitchcock, N. E., Gracey, M., and Gilmour, A. I. The growth of breast-fed and artificially fed infants from birth to twelve months. *Acta. Paediatr. Scand.*, 74:240-245, (1985).

Hofvander, Y., and Sjölin, S. Breast-feeding trends and recent information activities in Sweden. *Acta. Paediatr. Scand.*, suppl. 275:122-125, (1979).

Hofvander, Y., and Sjölin, S., WHO Collaborative study on breast-feeding. *Acta. Paediatr. Scand.*, 67:556, (1978).

Hood, L. F., and Oshea, G. K. Calcium binding by hydroxypropl distarch phosphate and un-modified starches. *Cereal Chem.*, 54:266, (1977).

Hurrell, R. F. Bioavailability of different iron compounds used to fortify rormulas and cereals: technological problems. In: *Nestle Nutrition Workshop Series. vol. 4: Iron nutrition in infancy and childhood.* (A. Stekel (Ed.) Raven Press, New York. 147:78, (1984).

Illingworth, R. S., and Lister, J. The critical or sensitive period, with special reference to certain feeding problems in infants and children. *J. Pediatr.*, 65:839-48, (1964).

Jakobsson, I., and Lindberg, T. Cow's milk as a cause of infantile colic in breast-fed infants. *Lancet*, ii:437-441, (1978).

Jansen, G. R. A consideration of allowable fibre levels in weaning foods. *Food Nutr. Bull.*, 2:38-47, (1980).

Jarrett, E. E. E. Activation of IgE regulatory mechanisms by transmucosal absorption of antigen. *Lancet*, ii:223-225, (1977).

Jelliffe, E. F. P. A new look at weaning multimixes in the contemporary Caribbean. *J. Trop. Pediat.*, 17:135, (1971).

Jelliffe, E. F. P. Infant feeding practices: Associated iatrogenic and commerciogenic diseases. *Pediatr. Clin. N. Amer.*, 24:49-61, (1977).

Jivani, S. K. M. The practice of infant feeding among Asian immigrants. Arch. Dis. Childh., 53:69-73, (1978).

John, T. J., Blazovich, J., Lightner, E. S., Sieber, Jr., O. F., Corrigan, J. J., and Hansen, R. Kwashiorkor not associated with poverty. *J. Pediatr.*, 90:730-735, (1977).

Johnston, F. E., and Marck, R. W. Obesity in urban black adolescents of high and low relative weight at one year of age. Am. *J. Dis. Child.*, 132:862, (1978).

Jundell, I. Mixed diet during the first year of life. *Acta. Paediat.*, 3:159-167, (1924).

Kerr, Jr., C. M., Reisinger, K. S., and Plankey, F. W. Sodium concentration of homemade baby foods. *Pediatrics*, 62:331-335, (1978).

King, J. M. Patterns of sugar consumption in early infancy. *Community Dent Oral Epidemiology*, 6:47-52, (1978).

Klackenberg, G., and Klackenberg-Larsson, I. The development of children in a Swedish urban community. A prospective longitudinal study. V. Breast-feeding and weaning: some social-psychological aspects. *Acta. Paediatrica Scandinavica*, suppl. 187:94-104, (1968).

Knotek, Z., and Schmidt, P. Pathogenesis, incidence and possibilities of preventing alimentary nitrate methemoglobinemia in infants. *Pediatrics*, 34:78-82, (1964).

Köhler, E. M., Köhler, L., and Lindquist, B. Use of weaning foods (beikost) in an industrialized society. Socio-economic and psychological aspects. *Acta. Paediatr. Scand.*, 66:665-72, (1977).

König, K. G. Caries prevention. *Ann. Nestle*, 44:1-10, (1986).

Kretchmer, N. Gastrointestinal and Immunologic Development. *Pediatrics*, 75:187-188, (1985).

LaRosa, J., and Finberg, L. Preliminary report from a conference entitled "Prevention of adult atherosclerosis during childhood." *J. Pediatr.* :317-318, (1988).

Lebethal, E., and Lee, P. C. Glucoamylase and disaccharidase activities in normal subjects and in patients with mucosal injury of the small intestine. *J. Pediatr.*, 97:389-393, (1980).

Lebenthal, E. Use of modified food starches in infant nutrition. *Am. J. Dis. Child.*, 132:850-852, (1978).

Lebenthal, E., Heitlinger, L., Lee, P. C., Nord, K. S., Hodge, C., Brooks, S. P., and George, D. Corn syrup sugars: In vitro and in vivo digetibility and clinical tolerance in acute diarrhea of infancy. *J. Pediatr.*, 103:29-34, (1983).

Li A. M. C., Baber, F. M., Yu, A. M. C., and Leung, V. S. The weaning diet of Hong Kong children. *J. Hong Kong Med. Assoc.*, 37:167-75, (1985).

Lozoff, B., Brittenham, G. M., Viteri, F. E., Wolf, A. W., and Urrutia, J. J. The effects of short-term oral iron therapy on developmental deficits in iron deficient anemin infants. *J. Pediatr.* 100:351, (1982).

Lozoff, B., Brittenham, G. M., Viteri, F. E., Wolf, A. W., and Urrutia, J. J. Developmental deficits in iron deficient infants: effects of age and severity of iron lack. *J. Pediatr.*, 101:948-952, (1982).

MacLean, W. C., Graham, G. G. Vegetarianism in children. *Am. J. Dis. Child.*, 134:513-518, (1980).

Maneely, G. R., and Dahl, L. K. Electrolytes in hypertension: The effects of sodium chloride. *Med. Clin. North Am.* 45:271, (1961).

Martin, J. Infant feeding 1975: *Attitudes and practice in England and Wales*. London, Office of Population Censuses and Surveys, Social Survey Division, Her Majesty's Stationery Office, (1978).

Martinez, G. A. Cited by Fomon, S. J. *Infant Nutrition, ed. 2*. Philadelphia; WB Saunders Co., p. 8, (1974).

Martinez, G. A., Dodd, D. A., and Samartgedes, J. A. Milk Feeding patterns in the United States during the first 12 months of life. *Pediatrics*, 68:863-868, (1981).

Martinez, G. A., and Nalezienski, J. P. 1980 Update: The recent trend in breast-feeding. *Pediatrics*, 67:260-263, (1981).

McMillan, J. A., Landaw, S. A., and Oski, F. A. Iron sufficiency in breast-fed infants and the availability of iron from human milk. *Pediatrics*, 58:686, (1976).

Milla, P. J. The weanling's gut. *Acta. Paediatr. Scand.*, suppl. 323:5-13, (1986).

Morris, C. E., FDA clears Aspartame. *Food Engineering*, 53:154-5, (1981).

Murthy, G. K., and Rhea, U. S. Cadmium, copper, iron, lead, manganese and zinc in evaporated milk, infant products and human milk. *J. Dairy Sci.*, 54:1001, (1971).

Oates, R. K. Infant feeding practices. *Br. Med. J.*, 2:762-4, (1973).

Olney, J. W. Brain lesions, obesity and other disturbances in mice treated with monosodium glutamate. *Science*, 164:719-21, (1969).

Orzalesi, M. Do breast and bottle-fed babies require vitamin supplements? *Acta. Paediatr. Scand.*, suppl. 299:77-82, (1982).

Oscai, L. B., and McGarr, J. A. Evidece that the amount of food consumed in early life fixes appetite in the rat. *Am. J. Physiol.*, 235:R141-44, (1978).

Oski, F. A. Is bovine milk a health hazard? *Pediatrics*, 75:182-186, (1985).

Oski, F. A., and Landaw, S. A. Inhibition of iron absorption from human milk by baby food. *Am. J. Dis. Child.*, 134:134-459, (1980).

Oski, F. A., Honig, A. S., Helu, B., and Howanitz, P. Effect of iron therapy on behavior performance in nonanemic, iron-deficient infants. *Pediatrics*, 71:877-880, (1983).

Persson, L. A., and Samuelson, G. From breast milk to family food, Infant feeding in three Swedish Communities. *Acta. Paediatr. Scand.*, 73:685-692, (1984).

Pisacano, J. C., Lichter, H., Ritter, J., and Siegal, A. P. An attempt at prevention of obesity in infancy. *Pediatrics*, 61:360-364, (1978).

Poley, J. R. Fat digestion and absorption in lipase and bile acid deficiency. In: *Lipid absorption: Biochemical and clinical aspects*, K. Rommel, H. Goebbel, R. Böhmer, (Eds.). Lancaster (England): MTP Press, :151-202, (1976).

Poskitt, E. M. E. Energy Needs in the Weaning Period. In: *Weaning: Why, What and When?* A. Ballabriga and J. Rey, (Eds.), Raven Press, New York (1987).

Poskitt, E. M. E. Obesity in the young child: whither and whence? *Acta. Paediatr. Scand.*, suppl. 323:24-32, (1986).

Powell, G. K. Enterocolitis in low birth weight infants associated with milk and soy protein intolerance. *J. Pediatr.*, 88:840-844, (1976).

Prentice, A. M. Variations in maternal dietary intake, birthweight and breast milk output in the Gambia. In: *Maternal Nutrition During Pregnancy and Lactation*, H. Aebi, and R. G. Whitehead (Eds.). Bern, Switzerland, Hans Huber, pp. 167-183, (1980).

Protein Advisory Group of the United Nations System. *Promotion of special foods (infant formula and processed protein foods) for vulnerable groups*. PAG Statement No. 23. Promotion of Special Foods, (1972).

Protein Caloric Advisory Group of the United Nations. *Guidelines on protein-rich mixtures for us as supplemental foods. The PAG Compendium (Vol E)*. New York: Worldmark Press Ltd., John Wiley :63, (1975).

Puyau, F. A., and Hampton, L. P. Infant Feeding Practices, 1966. Salt content of the modern diet. *Am. J. Dis. Child*, 111:370-373, (1966).

Räihä, N. C. R. Nutritional proteins in milk and the protein requirement of normal infants. *Pediatrics*, suppl. 75:136-141, (1985).

Rumeau-Rouquette, C., Crost, M. Breart, G., and Mazaubrun, C. Evolution de l'allaitement materneal en France entre 1972 et 1976. *Arch. Fr. Pediatr.*, 37:331-335, (1980).

Ransome-Kuti, O. Introduction of weaning foods into the infant's diet. In: *Nutritional adaption of the Gastrointestinal Tract of the Newborn*. N. Kretchmer and A. Minkowski (Eds.), Raven Press, New York (1983).

Rasch, C. A., Cotton, E. K., and Harris, J. W. et al. Blood loss as a contributing factor in the etiology of iron-lack anemia in infancy. *Am. J. Dis. Child.*, 100:627, (1960).

Reinhold, J. G. High phytate content of rural Iranian bread: A possible cause of human zinc deficiency. *Am. J. Clin. Nutr.*, 24:1204-6, (1971).

Reinhold, J. G., Faradji, B. Abadi, P., and Ismail-Beigi, F. Decreased absorption of calcium, magnesium, fzinc and phosphorus by humans due to increased fiber and phosphorus consumption as wheat bread. *J. Nutr.*, 106:493-6, (1975).

Reinhold, J. G., Nasar, A., and Hedayatti, H. Effects of purified phytate and phytate-rich bread upon metabolism of zinc, calcium, phosphorus and nitrogen in man. *Lancet*, 1:283-8, (1973).

Rey, J., Schmitz, J., and Amedee-Manesme, O. Fat absorption in low birth weight infants. *Acta. Pediatr. Scand.*, suppl. 296:81-84, (1982).

Roberts, I. F., West, R. J., and Ogilvie, D., et al. Malnutrition in infants receiving cult diets: A form of child abuse. *Br. Med. J.*, 1:296, (1979).

Robson, J. R. K. Food Faddism. *Pediatr. Clin. N. Amer.*, 24:189-201, (1977).

Rodriguez-Soriano, J. Adaptation of renal function from birth to one year. In: *Weaning, Why, What and When?* A. Ballabriga and J. Rey, (Eds.), Raven Press, New York (1987).

Rowland, M. G. M. The weanling's dilemma: Are we making progress? *Acta. Paediatr. Scand.*, suppl. 323:33-42, (1980).

Royal College of Physicians. Prevention of coronary heart disease. J. R. *Coll. Physicians Long.*, 10:213-75, (1976).

Saarinen, U. M., Siimes, M. A., and Dallman, P. R. Iron absorption in infants: high bioavailability of breast milk iron as indicated by the extrinsic tag method of iron absorption and by the concentration of serum ferritin. *J. Pediatr.*, 91:36, (1977).

Saarinen, U. M. Need for iron supplementation in infants on prolonged breast-feeding. *J. Pediatr.*, 93:177-180, (1978).

Saarinen, U. M., Backman, A., Kajosaari, M. and Siimes, M. A. Prolonged breast-feeding as prophylaxis for atopic disease. *Lancet*, ii:163-166, (1979).

Saarinen, U. M., and Kajosaari, M. Does dietary elimination in infancy prevent or only postpone a food allergy? *Lancet*, 1:166-7, (1980).

Sackett, W. W., Jr. Use of solid foods early in infancy. *General practitioner*, 14:98-102, (1956).

Sadowitz, P. D., and Oski, F. A. Iron status and infant feeding practices in an urban ambulatory center. *Pediatrics*, 72:33, (1983).

Salmona, M., Ghezzi, P., and Garattini, S. *Plasma glutamic acid levels in premature newborns*. Milan: Report of the Instituto di Ricerche Farmacologiche "Mario Negri," (1980).

Sanford, H. N., and Campbell, L. K. Desiccated beef as a food for premature and full term infants. *Arch. Pediat.*, **58**:504, (1941).

Schmitz, J., and McNeish. Development of structure and function of the gastrointestinal tract: Relevance for weaning. In: *Weaning: Why, What and When?* A. Ballabriga and J. Rey, (Eds.), Raven Press, New York, (1987).

Seward, J. F., and Serdula, M. K. Infant feeding and Infant Growth. *Pediatrics*, **74** suppl. part 2:728-762, (1984).

Shank, F. R., Park, Y. K., Harland, B. F., Vanderveen, J. E., Forbes, A. L., and Prosky, L. Perspective of food and drug administration on dietary sodium. *J. Amer. Diet. Assoc.*, **80**:29-35, (1982).

Shinwell, E. D., and Gorodischer, R. Totally vegetarian diets and infant nutrition. *Pediatrics*, **70**:582-586, (1982).

Shukla, A., Forsyth, H. A., Anderson, C. M., and Marwah, S. M. Infantile overnutrition in the first year of life: a field study in Dudley, Worchestershire. *Br. Med. J.*, **4**:507-15, (1972).

Shukla, A. P., Forsyth, H. A., Anderson, C. M., and Marwah, S. M. Infantile overnutrition in the first year of life: a field study in Dudley, Worcestershire. *Br. Med. J.*, **4**:507-515, (1972).

Siimes, M. A., Salmenperä, L. S., and Perheentupa, J. Exclusive breast-feeding for 9 months: risk of iron deficiency. *J. Pediatr.*, **104**:196-199, (1984).

Siimes, M. A., Vuori, E., and Kuitunen, P. Breast milk iron: A declining concentration during the course of lactation. *Acta. Paediatr. Scand.*, **68**:29-12, (1979).

Sjölin, S. Hofvander, Y, and Hillervik, C. Factors related to early termination of breast-feeding: A retrospective study in Sweden. *Acta. Paediatr. Scand.*, **66**:505-511, (1977).

Solomons, N. W., and Jacobs, R. A. Studies of the bioavailability of zinc in man. IV. Effects of heme and non heme iron on the absorption of zinc. *Am. J. Clin. Nutr.*, **34**:475-82, (1981).

Sommer, A., Tarwotijo, I., and West, K. P., Jr. Impact of vitamin A deficiency on infant and childhood mortality. In: *Vitamins and Minerals in Pregnancy and Lactation.* H. Berger (Ed.). Nestle Nutrition Workshop Series. Raven Press, New York. vol. **16**:413-419, (1988).

Stewart, C. A. The use of cereal thickened formulas to promote maternal nursing. *J. Pediatr.*, **23**:310-314, (1943).

Stolley, H., Kersting, M., and Droese, W. "Beikost" für Säuglinge im 1. lebensjahr. Eine ernährungsstudie in Familien. *Sozialpadiatrie in Praxis und Klinik*, **3**:418-420, (1981).

Stolley, H., Schlage, C. and Droese, W. Zur frage nitratgehalt inKarotten Für den Säugling in den ersten lebensmonaten. *Monatsschr Kinderheilkd*, **126**:100-1, (1978).

Superstein, S. Antigenicity of the whey proteins in evaporated cow's milk and whole goat's milk. *Ann. Allergy*, **18**:765-73, (1960).

Surjono, D., Ismadi, S. D., Suwardji, and Rohde, J. E. Bacterial contamination and dilution of milk in infant feeding bottles. *J. Trop. Pediatr.*, **26**:58-61, (1980).

Taitz, L. S. Infantile overnutrition among artificially fed infants in the Sheffield region. *Br. Med. J.*, **1**:315-316, (1971).

Thorogood, M., Clark, R., Harker, P., and Mann, J. L. Infant feeding and overweight in two Oxfordshire towns. *J. Roy. Coll. Gen. Practit.*, **29**:427-430, (1979).

Toenz, O., and Schwaninger, U. Infant Feeding practices in Switzerland 1978. Part II: Artificial feeding. *Schweiz Med. Wochenschr.*, **110**:1522-31, (1980).

Tung, T. C., and Tung, K. S. *Serum free amino acid levels after oral glutamate intake in infant and adult humans.* Taipei: Report of the Institute of Biochemistry, national Taiwan University (1979).

Underwood, B. A., and Hofvander, Y. Appropriate timing for complementary feeding of the breast-fed infant: A review. *Acta. Paediatr. Scand.*, suppl. 1294:2-32, (1982).

USRDA. *Recommended Dietary Allowances.* Committee on Dietary Allowances. Food and Nutrition Board. National Academy of Sciences. Washington DC, 9th ed. (1980).

Van Steenbergen, W. M. *et al.* Machakos project studies. Agents affecting health of mother, infant and child in rural area of Kenya. XXII. Bacterial contamination of foods commonly eaten by young children in Machakos, Kenya. *Trop. Geogr. Med.* 35:193-197, (1983).

Van Woelderen, B. F., and Goedhart, A. C. The importance of the type of milk feeding in later infancy. A Literature search. *Voeding* 48:1-8, (1987).

Vyhmeister, I. B., Register, U. D., and Sonnenberg, L. M. Safe vegetarian diets for children. *Pediatr. Clin. N. Amer.*, 24:203-210, (1977).

Walter, T., Kowalskys, J., and Stekel, A. Effect of mild iron deficiency on infant mental development scores. *J. Pediatr.*, 102:519-522, (1983).

Waterlow, J. C., and Thomson, A. M. Observations on the adequacy of breast-feeding. *Lancet*, ii:238-242, (1979).

Waterlow, J. C., Ashworth, A., and Griffiths, M. Faltering in infant growth in less developed countries. *Lancet*, ii:1176-1178, (1980).

Whitehead, R. G., Paul, A. A., and Ahmed, E. A. Weaning practices in the United Kingdom and Variations in anthropometric development. *Acta. Paediatr. Scand.*, 323:14-23, (1986).

Whitehead, R. G., Paul, P. A., Cole, T. J. A critical analysis of measured food energy intakes during infancy and early childhood in comparison with current international recommendations. *J. Hum. Nutr.*, 35:339-48, (1981).

Whitehead, R. G. The Human Weaning Process. *Pediatrics*, suppl. 75:189-193, (1985).

Whitington, P. F., and Gibson, R. Soy protein intolerance: four patients with concomitant cow's milk intolerance. *Pediatrics*, 59:730-732, (1977).

Whitten, C. F., Stewart, R. A. The effect of dietary sodium in infancy on blood pressure and related factors. *Acta. Paediatr.* Scnad., suppl. :279, (1980).

WHO. *Contemporary patterns of breast-feeding.* Report on the WHO collaborative study on breast-feeding. Geneva: WHO, (1981).

WHO. Technical Report Series No. 724, Geneva, *Energy and Requirements: report of a Joint FAO/WHO/UNU Expert Consultation.* pp. 64-66, (1985).

WHO. Programme for Control of Diarrhoeal Diseases: Vitamin A and Diarrhoea. *Update* 3:1-3, (1988).

WHO/UNICEF Joint statement. *Vitamin A for measles.* Weekly Epidem Res. 19:133-134 (1987).

Wiatrowski, E., Kramer, L. Osis, D., and Spencer, H. Dietary Fluoride Intake of Infants. *Pediatrics*, 55:517-522, (1975).

Wilkinson, P. W., and Davies, D. P. When and why are babies weaned? *Br. Med. J.*, 1:1682-1683, (1978).

Wilson, J. F., Lahjey, M. E., and Heiner, D. C. Studies on iron metabolism: V. Further observations on cow's milk-induced gastrointestinal bleeding in infants with iron-deficiency anemia. *J. Pediatr.*, 84:335, (1974).

Wood, C. B. S. How common is food allergy? *Acta. Paediatr. Scand.*, suppl. 323:76-83, (1986).

Woodruff, A. W., El Suni, A., Kaku, M., Adamson, E. A., Maughan, T. S., and Bundru, N. Infants in Juba, Southern Sudan: The first six months of life. *Lancet.* ii:262-264, (1983).

Yeung, D. L., Hall, J., Leung, M., and Pennell, M. D. Sodium intakes of infants from 1 to 18 months of age. *J. Am. Diet. Assoc.*, 80:242-4, (1982).

Zmora, E., Gorodischer, R., and Bar-Ziv, J. Multiple nutritional deficiencies in infants from a strict vegetarian community. *Am. J. Dis. Child.*, 133:141-144, (1979).

Zoppi, G., Andreotti, G., and Pajino-Ferrara, F. et al. Exocrine pancreas function in premature and full term neonates. *Pediatr. Res.*, 6:880, (1972).

9

Development in Infant Nutrition

L. J. Filer, Jr.

Department of Pediatrics
University of Iowa
College of Medicine
Iowa City, Iowa 52242

HISTORIC BACKGROUND

In The Windermere Lecture given before the British Paediatric Association in 1954, Alton Goldbloom succinctly encapsulated the evolution of the concepts of infant feeding (Goldbloom, 1954). This brief history reflects the scholarly and witty personality of Professor Goldbloom, who concluded his lecture by quoting from a short poem on the history of infant feeding attributable to Dr. John Ruhräh, pediatrician, historian and pioneer in the development of soybean formulas. The poem ends as follows:

"A hundred years will soon go by
Our places will be filled
By others who will theorize
And talk as long and look as wise
Until they too are stilled.
And I predict no one will know
What makes the baby gain and grow."

Ruhräh was president of the American Pediatric Society in 1925 and his presidential address on the history of pediatrics was extracted in part from his recently published book entitled *Pediatrics of the Past* (Ruhräh, 1925). The preface to this text considers it an anthology, chrestomathy and source book in that it provides a selection of the very best materials, specimen extracts from the foreign literature and basic original text. Much of the information provided relates to the early history of infant feeding, and Ruhräh, who frequently resorted to poetry to express his ideas, collected a series of pediatric poems for publication in this volume.

A more current, comprehensive and equally readable history of infant feeding from antiquity into the 20th century is found in the three volume series written by Thomas Cone (Cone, 1976; 1979 and 1985). While two of the three volumes contain the phrases "America or American Pediatrics" the reader soon realizes that the roots of infant feeding practice in the United States are derived from the experiences of physicians caring for infants and children in the U.K. and Western Europe.

One volume published to commemorate the bicentennial anniversary of the independence of the United States traces the laborious efforts of many, be they physician, scientist, industrialist or public citizen, to develop a safe and nutritious food supply for infants. Since formula products provide the major source of nutrients, including energy, during the first year of life, much of this historic review deals with changing physician's attitudes toward use of pasteurized rather than raw milk for infant feeding; the development of acidulated and powdered milk formulas; the process of producing evaporated milk and ultimately the growth of the infant formula industry to include special formulas from soybean protein for feeding the cow milk intolerant infant.

The history of the rationale for the fortification of infant formula products with vitamin D and ascorbic acid, public health measures that lead to the eradication of infantile rickets and scurvy, are indications of how recently our knowledge of infant feeding underwent change.

Cone did not review the most recent advance of public health importance in infant feeding, that of iron fortification of infant formula products. On a worldwide basis it is estimated that 43 percent of children from birth to four years of age have iron deficiency anemia (Viteri, 1989).

Prior to 1960 physicians were indifferent toward mild iron deficiency anemia and did not appreciate the importance of iron to the growth process, cognitive and psychomotor development, work capacity and performance, and infection. The critical need for iron during the first two years of life has recently been reviewed (Filer, 1989). Iron fortified formulas are extensively used in the United States where approximately 75 percent of formula fed infants receive iron-containing products (Fomon, 1987). The requirement that formula-fed infants enrolled in the public assistance program for women, infants and children (WIC) receive iron-fortified formula has been highly effective in reducing the number of infants with hemoglobin concentrations less than 11.0 g/dl (Yip, 1989).

Two studies, one from Costa Rica, the other from Chile, have independently shown impairment of psychomotor and cognitive development in association with hemoglobin concentrations less than 10g/dl (Lozoff, 1987; Walters, 1989). These highly congruent results should be of major concern to those responsible for the feeding and care of the world's children. Both studies indicate that iron deficiency in early life may result in irreversible damage to the central nervous system. If these conclusions are supported through longer term follow-up studies of infants given supplemental iron the need to provide bioavailable forms of iron during the initial years of brain growth and maturation will receive increased emphasis.

The effectiveness of ferrous sulfate to fortify infant formula products has been known for more than three decades (Marsh et al., 1959; Stekel et al., 1986). Unfortunately foods for infants cannot be fortified with ferrous sulfate because its presence produces off-flavors and unacceptable color changes. Heme iron, isolated from beef blood, has been used successfully to fortify cookies that are part of the school lunch program in Chile (Stekel et al., 1986).

The color changes produced in the finished cookie by this highly bioavailable form of iron were masked by the addition of chocolate.

Various forms of elemental iron have been incorporated into foods for infants. Feeding studies in growing pigs, a species whose gut is similar to that of the human infant, have shown that electrolytic iron with a particle size less than 40μ is bioavailable (Anderson *et al.*, 1974). Iron salts in the form of ferrous fumarate and ferrous succinate have been shown to be bioavailable; however, the technical problems associated with use of these components to fortify foods for infants is unclear (Ziegler, 1989a; Hurrell *et al.*, 1989).

Means to eradicate nutritional iron deficiency have been developed and it is essential that this technology be translated into public policy to minimize, if not prevent, the sequelae of iron deficiency.

As predicted by Ruhräh, interest in weight and length gain during early infancy will continue for at least 100 years. Nelson and coworkers have recently published reference data for gain in weight and length of breast and formula-fed term infants over the first four months of life, or the period of the neonatal growth spurt (Nelson *et al.*, 1989). These data on over 1100 healthy infants indicate that the sex-related difference in body weight is greater than the difference related to mode of feeding. For the first six weeks of life no statistically significant difference was noted in gain of weight or length of breast and formula-fed infants. From six to 16 weeks of age, however, formula-fed infants gain more in weight and length than breast-fed infants. As we enter the last decade of the 20th century, the wisdom and insight of Ruhräh becomes increasingly apparent.

LOW-BIRTH-WEIGHT INFANTS

Four decades ago Powers reported that low-birth-weight infants (LBW-infants), or as they were classified then premature infants, fed one-half skimmed milk with ten percent added dextri-maltose gained body weight more rapidly than LBW-infants fed human milk (Powers *et al.*, 1948). Similar results had been reported one year earlier by Gordon and Levin (Gordon *et al.*, 1947).

It was concluded from these studies that the LBW-infant had an increased requirement for dietary protein and that human milk did not meet this demand. However, it was uncertain whether the increase in weight gain was a function of dietary intake of protein or electrolytes, specifically sodium, with the latter contributing to an increase in extracellular water and in some infants clinical evidence of edema (Kagan *et al.*, 1955). Since the composition of the weight gain of formula versus human milk fed LBW-infants was unknown it was impossible to consider one feeding superior to the other.

Table I. Protein-energy ratios of formulas for feeding LBW-infants		
Reference	Year	Protein/Energy Ratio g/100 Kcal
Hess and Lundeen	1949	3.0
Keitel *et al.*	1959	2.8
Snyderman and Holt	1961	2.8
Falkner *et al.*	1962	2.8
Pediatric Nutrition Handbook	1985	
Enfamil Premature		3.0
Similac Special Care		2.7
SMA Preemie		2.5
Ziegler *et al.*	1981	
Advisable Intake		
Birthweight 800-1200 gm		3.1
Birthweight 1200-1600 gm		2.7

Physicians caring for premature infants prior to 1970 focused on the need for rapid infant growth, which they considered important for control of the cost of hospitalization and nosocomial infection (Kietel *et al.*, 1959; Snyderman *et al.*, 1961; and Falkner *et al.*, 1962). There was considerable discussion about the question "is bigger better" and a number of studies were carried out to investigate the relative physiological effects of intrauterine versus extrauterine maturation.

In 1977 the Committee on Nutrition of the American Academy of Pediatrics suggested that the optimal diet for the LBW-infant may be defined as one that supports a rate of growth approximating that of the third trimester of intrauterine life (American Academy of Pediatrics, Committee on Nutrition, 1977). Such an optimal diet implies that postnatal changes in body composition of the premature infant should resemble those of the normal fetus (Ziegler *et al.*, 1976). On the basis of changes in body composition of the growing fetus, Ziegler and coworkers reported that the ratio of dietary protein to energy intake was critical and recommended an advisable intake of 2.7 to 3.1 grams of protein per 100 Kcal of energy for LBW-infants of varying birthweights (Table I) (Ziegler *et al.*, 1981). Feeding a formula that provides a protein-energy ratio of this magnitude should result in a daily weight gain comparable to that achieved by the fetus in-utero.

Studies from the University of Toronto demonstrating that the composition of weight gain and resultant body composition of formula-fed premature infants differs from that of a comparable placentally nourished fetus support the recommendation advanced by Ziegler and coworkers (Reichman *et al.*,

1981). When the protein-energy ratio was less than 2.7, as it is in human milk, (1.86), the daily rate of gain is less and body composition is primarily fat rather than protein and water. The critical nature of the ratio of dietary protein to energy had been described in animal studies as early as the 1930's. Rats or pigs fed low protein diets were fatter than animals fed diets adequate in protein content (Filer *et al.*, 1966; McCracken, 1975).

Recent clinical studies on the effect of varying the protein-energy ratio on body composition of LBW-infants and term male infants provide strong support for the recommendations advanced by Ziegler (Kashyap *et al.*, 1988; Bell *et al.*, 1988; Fiorotto *et al.*, 1989). On the basis of the current data base it is recommended that the protein content of formula products designed for feeding LBW-infants not exceed 3 g per 100 Kcal. Increasing the energy density of formulas for feeding LBW-infants by the addition of carbohydrates or fat in an effort to increase weight gain cannot be condoned. Such additives distort the protein-energy ratio and result in the deposition of body fat, not physiological growth.

Sixty years ago Hess used a mixture of human milk plus cultured skimmed cow milk (4:1) for feeding LBW-infants at the Michael Reese Hospital (Hess & Lundeen, 1949). This process extended the available supply of human milk and provided a formula for feeding premature infants with a protein-energy ratio of 3.0. Thus, Hess had arrived unknowingly at a formulation that met a major nutritional requirement for the premature infant; i.e., an appropriate balance between dietary energy and protein.

INFANT FEEDING

The National Center for Health Statistics estimates that 3,913,000 infants were born in the U.S. in 1988, the largest number of births reported since 1964 (Anonymous, 1989). With but few exceptions these infants were breast-fed or fed heat processed infant formula products. According to market research data collected by Ross Laboratories, 97 percent of infants are breast or formula-fed in the first six months of life (Martinez & Kreiger, 1985; Martinez *et al.*, 1985; Martinez, 1986). Approximately one-half of these infants continue to receive human milk or commercial formula during the latter half of the first year of life. It is difficult to decide what or who directs infant feeding practices during these early months. According to Sarett and coworkers, mothers who elect to breast-feed make this decision in the second trimester of pregnancy (Sarett *et al.*, 1983). As shown in Table II the decision to breast-feed is influenced by ethnicity and socioeconomic factors (Ryan and Martinez, 1989). This sociodemographic pattern parallels that of access to health care delivery services. It may also reflect physician or other health-care professional in-

Table II. Percent of infants breast-fed in hospital and at 6 months of age--1987							
	In Hospital				Age 6 Months			
	Employed		Non-working		Employed		Non-working	
	White	Black	White	Black	White	Black	White	Black
Variable								
All Mothers	59	33	62	21	11	6	29	8
Family Income ($)								
< $ 7,000	41	19	42	16	6	4	11	4
> $25,000	65	48	74	44	13	9	39	20
Maternal Education								
High School or less	48	24	54	17	6	4	21	6
College	72	45	80	41	17	9	44	17
Adapted (Ryan & Martinez, 1989)								

fluences on selection of method for infant feeding. Societal trends such as increasing numbers of women in the work force, the increase in media coverage of health messages, the availability of convenient forms of formulas resembling human milk in nutritional value and public assistance programs (WIC) strongly influence infant feeding practices, especially infants from 6 to 12 months of age. Joffe and Radius (1987) have suggested that personal experience, including contact with young women who have successfully breast-fed their infants, may be a major factor in the promotion of breast-feeding by adolescents.

In 1982 the Academy of Pediatrics issued a policy statement on the promotion of breast-feeding (AAP, 1982). This document placed emphasis on the role of education in the promotion of breast-feeding. The document recommended that the educational process be initiated within the school system to include schools training health professionals. Furthermore, the Academy recommended education of the public to the advantages of breast-feeding *via* television, newspapers, magazines and radio.

A similar position on the promotion of breast-feeding was taken by the American Dietetic Association (ADA) in 1986 (Anonymous, 1986). Health care professionals, breast-feeding support groups and the public were targeted for educational and training programs. If breast-feeding was not an option, the ADA position paper recommended that appropriate alternative feeding methods should be made available to mothers.

Physician and maternal attitudes toward use of whole cow milk for feeding infants in the latter half of the first year of life have changed dramatically within the last two decades. An increasing number of physicians have become aware of the fact that cow milk provides a high renal solute load

(Ziegler & Fomon, 1989), is low in iron content and commonly provokes gastrointestinal blood loss in normal infants (Ziegler, 1989b; Ziegler *et al.*, 1989). For some infants this blood loss may be nutritionally significant.

Mothers who have elected to breast-feed their infants perceive infant formula as the ideal substitute for human milk. How much of this perception is physician influence *versus* parental or peer group endorsement is unknown.

At the present time it appears as though the mother is playing an increasingly important role in directing infant feeding practices. More hospitals are providing mothers who do not plan to breast-feed their infant the opportunity to select the formula to be used upon discharge. Physician control of infant feeding practice is further eroded by state WIC programs. Approximately 31 percent of all infants are enrolled in the WIC program with enrollment growing at a rate approximating 10 percent per annum (Martinez, 1989). Since 1987 the choice of formula for these infants is dictated in 44 states and the District of Columbia by state purchasing agents who frequently select formula on the basis of low bid. These trends, coupled with the large number of mothers who are breast-feeding, are indicative of the importance of the mother in directing infant feeding.

The Infant Formula Act mandated by the Congress in 1980 positioned infant formulas as the most highly regulated and controlled food in the marketplace (Cook, 1989). Food and Drug Administration regulations, as applied to infant formulas, control nutrient levels, quality control procedures and product labeling. The rigidity of such regulations makes it difficult to demonstrate clinical or nutritional differences among the several brands of formula products available for purchase. Thus, FDA regulations have focused the purchasing practice of mothers as it has in the WIC program upon considerations of price rather than nutritional or clinical advantages.

It should come as no surprise that physician control of infant feeding is being eroded, a situation not unlike that faced by infant formula producers and the medical profession at the turn of the century (Apple, 1980).

Two decades ago it was evident that infant feeding practices, in hospital and home, were driven by convenience, conservation of time and reduction in labor costs (Filer, 1971). Infant formula manufacturers were providing a variety of nutritionally sound products in ready-to-feed, disposable units for hospital and home use. Hospital formula rooms were being replaced by storerooms and infant formula products were sold primarily through supermarket chains. This simplification of the practice of infant feeding represented the culmination of major advances in knowledge of infant nutrition and the technology necessary to formulate, package and deliver a product of high quality. Twenty years later it appears as though the innovations in infant feeding initiated by formula manufacturers coupled with changes in the role of women in society, and increasing federal and state regulation of the formula industry, including public assistance, have modified the role of the physician in directing infant feeding. Physicians caring for infants, however, should continue to concern themselves with the nutritional quality of new protein sources, the safety of intentional or unintentional food additives and the newer trace elements.

CONDITIONALLY-ESSENTIAL NUTRIENTS AND TRACE ELEMENTS

Within recent years taurine and carnitine have been added to infant formulas. Taurine has been added to both milk-based and soy-protein-based products with the addition of carnitine limited to soy formulas since carnitine occurs naturally in cow milk formulas. The rationale for supplementation of the infants' diet with taurine and carnitine has its origin within the concept of a "conditionally-essential" nutrient. This terminology implies that the essential nature of the nutrient for man is yet to be defined and that the nutrient can be synthesized to some degree by healthy individuals. Furthermore, a diet comprised of a variety of foods provides an exogenous source of the nutrient. In the case of the infant whose sole source of food is human milk or infant formula, such feedings need to be nutritionally complete. In this sense the diet of the breast-fed infant is supplemented with vitamin D and iron and the diet of formula fed infants is supplemented with a variety of vitamins and minerals. Low-birth-weight infants whose limited body stores of nutrients are readily compromised by growth are further limited in the volume of milk ingested at each feeding. Such physiological events accentuate the need for conditionally-essential nutrients.

TAURINE

The rationale for adding taurine to infant formula products primarily stems from the observation that the taurine concentration of plasma and urine of formula fed infants is less than that of the breast-fed infant. Infants fed formula containing added taurine (30 μM/dL) resemble breast-fed infants with respect to plasma and urine concentrations of taurine (Chesney, 1988).

Taurine, a β-amino acid, is not incorporated into tissue proteins; however, it exists in high concentrations within the intracellular water of many organs--brain, myocardium, liver, kidney, muscle and red blood cells. In addition to its function of regulating cell volume, taurine has been shown to protect the integrity of cell membranes and function as a biological antioxidant. An excellent review of the role of taurine in infant feeding has been published by

Gaull (1989). While Chesney did not conclude that taurine was required for infant nutrition, Gaull concluded that present experimental evidence suggests that the provision of taurine to infants and older children with cystic fibrosis was prudent.

CARNITINE

Carnitine, like taurine, is synthesized endogenously; low-birth-weight infants, however, term infants and adults with genetic, infectious and injury-related illnesses lack the capacity to meet their carnitine requirements from endogenous sources (Rebouche, 1988).

Primary dietary sources of carnitine are milk, dairy products, meat, poultry and fish. Vegetables, fruits and grains provide little carnitine, thus plasma concentrations of carnitine in vegetarians are lower than those of adults or children on a mixed diet (Lombard et al., 1989).

Infants fed soy-protein-based formulas without added carnitine have plasma free and total carnitine levels, one-third those of infants fed a carnitine supplemented formula (Olson et al., 1989). The lack of a dietary source of carnitine alters lipid metabolism in these infants as manifest by an increase in serum free fatty acid concentrations and an increase in urinary excretion of the medium-chain dicarboxylic acids; adipic acid, sebacic acid and suberic acid (Olson et al., 1989). These biochemical changes are a manifestation of the important role that carnitine plays in the regulation of cellular metabolism, i.e. the entry of long-chain fatty acids into mitochondria and the removal from mitochondria of short- and medium-chain organic acids. On the basis of these biochemical findings, L-carnitine has been added to commercially produced soy formulas at a level of 86 μmol/L.

SELENIUM

Unlike taurine and carnitine, selenium is not endogenously synthesized, thus infants are dependent upon a dietary supply of this essential element. Two diseases of childhood have been shown to be associated with selenium deficiency: Keshan disease and Kashin-Beck disease. The former is a cardiomyopathy affecting children 2 to 10 years of age; the latter, an osteoarthritis that occurs in the preadolescent or adolescent years. The selenium concentration of human milk obtained from areas of the Peoples Republic of China, where Keshan disease is endemic, approximates 3 micrograms per liter (Levander, 1989). The concentration of selenium in the serum of infants is proportional to its concentration in their diet (Smith et al., 1982). Other factors excluding bioavailability of selenium from the diet are equally important. Litov and coworkers have demonstrated that human milk or formula that contains 13 to 15 micrograms of selenium per liter will maintain an adequate selenium status in infants (Litov *et al.*, 1989). Levander (1989) has recommended a daily dietary intake of selenium for infants of 9 micrograms per day.

Fortification of infant formula products with selenium has recently been undertaken by one manufacturer who has added selenium in the form of selenite to a soy-based-infant formula (Irons, 1989). This step may herald another advance in infant feeding that will require three or more decades to appreciate.

FUTURE

Advances in biotechnology or genetic engineering have made it possible to make substantial changes in milk composition to the point of producing new products in milk (Bremel, 1989; Simons *et al.*, 1987). While most of these studies have been limited to the lactating mouse or sheep, it ultimately will become feasible to carry over these technologies to the cow. Through alterations in genetic coding it will be possible to eliminate or reduce the concentration of specific milk proteins such as beta lactoglobulin or proteins associated with enzyme systems that control the synthesis of milk fat or lactose. It is conceivable that the enzyme systems that control the molecular structure of triglycerides could be reprogrammed to produce a triglyceride resembling that of human milk fat. The high digestibility of human milk fat relative to cow milk fat is a function of its triglyceride structure (Filer *et al.*, 1969). The directed synthesis of a new molecular species of triglyceride within the mammary gland, along with changes in protein species and lactose concentration, could improve cow milk for infant and child feeding.

Bremel (1989) has forecast that genetic engineering, including the development of transgenic dairy cattle, sheep and goats, could launch the production of specialty milks in the first decade of the 21st century. Such products could be designed to facilitate growth of specific cells or organs such as the gastrointestinal tract; to confer immunity or to be hypoallergenic without the necessity for extensive hydrolysis of intact protein. Since alternative means for infant and child feeding are highly dependent upon milk from ruminant animals, biotechnology provides one approach to tailor-make more nutritious and clinically acceptable products.

REFERENCES

American Academy of Pediatrics Committee on Nutrition, Nutritional needs of low-birth-weight infants. *Pediatrics*, 60:519, (1977).
American Academy of Pediatrics Policy Statement, The promotion of breast-feeding. *Pediatrics*, 69:654-661, (1982).
American Academy of Pediatrics, *Pediatric Nutrition Handbook*, Appendix L, p. 371, (1985).

Anderson, T. A., Filer, Jr., L. J., and Fomon, S. J. *et al.*, Bioavailability of different sources of dietary iron fed to Pitman-Moore miniature pigs. *J. Nutr.*, **104**:619-628, (1974).

Anonymous, Position of the American Dietetic Association: Promotion of breast-feeding. *J. Am. Dietetic Assoc.*, **86**:1580-1585, (1986).

Anonymous, *Monthly Vital Statistics Report*, vol. 37, no. 13, July 26, 1989.

Apple, R. D., "To be used only under the direction of a physician," Commercial infant feeding and medical practice 1870-1940, *Bull. Hist. Med.*, **54**:402-417, (1980).

Bell, E. F., Rios, G. R., and Ungs, C. A., *et al.*, Influence of energy and protein intake on energy utilization and body composition of small premature infants. *Pediatr. Res.*, **23**:479A, (1988).

Bremel, R. D. *Alteration of milk composition using molecular genetics*, Proceedings Dairy Research Conference Center for Dairy Research Milkfats--Trends and Utilization, University of Wisconsin--Madison, pp. 101-105, (1989).

Chesney, R. W. Taurine: Is it required for infant nutrition, *J. Nutr.*, **118**:6-10, (1988).

Cone, T. E. *200 years of feeding infants in America*, Ross Laboratories, Columbus, OH, (1976).

Cone, T. E. *History of American Pediatrics*, Little Brown & Company, Boston, (1979).

Cone, T. E. *History of the care and feeding of the premature infant*, Little Brown & Company, Boston, (1985).

Cook, D. A. Nutrient levels in infant formulas: technical considerations, *J. Nutr.*, **119**:1773-1778, (1989).

Falkner, F., Steigman, A. J., and Cruise, M. O. The physical development of the premature infant, *J. Pediatr.*, **60**:895-906, (1962).

Filer, Jr., L. J. Infant feeding in nineteen seventies, *Pediatrics*, **47**:489-490, (1971).

Filer, Jr., L. J. *Dietary Iron: Birth to Two Years*, (L. J. Filer, Jr., Ed.) New York, Raven Press Ltd., (1989).

Filer, Jr., L. J., Mattson, F. H., and Fomon, S. J. Triglyceride configuration and fat absorption by the human infant, *J. Nutr.*, **99**:293-298, (1969).

Filer, Jr., L. J., Owen, G. M., and Fomon, S. J. Effect of age, sex and diet in carcass composition of infant pigs. In: *Swine in Biomedical Research* (L. K. Bustad & R. W. McClellan, Eds.) Frayn Printing Co., Seattle, WA, p. 141, (1966).

Fiorotto, M., Brown, B., Fraley, K., and Klish, W. Effect of diet on the composition of growth of human infants birth to 4 months, *Pediatr. Res.*, **25**:112A, (1989).

Fomon, S. J. Reflections on infant feeding in the 1970s and 1980s, *Am. J. Clin. Nutr.*, **46**:171-182, (1987).

Gaull, G. E. Taurine in pediatric nutrition: review and update, *Pediatrics*, **83**:433-442, (1989).

Goldbloom, A. The evolution of the concepts of infant feeding, *Archives Dis. Childhood*, **29**:385-390, (1954).

Gordon, H. H., Levine, S. Z., and McNamara, H. Feeding of premature infants, a comparison of human and cow's milk, *Am. J. Dis. Child.*, **73**:442-452, (1947).

Hess, J. H., and Lundeen, E. C. *The Premature Infant, Medical & Nursing Care, 2nd Edition*, J. B. Lippincott Col., Philadelphia, 1949, p. 121.

Hurrell, R. F., Furniss, D. E., and Burri, J. *et al.*, Iron fortification of infant cereals: a proposal for use of ferrous fumarate or ferrous succinate, *Am. J. Clin. Nutr.*, **49**1274-1282, (1989).

Irons, D. S. Personal Communication, (1989).

Joffe, A., and Radius, S. M. Breast versus bottle: correlates of adolescent mother's infant-feeding practices, *Pediatrics*, **79**:689-695, (1987).

Kagan, B. M., Hess, J. H. and Lundeen, E. *et al.*, Feeding premature infants--a comparison of various milks, *Pediatrics*, **15**:373-382, (1955).

Kashyap, S., Forsyth, M., and Zucker, C., *et al.*, Effects of varying protein and energy intakes on growth and metabolic response in low-birth-weight infants, *J. Pediatr.*, **108**:955-963, (1988).

Kietel, H. G., Ting, R., and Schlitt, L., *et al.*, The clinical and laboratory findings of premature infants fed a concentrated form of low-solute-content breast-milk substitutes, *Am. J. Dis. Children*, **98**:607-608, (1959).

Lazoff, B., Brittenham, G. M., and Wolf, A. W., *et al.*, Iron deficiency anemia and iron therapy effects on infant developmental test performance, *Pediatrics*, 79:981-995, (1987).

Levander, O. A., Upper limit of selenium in infant formulas, *J. Nutr.*, 119:1869-1873, (1989).

Litov, R. E., Sickles, V. S., Chan, G. M., Hargett, I..R., and Cordano, A., Selenium status in term infants fed human milk or infant formula with or without added selenium, *Nutr. Res.*, 9:585-596, (1989).

Lombard, K. A., Olson, A. L., Nelson, S. E., and Rebouche, C. J., Carnitine status of lactoovovegetarians and strict vegetarian adults and children, *Am. J. Clin. Nutr.*, 49:301-306, (1989).

Marsh, A., Long, H., and Stierwalt, E., Comparative hematologic response to iron fortification of a milk formula for infants, *Pediatrics*, 24:404-412, (1959).

Martinez, G. A., *Milk feeding trends in the United States 1955-1985*, Personal Communication, (1986).

Martinez, G. A., Personal Communication, (1989).

Martinez, G. A., 1984 Milk-feeding patterns in the United States, *Pediatrics*, 76:1004-1008, (1985).

Martinez, G. A., Ryan, A. S., and Malec, D. J., Nutrient intake of American infants and children fed cow's milk or infant formula, *Am. J. Dis. Child.*, 139:1010-1018, (1985).

McCracken, K. J., Effect of feeding pattern on the energy metabolism of rats given low-protein diets, *Br. J. Nutr.*, 33:277-289, (1975).

Nelson, S. E., Rogers, R. R., Ziegler, E. E., and Fomon, S. J., Gain in weight and length during early infancy, *Early Human Development*, 19:223-239, (1989).

Olson, A. L., Nelson, S. E., and Rebouche, C. J., Low carnitine intake and altered lipid metabolism in infants, *Am. J. Clin. Nutr.*, 49:624-628, (1989).

Powers, G. F., Some observations on the feeding of premature infants based on twenty years' experience at the New Haven Hospital, *Pediatrics*, 1:145-158, (1948).

Rebouche, C. J., Carnitine metabolism and human nutrition, *J. Applied Nutr.*, 40:99-111, (1988).

Reichman, B., Chessex, P., and Putet, G., *et al.*, Diet, fat accretion and growth in premature infants, *New Eng. J. Med.*, 305:1495-1500, (1981).

Ruhräh, J., *Pediatrics of the past*, Paul B. Hoeber Inc., New York, (1925).

Ryan, A. S., and Martinez, G. A., Breast-feeding and the working mother: a profile, *Pediatrics*, 83:524-531, (1989).

Sarett, H. P., Bain, K. R., and O'Learly, J. C., Decisions on breast-feeding or formula feeding and trends in infant-feeding practices, *Am. J. Dis. Child.*, 137:719-725, (1983).

Simons, J. P., McClenaghan, M., and Clark, A. J., Alteration of the quality of milk by expression of sheep β-lactoglobulin in transgenic mice, *Nature*, 328:530-532, (1987).

Smith, A. M., Picciano, M. F., and Milner, J. A., Selenium intakes and status of human milk and formula fed infants, *Am. J. Clin. Nutr.*, 35:521-526, (1982).

Snyderman, S. E., and Holt, L. E., The effect of high caloric feeding on the growth of premature infants, *J. Pediatr.*, 58:237-240, (1961).

Stekel, A., Monckeberg, and Beyda, V., *Combating iron deficiency in Chili: A case study, A Report of the International Anemia consulatative Group (INACG)*, Washington, DC, (1986).

Viteri, F. E., Influence of iron nutrition on work capacity and performance. In: *Dietary Iron: Birth to Two Years* (L. J. Filer, Jr., Ed.) Raven Press Ltd., New York, pp. 141-160, (1989).

Walter, T., Effect of iron deficiency anemia in infant psychomotor development. In: *Dietary Iron: Birth to Two Years*, (L. J. Filer, Jr., Ed.) Raven Press Ltd., New York, pp. 161-175, (1989).

Yip, R., The changing characteristics of childhood iron nutritional status in the United States. In: *Dietary Iron: Birth to Two Years*, (L. J. Filer, Jr., Ed.) Raven Press Ltd., New York, pp. 37-56, (1989).

Ziegler, E. E., Bioavailability of iron from infant foods: studies with stable isotopes. In: *Dietary Iron: Birth to Two Years*, (L. J. Filer, Jr., Ed.) Raven Press Ltd., New York, pp. 83-88, (1989).

Ziegler, E. E., Intestinal blood loss by normal infants fed cow's milk. In: *Dietary Iron: Birth to Two Years* (L. J. Filer, Jr., Ed.) Raven Press Ltd., New York, pp. 75-80, (1989).

Ziegler, E. E., Bega, R. L., and Fomon, S. J., *Textbook of Pediatric Nutrition* (R. M. Suskind, Ed.) Raven Press Ltd., New York, pp. 29-39, (1981).

Ziegler, E. E., and Fomon, S. J., Potential renal solute load of infant formulas, *J. Nurt.*, 119:1785-1788, (1989).

Ziegler, E. E., Fomon, S. J., and Nelson, S. E., *et al.*, Cow milk feeding in infancy: further observations on gastrointestinal blood loss, *J. Peds.*, 116:11-18, 1990.

Ziegler, E. E., O'Donnell, A. M., Nelson, S. E., and Fomon, S. J., Body composition of the reference fetus, *Growth*, 40: 329-341, (1976).

10

The Infant Food Industry as a Partner in Health

Fred T. Sai[1]

The World Bank
1818 H Street NW
Washington, DC 20433

---

1   Although the author is employed by the World Bank, this paper reflects the view of the author alone, and should not be taken to reflect the official policy of the Bank.

INTRODUCTION

The infant food industry has been credited by some experts, such as Aykroyd (1971) with making a significant contribution to the improvement of infant survival and health in the industrialized societies during the early years of this century. Others such as Vahlquist (1981) doubt this, maintaining instead that the improvements were due to general environmental improvements and economic and social changes which benefited the lower strata of society. The chances are that both positions are correct and that the food industry's contribution worked synergistically with general social, economic and environmental development. The changes in women's lifestyles - their ability to join the work force, enjoy more leisure and mobilize for more forceful political and social involvement would perhaps have proved more difficult and slower had not the time-consuming tasks of infant and young child feeding been made easier by the availability of nutritionally satisfactory and safe breast milk substitutes and almost ready-to-use weaning foods.

Yet the entry of industry into this field has not been without controversies of various kinds. Initial controversies were based mainly on scientific issues, such as which ingredients were best for infant feeding and in what proportions, and how best to prepare the foods to avoid problems of diarrhoea and vomiting. The sciences of biochemistry, nutrition and bacteriology helped to resolve these questions. Other controversies concerned the economics of the products, and still others were more political -challenging industry's motives and practices. As the products became available in less developed countries, (LDC), many of the controversies resurfaced and in the last 15-20 years, the infant food industry has faced concerted criticism of its marketing practices in relation to breast milk substitutes, criticism that is based on the science, politics and ethics of marketing such foods in poor communities.

DEFINITIONS

The infant food industry is relatively young - less than 100 years old. Definition of the term infant food industry is itself a matter which has not been completely settled. For some the infant food industry represents only those manufacturers who use non-milk products for producing feeds for infants and young children. To others the infant food industry would include all manufacturers who use milk products which they modify or reformulate for the feeding of infants -- the word infant here being a child under one year old. Finally there is the group of companies that processes milk plus other foods for infants and young children generally. For the purposes of this paper, infant foods include dietary products which wholly or partially replace breast milk in the feeding of infants and those used as supplements to breast milk or formula until the child is able to eat the ordinary household diet. Therefore it includes weaning foods, as well as fruit and fruit juices and vegetable preparations.

HISTORY OF ARTIFICIAL FEEDING

That breast milk is best for the human infant has been emphasized over generations throughout history. Cone (1976) describes early efforts to feed young infants with alternatives to the breast and how unsatisfactory such efforts proved to be. The hazards of artificial feeding were so severe that wet nursing was really the only alternative that physicians advised until the late 18th and 19th Centuries, and many recommendations were made in the 17th Century and even before on how wet nurses should be selected. It was generally advised that not only should the women be physically strong but also morally upright, since it was believed in those days that moral character could somehow be transmitted through the breast milk. Artificial feeding, called dry nursing in those times, was used in foundling hospitals with disastrous consequences. In Paris, for example, it was stated that 85% of foundlings who were dry nursed died. In a Dublin hospital, 99.6% of infants admitted in the late 1700s died. With such figures as a reminder the contribution of the infant food industry to child survival must have been invaluable in the circumstances of those hostile to the industry.

An English physician, Hugh Smith, writing in the late 18th century, was the first to recommend cow's milk as the best substitute for breast milk. However, others claimed that cow's milk was too thick, or too rich, for infants to digest, and suggested various ways to dilute the milk or add elements considered to make it more like human milk. During the 19th century considerable attention was paid to analyzing the content of breast milk in order to derive formulas for making cow's milk as much like human breast milk as possible, and these analyses laid the foundation for the development of the infant food industry. One scheme in particular, the Rotch system, became very influential, especially in the United States, and laboratories were established in many cities, and in London, to prepare formulas according to this system. Although the results for infant feeding were better than with any other system, it is probable that this success was in great part due to the requirement that the milk used in the laboratories should be much purer than that generally available to the public at large.

The milk available to most people, especially in cities, was often produced by diseased cows in very unsanitary conditions, frequently diluted with water, and stored in the open without, of course, the benefit of coolers or ice boxes.

Yet, whether to boil such milk for use by infants was again a matter of great controversy. The "germ" theory of disease was gaining currency but not universally accepted, and though some recommended boiling milk in order to destroy germs and bacteria, others were of the opinion that boiling milk destroyed some of its beneficial qualities and that infants fed on boiled milk did not thrive well.

The milk industry, if such it may be called in the 19th century, was completely unregulated and conditions of production, transport and storage extremely dirty. Cone describes the way in which half of New York's milk supply was produced in the 1830's. The cows were kept in sheds next to distilleries, fed distiller's mush and milked by city tramps. Not surprisingly, the milk was heavily contaminated. Similar conditions were common throughout the country well into the early part of the 20th century. The quality of milk began slowly to improve as a result of several developments in the late 1800's and early 1900's. Pasteurization increased the life of milk and protected against milk borne disease; and public demands for improvements led to the production of "certified" milk whose content and handling met certain standards. The effect of these changes can be seen in such evidence as the decline in mortality among infants in some foundling hospitals in New York State. Fatalities dropped from 51 to 18 percent in the first year after these hospitals were supplied with pure and pasteurized milk (Cone, op cit).

The latter part of the 19th century also saw the beginnings of the proprietary infant food industry. In 1867 a chemist named Justus von Leibig marketed his "perfect" infant food containing wheat flour, cow's milk and malt flour cooked with bicarbonate of soda. This was soon followed by a wide variety of infant foods which fell into three main groups: dried cow's milk, cereal and sugar; malted carbohydrates, and pure cereal to be used with fresh cow's milk. They were heavily criticized as being inferior to breast milk but the greatest harm from most of these foods was their use as an infant's only food source. This deficiency was made worse by the fact that the introduction of solid foods was generally not recommended until late in the first year of life, and even then, many fruits and vegetables now recommended after six months of age were advised against until a child was two or three years of age. This proscription was due to fears of diarrhoea, and it was not until the 20th century that diarrhoeal disease was understood to be generally of bacterial origin.

1928 saw the beginning of what can be properly considered an infant food industry with Gerber's introduction of strained foods. At about this time also, with the advent of better understanding of biochemistry and bacteriology, it was possible to produce various powder and liquid formulae for infant and young child feeding which were nutritionally sound. These developments helped to usher in the period of large scale recourse to artificial feeding and the decline in breast feeding which was to create a major controversy in the 1970s.

Whilst health professionals were prepared to sing the glories of breast-feeding they did not, on the whole, take any steps to prevent a wholesale stampede to artificial feeding perhaps because in industrial countries formula feeding had satisfactory results in terms of child health and development. There have been occasions when some of the foods have been found to be deficient in one respect or another and these have created problems; but after a short controversy these problems have been resolved. Such an issue was the pyridoxine deficiency in S.M.A.[2]

Before the science of nutrition was well established, rickets and infantile scurvy were common conditions in children. The latter in particular was found to be more common in babies who were artificially fed. It was later discovered that this problem could be resolved by the addition of fresh foods, especially citrus fruits, and later still with the addition of vitamin C.

THE INTERNATIONAL BREAST-FEEDING CONTROVERSY

Throughout, however, evidence accumulated that even in the best hands there were, and are, medical conditions that are more common in formula-fed children than in children who were wholly breast-fed. Diarrhoea, for example, is more common among children who are artificially fed. Breast milk is believed to contain protective agents that help lower the incidence of diarrhoea. It is also considered to provide immunologic protection against some ailments common during the first few months of life.

But it was when formula feeding became a major method of child feeding in some developing countries, contrary to what many doctors in those countries were advising, that an international controversy really arose. Like many major controversies, this one started mildly enough. Between about 1968 and 1977, the Protein Advisory Group (PAG) of the U.N. was concerned about reports that promotional advertising of breast milk substitutes was to blame for the accelerating decline in breast-feeding in some developing countries and further, that, due to poverty and lack of adequate water supply, formula was often being used wrongly with serious adverse consequences. The PAG, believing that industry and concerned scientists could work

2   Synthetic Milk Adopted. One of the first infant formulas marketed by Wyeth.

together to resolve problems and, in fact, work towards the development and responsible marketing of infant foods more suited to LDC conditions, convened meetings and prepared statements providing guidelines for such a development.

Some scientists, however, felt this approach was too soft and that industry could not be depended upon to be a true partner. They took the issues to the public - in particular to U.S. consumer advocates. A paper was written for the British charity "War on Want," entitled, "The Baby Killers." It claimed that many deaths from malnutrition and diarrhoea in developing countries were directly due to the feeding of infants with manufactured formula given incorrectly and in unsanitary circumstances because of poverty, attended by absence of good water supply, good cooking sources and refrigeration. Matters came to a head in 1973 when a Swiss group translated "Baby Killers" and re-titled it, "Nestle Kills Babies" thus directly accusing the company. This article alleged that Nestle was killing babies in the developing world by unethical marketing practices. The company was pushing baby formula without considering the fact that the people who were purchasing it had little money, poor water supplies and sanitation and limited appreciation of how to use formula correctly. It was implied that making the formula available enticed mothers to give up breast-feeding and to choose artificial methods. Nestle took the matter to court, as it felt its corporate image was being tarnished. Although Nestle won the libel case it attracted so much negative publicity that it was a pyrrhic victory and the ground was laid for a major controversy which was to last 10 years and in which quite frequently it was obvious that the protagonists had interests other than infant nutrition alone to pursue.

THE BASIS OF THE DISPUTE

No controversy surrounding the infant food industry or indeed surrounding any industrial issue in recent times has had greater international significance or impact than the controversy which led to the "Nestle Boycott." In essence this was fought between industry, particularly Nestle, on the one hand, and those that came to be called "activists," including representatives of consumer organizations, church groups, physicians and scientific and research organizations on the other. A great deal has been written about this controversy which raged from 1973 to 1984. The interested reader is directed to an extensive library kept by the American Public Health Association on the subject. Those who have less time are advised to read "The Politics of Baby Foods" by Andrew Chetley which deals with the subject from the point of view of the activists, and "Infant Feeding: Anatomy of a Controversy 1973 to

1984," edited by John Dobbing, which describes the controversy from the point of view of industry, particularly that of Nestle. A third book: "Out of the Mouth of Babies" by Fred D. Miller, is an interesting discussion of some basic philosophical issues underlying the controversy, rather than an account of the controversy itself.

The basis of the dispute can be simplified as follows:

1) There was a worldwide decline in the practice of breast-feeding beginning first with the more advanced countries and more recently in some of the developing countries;

2) infant mortality rates are very high in the developing countries, and a large proportion of the mortality is due to diarrheas, some of which are associated with early weaning or early recourse to formula feeding;

3) industry was aggressively promoting formula foods and artificial feeds of various kinds in LDCs and entrapping mothers into buying and using them; and

4) mothers in developing countries, poor and illiterate, living in insanitary environments, were becoming passive associates of industry in the killing of their infants.

That by 1970 breast-feeding in the more advanced world had declined almost to the point of becoming insignificant in child nutrition has to be accepted. The question of whether this was simply a response to marketing rather than to other causes remains to be determined. Chetley notes that 38 percent of infants were breast-fed upon discharge from hospitals in the United States in 1946 against 18 percent in 1966. In Sweden in 1944, just under 90 percent of children were breast-fed at two months of age; by 1970 the figure had dropped to under 40 percent. In Poland, 80 percent of infants were breast-fed at 3 months in 1937 and by 1971 the figure was 30 percent. In the United Kingdom 40 percent of 3 month olds were being breast-fed in 1947 and by 1968 it was just over 10 percent. Many experts were concerned at the trend and advocated measures to reverse it, but it was when the pattern spread to the developing countries of Asia, Africa and Latin America that many more became convinced that it presented a significant threat to infant survival. In Singapore, to quote Chetley again, over 80 percent of babies were breast-fed at birth in 1951, by 1971 the figure had dropped to just 30 percent. In Brazil 96 percent were breast-fed at one month of age in 1940; in 1974 only 39 percent were breast-fed. On the other hand a major WHO study, which documented the trend in seven LDCs, found that breast-feeding was prolonged and almost universal among rural women and the economically disadvantaged in cities (World Health Organization -WHO-, 1981,a).

The reasons for the decline have not really been scientifically analyzed. It is possible that a major reason was the convenience of these foods for the life-styles of women in developed countries. Second, was the fact that health professionals themselves, lacking in knowledge of human nutrition or excessively enamored of the benefits of technological interventions in human life, either passively stood by and watched these changes occur or, in some cases, actively assisted with the changes themselves. Some of the ways in which the medical profession actively or passively assisted concerned practices that took place in delivery rooms and within hospitals generally. Technological interventions such as the use of anaesthesia during delivery, and the separation of infants from mothers at birth, did not help mothers to initiate nursing satisfactorily. Within the hospital nurseries, artificial feeding of the baby helped to create an atmosphere of tranquillity that was helpful for, and encouraged by staff going about their tasks.

Even if industry was not causing the problem the view was that by actively or aggressively promoting substitutes directly to mothers, and by its seduction of the health professionals through various routes - lavish entertainment, travel, free gifts, etc. - industry was unethically deriving its profits from the suffering of others. Once the controversy left the arena of scientific debate and became a media and aggressive populist cause, rapid and easy solution became unlikely.

THE NESTLE BOYCOTT

Early in the controversy, the major infant food manufacturers sought to form a group to fight the attack together. This group, the International Council of Infant Food Industries (ICIFI) proved to be unable to prevent an escalation of the controversy or to handle it successfully. Its commitment to work for the implementation of the PAG guidelines did not satisfy industry critics. In the U.S. the battle against industry was fought in the boardrooms and in the courts. The atmosphere convinced three major U.S. companies to concede the demands of critics to eliminate direct promotion to mothers, including the use of mother-craft "nurses."

Nestle was the outside U.S. corporation to be targeted. A boycott against its products was launched in July 1977. The lead group of the boycott was the Infant Formula Action Coalition (INFACT) which made the following demands of Nestle (Dobbing, 1988).

1) Stop all promotion of infant formula
2) Stop mass media advertising of formula
3) Stop distribution of free samples to hospitals, clinics and homes
4) Discontinue service of milk nurses

5) Stop promotion to the medical profession
6) Assure that infant formula does not reach "people who do not have the means or facilities to use it safely"

Negotiations between INFACT and Nestle failed to resolve the issues. The controversy became so intense that the U.S. Congress became involved, and held committee hearings chaired by Senator Kennedy. The Kennedy Committee Hearings did not resolve the problem. In fact, in some ways they heightened it. An expert witness for Nestle made the mistake of presenting the controversy as a dispute between leftists who wanted to limit the powers of multinational corporations, and the needs of the free market. This met with widespread condemnation and showed Nestle in a very poor light. Within a few weeks the boycott of Nestle products had become a world-wide issue. This boycott was very noisily broadcast in Europe, although the extent to which it was supported in developing countries has not been really documented. Many efforts were made to try to resolve the problem. Nestle gave out different instructions to its sales people, made promises of changing its promotional tactics and materials, and so on, but to no avail.

In October of 1979 WHO and The United Nations International Childrens Emergency Fund (UNICEF) convened a meeting to help find a solution. The meeting entitled, "Infant and Young Child Feeding" took place in Geneva. The present writer chaired the meeting which brought together about 150 people representing governments, industry, scientists and the consumer's organizations or activists. This was the first time that under an international organization, at any rate the WHO, that such diverse groups had been brought together as equals to discuss a major problem. Everybody at the meeting had the same status. After the issues were debated in plenary sessions, there were discussions in four working groups. As can be imagined, the group that dealt with industry's sales practices had the most serious problems. The question of withholding information to an individual or group because they were judged incapable of using such information correctly was an ethical issue to which no answer was found. The meeting did its work reasonably well and recommended the drawing up of a code of marketing for breast milk substitutes. This recommendation was adopted, and in May 1981 after a great deal of discussion and negotiation, the WHO International Code of Marketing of Breast-milk Substitutes was finally presented for approval to all member governments of the WHO. In the end, approval was nearly unanimous, with the United States the only country casting a negative vote. The interested reader should study the code. (WHO, 1981,b)

THE WHO INTERNATIONAL CODE

The aim of the code is stated as:

> "to contribute to the provision of safe and adequate nutrition for infants, by the protection and promotion of breast-feeding, and by ensuring the proper use of breast milk substitutes, when these are necessary, on the basis of adequate information and through appropriate marketing and distribution,"

and its scope as:

> "The Code applies to the marketing, and practices related thereto, of the following products: breast-milk substitutes, including infant formula; other milk products, foods and beverages, including bottle-fed complementary foods when marketed or otherwise represented to be suitable, with or without modification, for use as a partial or total replacement of breast-milk; feeding bottles and teats. It also applies to their quality and availability, and to information concerning their use."

The Code addresses governments and charges them with the responsibility to ensure that all aspects of marketing of breast-milk substitutes conform with the guidelines in the Code. These are meant to include clear information on

1) the benefits and superiority of breast-feeding
2) maternal nutrition and the preparation and maintenance of breast-feeding
3) the negative effect on breast-feeding of introducing partial bottle feeding;
4) the difficulty of reversing the decision not to breast-feed;
5) where needed, the proper use of infant formula.

The Code also details what is permitted or not in the relationship between the representatives of industry and the general public and mothers, with the health care system and with health professionals. It deals with labelling, quality control and implementation and monitoring of compliance.

Once the Code was accepted, the question was then one of implementation and monitoring arrangements. The activists maintained at the beginning that industry, including Nestle, could not be depended upon to monitor what was happening. Nestle had, prior to the approval of the code, constituted a committee for monitoring compliance. This committee under Senator Muskie had assisted in examining reports of violations of the Code, and made reports of its findings. The Muskie Commission worked well and its work was respected. The activists undertook their own monitoring. WHO has some staff who receive reports from countries and interested parties. With the finalization of the Code and the initiation of monitoring, efforts were directed towards resolving the controversy with Nestle. UNICEF and the United Methodist Church played a laudable role in finally bringing the warring factions together and the boycott against Nestle was lifted in October 1984.

NEED FOR A MORE BALANCED VIEW

The controversy over infant feeding has two main contributing strands. The first concerns the relative merits of breast-feeding and artificial feeding. The second concerns the role of the marketing of infant foods in breast-feeding declines.

With regard to the first, virtually everyone agrees that breast-feeding provides the optimal diet for infants until four to six months of life, and has, in addition, other benefits such as giving immunologic protection, providing a natural form of contraception for some period of time post-partum, and contributing to the emotional bonding of mother and infant. It is also less costly. A government study in the U.S. reviewed the literature on the role of feeding mode on infectious disease morbidity and mortality in LDCs, and found that it supported an association between bottle feeding and infectious disease. It also suggested, however, that other factors such as water source and sanitation may be more important factors in infant health Many of the studies used as evidence of the harmful effect of commercial formula do not, in fact, identify what is in the bottle being fed to the baby, or make it clear that many traditional substitutes and supplements are prepared and stored under the same circumstances that are prejudicial to the safe preparation of formula.

This brings me to the question of whether the marketing of commercial formula has caused the declines in breast-feeding and, by implication, the malnourished conditions of many infants and children in the Third World. A related question is whether formula is used as a substitute for breast milk, or, rather, as a substitute for preparations that would otherwise have been used. Throughout developing countries, there are many ways of feeding children, which would appear to pose a great deal more danger to the health of an infant than any nutritionally adequate, well prepared formula. The concern expressed that these formulae are promoted to women who have neither the money nor the knowledge to handle them properly requires a little more examination. The WHO study of breast-feeding referred to earlier revealed that the vast majority of mothers felt that breast-feeding was superior to bottle feeding. The researchers divided mothers into three groups based on this breast-feeding pattern. In Category III, which included most of the urban poor groups, all the rural, and one economically advantaged group, breast-feeding was prolonged and almost universal. In no group in this category did more than 2 percent of mothers fail to initiate breast-feeding, and 50 percent of mothers were breast-feeding at 18 months post partum. The report comments, "Certainly it is interesting to note that the social and economic groups that were less favored as regards general health, nutrition and environmental conditions were the very ones in which breast-feeding was most prevalent and prolonged, and presumably most successful" (WHO, 1981a, p. 146). In conjunction with another of the report's findings that there was fairly widespread knowledge of commercial formula, this would seem to indicate that the very groups about which most concern has been expressed are in fact choosing to breast-feed. Yet these, too, are the same groups in which experience of previous child loss is high. It does not seem logical therefore to conclude that the marketing of infant formula is the prime cause of malnutrition and mortality in these groups.

Why was so little attention paid to some of these findings? Why did the case against the infant food industry seem so unassailable? Probably the first reason is that the death of infants is such an emotional issue that rational and objective balancing of the evidence was a casualty of the impulse to find some target for action, if not blame. Second, industry played into the hands of critics in many ways. Although some groups were prepared to use the infant food issue as a stick with which to beat multinational corporations, industry's questioning the motives of their critics rather than rebutting the charges, was a disastrous ploy. Third, the companies' attempts to form an industry group foundered as a result of their reluctance to share information that might erode their competitive advantage vis-a-vis each other. This again, gave credence to the view that they were interested in profits, rather than infant health. Fourth, industry was slow to appreciate the importance of perception as against reality, and the perception of them as unethically promoting harmful substances was enhanced by dubious practices such as dressing sales persons as "nurses."

LESSONS FROM THE CONTROVERSY

This controversy, long and difficult though it was, proved that the time had come for health workers, industry and consumer representatives to forge a different kind of cooperative relationship. The confrontation has been costly in money, time and energy. Some of the statements made and the stance by some of the activists have unwittingly silenced more considered opinion from LDCs. Most of the time the position of the opponents of industry was "if you are not with us you are against us." In such a climate, scientific work suffers. Industry had made mistakes, some of them callous and stupid, but mainly through a lack of appreciation of the extent of corporate responsibility. It has learnt some important lessons. Among these are the need to appreciate the problems created by or in using these products within different economic, social and cultural environments, to be careful of pursuing "modern trends" in all circumstances, and to really involve both their shareholders and consumers in a reasonable dialogue. The relationship with health workers, the question of bribery by gifts, supports and grants, are areas which require very careful consideration.

There is no doubt that the infant food industry has a role to play in LDC development. What that contribution is needs to be examined on a case by case basis. One casualty in this controversy has been a loosening of the collegial spirit between scientists in the field and those in industry. During the mid-sixties when protein deficiency was a major consideration of the Protein Advisory Group and others, industry was being advised to put money into weaning foods. It is documented that at times industry lost large amounts of money in research which yielded very little in the end. Nestle lost money over projects in Brazil and Glaxo lost money in efforts in Nigeria. For the best cooperation or collaboration what one would suggest is that industry and the scientific community plus the government form some kind of a child nutrition coordinating group in each country to examine the problem and potential for solution. Such groups should include university research groups.

It is also important to examine further the criticism of health workers being so gullible or so easily seduced that the promotion mechanisms have pushed them into a situation of expounders of what industry requires. In fact, some people have such disdain for doctors that at one stage during the development of the Code, there were questions of what kind of gift to a doctor might be considered as seduction for him to do what industry wants; leading to efforts to limit these to a percentage of his salary. Those who maintain this view should seek much more promising avenues for making the profession ethical if indeed it is so bad, rather than having band-aid solutions.

During the whole confrontation, very little attention was paid to some issues which would appear to me to be basic. "When is it right to withhold information from anyone?" Who has the right to decide that because a person is illiterate she is unable to follow simple instructions and who decides that women are not aware of their true needs. For those of us in family planning and in preventive health generally, our axiom is that illiteracy and idiocy are not synonymous and that individuals do things that in their sights and circumstances will maximize their opportunities. It is for this reason that we are told often over and over again that we are presenting family planning in such a way that it does not accord with what people perceive as their own best or better interest. If that is true, how is it that we maintain that the same people are so ignorant that they cannot perceive what is good for their own children? If they are so easily persuaded to use infant formula why are they not so easily persuaded to adopt family planning? This sort of question was never addressed and I am sure that it cannot be addressed unless the atmosphere of violent criticism of anyone who holds a view contrary to "the industry is doing wrong - let's go get them" kind of approach is removed. That approach is frightening - too frightening to pursue. What is needed for the future is for there to be a spirit of genuine cooperation and collaboration. It is my view, as I stated at the beginning of the October 1979 meeting that there can be no final solution to the problems of infant and young child feeding in the LDCs to which industry will not make large inputs from the application of industrially-based technologies. If that is accepted then it is incumbent on all of us to find ways and means of providing the machinery and the processes by which academics, professional health workers, Ministries of Health and consumer representatives can come together and evolve approaches to resolving problems of food and nutrition and for planning towards a better future and better future ways of handling issues relating to children.

The atmosphere of confrontation and recrimination, if not open warfare, that surrounded the Breast-milk Substitute Controversy has achieved certain things, as stated above, but it has also helped to stifle what was beginning to appear as a rational collaboration between industry, the international scientific community and, in some countries, with the scientists of the countries. I believe also that the controversy, for a time, so overshadowed everything else in infant and young child nutrition that there was a tendency for people to think that once this is sorted out, everything that is related to infant and young child nutrition would be solved. There is no such prospect in the developing countries and problems of infant and young child nutrition remain as important as ever. What is more, although with the small improvements in economic conditions the rates of problems may be coming down, with population growth the actual numbers of malnourished children in some parts of the world are increasing. As UNICEF pointed out in their State of the World's Children 1989 message, the current economic crisis and the need for structural adjustments leading on to cuts in social sector expenditure are helping to make this situation much more difficult. In addition, we have to accept that there is increasing urbanization, there is a call for increasing women's participation in the work place, there is a noticeable attention to child birth at young ages and a call to make the young mothers return to school or to their training. All of these are situations which may exacerbate the problems of infant and young child nutrition. We need to increase the choices open to mothers, to ease their lives, not constrain them.

In such circumstances, it is necessary to anticipate the fact that industry will have to be a partner to scientists, physicians and the population at large in all of the development approaches and particularly in the area of weaning foods and supplementary foods or even substitute foods for those who cannot breast-feed. In the case of breast milk substitutes in particular, there are some questions which are still waiting for answers. First, to what extent do mothers breast-feed and what is the direction of change? To what extent do they supplement and what do they use? Are the substitutes/supplements nutritionally sound? Do commercial formulas substitute for breast milk or substitute for other substitutes which would have been used anyway? Are commercial formulas used as substitutes or supplements to breast-feeding or are they used as weaning foods? If they are used as supplements, are they displacing, more or less, nutritional elements? Under what conditions really is the use of formula dangerous and would the danger exist without the use of formula? What is the relative role of maintained breast-feeding and improved conditions in protecting nutritional status? These questions, as well as a question which was posed over and over in Geneva and not really dealt with, namely, when does growth faltering start in the fully breast-fed infant and what does one do about it, should be tackled on a coordinated basis.

NEED FOR COORDINATING ARRANGEMENTS

Many of these questions will be best addressed if there is a calm atmosphere in which issues are debated freely and approaches sought jointly. At the international level, naturally the WHO and UNICEF provide flora for debate on these issues. Even with those organizations, debates are often not removed from politics. I am aware that a sub-committee on nutrition of the Advisory Committee on Coordination of the UN System, with its expert advisory group of nutrition scientists is trying to do a good job of identifying some of the issues and discussing them. I believe, however, that this committee is too much of a committee of UN staffers and not enough of a committee of experts and concerned citizens. What is probably needed at the international level is a standing committee composed under the mandate of UNICEF and WHO jointly, which brings together experts in nutrition science, experts in child health and development, representatives of international consumer organizations and one or two individuals who have shown from their approaches in the development field their concern for harmonious development. The international professional associations, such as that of pediatricians and that of nutritionists, do not appear to examine these issues vigorously enough. It is suggested that the questions of infant and young child nutrition be made a major program activity of these organizations in the future at every one of their congresses.

Irrespective of what happens at the international level, it is at the national level that problems are likely to be finally resolved and progress made. It is good that the International Baby Food Coalition is helping to monitor the implementation of the Code. But putting every infraction of the Code on the shoulders of industry is unlikely to lead to satisfactory development. It is timely that efforts are made to help developing countries, not only to develop and implement the Code in relation to their own circumstances, but also to try to develop the capability for monitoring adherence to it, not only by international corporations, but also by corporations which are indigenous. Some of the indigenous corporations have proved to be less respectful of international accords than even the international corporations which are exposed to the world view through the international media.

At the national level, therefore, structures needed should include a sub-committee on infant and young child nutrition where there are food and nutrition councils. This sub-committee should be charged with the responsibility for advising government, industry and the universities of the major issues in infant and young child nutrition, as perceived within the borders of the country. Naturally, the committee should be composed of representatives of all of the interested parties. It should have active secretariats based in either the nutrition council itself or, where possible, in a national research institution. Such a committee should help the regulatory agency of the country to examine the implementation of the Code as well as any other regulations that pertain to infant feeding.

Regionally, there may not be any need to create another structure. However, by the use of existing professional associations and under the auspices of the Regional World Health Organization concerned, it should be possible for a periodic assessment of what is happening in infant and young child nutrition in the countries of each region. Again the subject should be on the regular agenda.

CONCLUSION

In the 100 or more years since the baby food industry has been in existence, it has provided much assistance to women and to families in many circumstances. The baby food industry is here to stay. In its approaches, however, to the developing countries, it has often tried methods which would not accord with the realities of those developing countries. The controversies that have arisen recently over industry's behavior in LDCs have helped to sharpen some of these lapses. In some instances, the accusations have been correct. In others, they have not been so truthful. Yet, all sides in these controversies should be interested in one thing only. The safe, effective nutrition of infants and young children throughout the world. This can only be fulfilled when development has reached and touched the lives of the billions that are left behind the development process at the present time. It can also be facilitated by better approaches to infant and young child nutrition, approaches which depend on biologically ascertainable facts and accepted improvements in the ways of infant and young child feeding assisted, when necessary, by industrial products.

Industry can play a part as a partner to families but the part they play needs to be regulated very well. Who regulates and who monitors compliance of the regulations should be a matter within the hands of competent national authorities. Industry is being called upon to be a partner and assist national authorities to develop the necessary competencies. Industry, by assisting with training and research in the universities on a completely altruistic basis should be making a major impact to the development effort in many countries. Attacks on the motives of industry are justified when bad motive can be proved, but shrill attacks which do not derive from facts can only be unhelpful to the developing countries themselves.

Full and complete breast-feeding is accepted as the best start for the human infant. There is no question about that in the mind of anyone. However, there are circumstances in which full and complete breast-feeding cannot be guaranteed and "the breast is best" message falls short of what is realizable. Under such circumstances, the products of industry need to be given their proper place. It is good that the international consumer movement and activists have found the baby food industry a target for their wrath and their complaint about bad business practices. Let us hope that the lessons that have been learned from this controversy will help avoid similar controversies in the future.

REFERENCES

Aykroyd, W. R.: Nutrition and Mortality in Infancy and Early Childhood: Past and Present Relationships. *Amer J. Clin Nutr.*, 24:480-87 (1971).

Chetley, A.: *The Politics of Baby Foods.* Frances Pinter, London (1986).

Cone, T.E.: *200 Years of Feeding Infants in America.* Ross Laboratories, Columbus, Ohio (1976).

Infant Feeding. *Anatomy of a Controversy 1973-1984.* J. Dobbing, ed. Springer-Verlag, Berlin, Heidelberg, New York (1988).

Miller, F.D.: *Out of the Mouths of Babes: The Infant Formula Controversy.* The Social Philosophy and Policy Center, Bowling Green State University, Bowling Green, Ohio (1983).

Muller, M.: *The Baby Killer.* Third Edition, War on Want, London (1977).

Vahlquist, B.: *Introduction to the Report on the WHO Collaborative Study on Breastfeeding, Contemporary Patterns of Breastfeeding*, pp. 1-10. WHO, Geneva (1981).

World Health Organization: *Contemporary Patterns of Breastfeeding.* Report on the WHO Collaborative Study on Breastfeeding. WHO, Geneva (1981).

World Health Organization: *International Code of Marketing of Breast Milk Substitutes.* WHO, Geneva (1981).

11

Direct Intervention Programmes to Improve Infant and Child Nutrition

Mahshid Lotfi[1]
and John B. Mason[2]

United Nations
Administrative Committee on Coordination
Subcommittee on Nutrition
Geneva, Switzerland

1   Dr. M. Lotfi is consultant to the UN ACC Sub-Committee on Nutrition (ACC/SCN).
2   Dr. J. B. Mason is Technical Secretary of the ACC/SCN.
     The views expressed are those of the authors and not of the ACC/SCN.

INTRODUCTION

Adequate nutrition is closely related to good health, physical and mental development and the state of well-being of individuals and populations. It is now increasingly recognized that nutritional improvement and economic growth and pattern of a society are interrelated. Economic development is necessary for sustained improvement in nutrition, but waiting for this may be regarded as unacceptable - interim measures are needed. Conversely, malnutrition is likely to affect adversely the level and pace of development by its influences on physical working capacity, learning ability and on the general alertness and vitality of individual members of a society. Thus by regarding malnutrition as an important development problem, consequences of malnutrition for national development are clearer now than ever before.

Information now becoming available indicates substantial improvement of nutrition in some regions (*e.g.* South East(SE) Asia, ACC/SCN, 1987a) and countries (ACC/SCN, 1989a). This is usually linked with favorable economic conditions, and frequently with vigorous nutrition programmes, although the relative effects of these factors are difficult to disentangle. Thus, for example, in SE Asia, Thailand and Indonesia have shown evidence of improved nutrition and child survival (ACC/SCN, 1989a), associated with both programmes and economic growth. In Latin America, the good nutritional situation of children in, for example, Chile, Costa Rica and Cuba, is ascribed to vigorous and sustained health and nutrition activities (Horwitz, 1987). On the other hand, many countries are badly affected by economic stress, some showing evidence of nutritional deterioration (Cornia *et al.*, 1987, 1988 ; ACC/SCN, 1987a, 1989a); it may be particularly important to have effective nutrition programmes in these cases; at a minimum to protect nutrition while grappling with economic problems.

According to a World Bank report, even under the best conditions growth in economy of many poor nations is not fast enough to improve substantially, in short run, nutrition situations in these societies. At the same time, hunger and malnutrition remain probably the most widespread causes of human suffering in the world. Some 150 million children are estimated to be undernourished in developing countries (ACC/SCN, 1988). Many millions suffer from specific mineral and vitamin deficiencies such as vitamin A, iodine, and iron, prevalent in many developing countries. Severe vitamin A deficiency is a major cause of those 40 million people estimated to be blind globally and even moderate deficiency appears to contribute to child death and lowered resistance to disease. Iodine deficiency affects nearly 200 million people.

Again, iron deficiency anemia affects nearly one in two women in reproductive age in developing countries, and may have far-reaching effects on psychological function and cognitive development in children (ACC/SCN, 1987a). Still other micronutrient deficiencies exist contributing to the overall picture of malnutrition and malfunctioning of the body. Some of these reappear forming a significant health problem, notably vitamin D and calcium deficiency (Fraser, 1989).

It follows that while addressing underlying causes of poverty and underdevelopment, in any given society, must remain the main goal for governments and policy makers in the poorer countries of the world, as Berg (1987) has pointed out, malnutrition problems need to be dealt with, concurrently and continuously, in a more specific and direct manner in order to decrease much economic and human waste in a shorter period of time.

On the other hand, economic crisis, economic recession and rising debt, currently afflict many developing countries. As a result, major shifts in economic policy, in the form of structural adjustment programmes, have been employed by governments to respond to such crises. The implementation of these programmes are shown to not infrequently coincide with substantial nutritional deterioration, particularly in the short run, among the poorest. These adverse effects have in many affected countries reversed the stable or even improving trends in malnutrition and infant mortality rates. This outcome - according to a statement issued by the SCN following the Symposium on "Economic Recession, Adjustment Policies and Nutrition" - is not inevitable if appropriate measures are taken (ACC/SCN, 1986). Indeed, intervention is needed, to prevent the poor and vulnerable groups, dying and wasting, while one hopes for sound economic development to occur. Compensatory measures to avoid negative effects of such policies have been introduced to intervene with nutrition/health positive consequences (Cornia *et al.*, 1987).

Over 30 years of experience has now accumulated in the planning and implementation of nutrition interventions and food-related programmes in the world. However, the compensatory programmes in response to negative changes in economic circumstances, are rather new efforts. According to Berg (1987), special attention should be paid to the potential applicability of nutrition programme experience to the design and support of structural adjustment programmes.

Experience of large-scale nutrition programmes is, therefore, now more relevant than ever. In this chapter we aim to describe some of this experience, in terms of the types of activities undertaken - giving some details of six illustrative programmes - and comment on programme design and the level of effort that seems likely to be effective, especially in terms of protecting or improving child nutrition, in different circumstances.

Drawing on experience inevitably needs selection of programmes. Particularly important is the experience of large-scale programmes, covering substantial numbers of people and being managed as routine government programmes. Material is drawn from several sources. The ACC/SCN organized a workshop in August 1989 on "Managing Successful Nutrition Programmes," and the information presented at this workshop - shortly to be published (ACC/SCN, 1989 b) - has been drawn upon. External assistance to large-scale nutrition programmes has been sustained for many years by the World Bank, and a review of this experience (Berg, 1987) has been invaluable. A most useful review on "Comparative Analysis of Nutritional Effectiveness of Food Subsidies and other Food-related Interventions" by Kennedy and Alderman (1987) has been extensively used. Other sources are quoted below.

TYPES OF ACTIVITIES

A variety of strategies are used by governments to achieve nutrition goals. With direct intervention programmes, what types of activities have so far been used?

Broadly speaking, efforts of these kinds have resulted in the planning and development of specific projects at three levels - individuals, family and the entire community and/or nation - as described by Kennedy and Alderman (1987). Some examples of these interventions are given in Table I.

Direct nutrition programmes conventionally may refer primarily to some or all of the individual level activities shown in Table I. We will not attempt here any detailed comparisons of the effectiveness, under different circumstances, of interventions at the different levels. Comments are given by Austin et al. (1978), Austin and Zeitlin (1981), Kennedy & Alderman (1987), however, this remains an important area of policy research. We focus here mainly on individual level intervention.

Although the mass coverage of an intervention might theoretically include all individuals and families, a localized and well-targeted intervention which focuses on a specific section of the community, usually those most needy of nutritional support, has repeatedly shown greater impact and higher cost-effectiveness. Planning and organizational capacity, the degree to which monitoring and necessary management can be applied, and the available resources both financial and human - as will be considered later - are just some of the factors responsible for choice and success/failure of any intervention.

Table I. Examples of some direct intervention programmes to improve nutrition at individual, family and national level

Individual Level	Family Level	Community or National Level
Growth monitoring	Family targetted food subsidy	Non-targetted food subsidy
Supplementary feeding for infant, child, PNW, *etc.*	Supplementary foods for poor families	Mass-feeding in famine/drought *etc.*
Breast-feeding campaigns Weaning food preparation ORT Immunization	Income transfer: Food stamps/coupons Poverty relief	Nutrition oriented food policies: Import/export policies Cash crop expansion Agric. price policies
Micronutrient suppl.	Income generating projects: Food for work Home Nutr. garden	Technological changes Fortification of centrally processed foods
Therapeutic feeding for severely malnut	Nutr/health education and counselling	Nutr/health education through mass media
Nutrition/health education and counselling	Health services	Community Nutr. gardens
		National School Feeding Programmes

PNW = Pregnant and Nursing Woman
ORT = Oral rehydration therapy
Source: Based on structure from Kennedy and Alderman (1987). See references.

In practice, most programmes are targeted towards those defined as nutritionally most vulnerable *i.e.* infants, young children and pregnant and nursing women. The reason for exclusion of other malnourished subjects in need of such support is to optimize use of resources. This resource insufficiency has proved a real constraint, even in more advanced countries where nutritional intervention programmes have been functioning. For example, in USA, the women, infants and children (WIC) programme in operation since 1974, has been able to register only half of those eligible for the services because of insufficient funding (Kennedy and Summer, 1989).

Table II summarizes the general characteristics of a series of 13 large-scale projects. These were chosen from available material to illustrate project characteristics in a variety of circumstances; the Table also draws attention to

Table II. Programme characteristics

Project/Country	Duration	Component	Coverage			Target Group/Method	Objective
			Population Served	Number of Beneficiaries	% Covered or Monitored by Project		
Botswana Drought Relief Programme	1982 - June 1988	Intensive supplementary feeding: direct feeding take-home rations cash for work projects Agricultural relief & recovery programmes	National scale 70% population covered	550,000 (June 87 - May 88)	Very high coverage of specific vulnerable groups (about 100%) plus 74,000 workers were covered (in 1985/86) in labour-based relief activities	Vulnerable members of the community. Individuals by age group, sometimes by weight-for-age. Area targetting by wt/age from national nutrition surveillance data.	Preservation of human life
Costa Rica NNHCP	Late 1974 -	School feeding Food distribution programme (milk oil) Centers for education & nutrition Centres for comprehensive child care	—	498,000 in 1983	—	Children and PNW attending nutrition centres.	Eradication of third degree malnutrition
Costa Rica ISDP	1970-79	Anemia control Rural health intervention. Treatment & follow up in clinics. Health and Nutrition education.	—	In 1983 777,000	58%	Children and PNW in all rural and semi-urban areas/both by age and sex and area targetting.	Promoting mother and child health and survival

GM = Growth Monitoring; PNW = Pregnant and Nursing Women; WA = Weight for Age; IDD = Iodine Deficiency Disorders; ORT = Oral Rehydration Therapy; — = No Data

Table II. (Continued) Programme characteristics

Project/Country	Duration	Component	Population Served	Coverage		Target Group/Method	Objective
				Number of Beneficiaries	% Covered or Monitored by Project		
India TINP	Oct 1980 –March '89	GM of all 6–36 month old children. Short-term selective supplementary feeding. Nutrition education. Anemia Control & other micro-nutrient therapy (Vitamin A, iron, folic acid). Institutional building. Health services (immunization deworming, water supply)	43% of static rural population 17.2 million of 6 districts	1.1 million children 6–36 month old plus 0.28 million PNW Approx 1/2 rural Tamil Nadu	Over 90% for GM 95% of which were fed (Also PNW were selectively fed) 1/3 of all children weighed were fed. (By the end of prog. only 1/4 needed to be fed)	6–36 month old children plus PNW. Individual children selected for feeding based on GM.	To reduce malnutrition and high mortality of years and to improve health and nutritional status of vulnerable groups including PNW
Tanzania JNSP	1984–89	GM, Nutr. Educ. Maternal & child health Water & environmental sanitation Household food security Income generating promoting regular & frequent feeding Home gardens Immunization	As pilot in 6 districts of Iringa region with 1.2 million population. 168 villages in 1984 610 villages in 1987	46,000 children < 5 years old (250,000 total target popnl receiving goods and services from programme)	In 1984 30,600 < 5 years old children and in 1988 332,000 weighed. About 80% of the villages reported regularly for GM	Different components targeted at appropriate age/sex groups.	To improve maternal nutrition & child growth & development, to decrease infant & young child mortality & morbidity and to improve capabilities at all levels of society to assess and to analyse nutrition problems and to design appropriate action
Zimbabwe SFPP	1981-	Supplementary feeding. Nutrition Education. Food Production Community mobilization GM	National scale (initiated on a pilot scale now covers most districts in the country)	—	—	For most components the whole community was targeted. For feeding less than 5 year old underweight children and their families.	To increase awareness of nutrition problems. To meet the demand for nutritious foods by encouraging communities to work together

Table II. (Continued) Programme characteristics

Project/ Country	Duration	Component	Coverage			Target Group/Method	Objective
			Population Served	Number of Beneficiaries	% Covered or Monitored by Project		
India ICDS	1975-	Supplementary feeding GM Immunization Health check ups Nutrition & health education Non-formal pre-school education Referral services.	March 1989 1,952 blocks with 165 million population. 28 million children 0-6 years old and 6.6 million PNW.	For supplementary feeding 13.6 million Beneficiaries included 11.4 million 0 - 6 year olds and 2.2 million PNW in 1989.	40% of targeted 0-6 year olds 30% of targeted PNW.	Area by socio-economic criteria. 0-6 year olds selected by MUAC <13.5 cm & ≤WA grade II and below also pre-school education children attending anganwadis and poor women.	-To improve the nutrition and health status of children aged 0-6 years and PNW. -To reduce mortality, morbidity, malnutrition & school drop out
Indonesia UPGK	1974-	GM Nutrition & health education. Vit A to children Iron to PNW Home nutrition gardens Health services.	National 58,355 villages (in 1981 20,000) 25.5 million children 81% of all <5 years old in Indonesia	17 million children for GM	98% in W. Java; 85% in Sulawesi; 81% in S Sumatra For GM active long term participation 77% of all < 5 years olds covered.	<5 year old children, PNW; children identified at risk by GM get special attention.	To improve nutrition status & health of years old and PNW through modification of nutritional related behaviour of mother and increasing community participation in programme.
Philippines ASNP	1983-	Supplementary feeding in schools supported by income generating activities of the school and families. Nutrition education Food production Environmental sanitation.	1047 elementary schools in 11 regions of the country.	—	—	Moderately and severely underweight schoolchildren selected.	To develop local capability to undertake a self-sustaining nutrition programme
Thailand National Nutrition Programme	1982-2001	GM Nutrition education Supplementary feeding Food Production School Nutrition programme ORT Immunization Antenatal care Control of anemia and IDD	National	In 1982 1 million In 1989 2.5 million	85% of all < 5 year olds 98% of rural villages attended GM during Jan-Mar 1989.	Preschool & school children Pregnant women; underweight children selected.	To improve nutritional status of mothers, infants, preschool and school children were the objectives for 1987-91.

Table III. Frequency (%) of types of activities to improve nutrition (n=15)		
Component	Number	Frequency %
Nut. Education	14	93
Health Services	11	73
Supplemental Feeding Programme (SFP)	12	80
Growth Monitoring (GM)	10	67
Micronut. Suppl.	4	27
Nut. home gardens	3	20
Sources: see Table II. Information on Chile and Cuba from Horwitz (1987).		

similarities between projects. The components of these projects are summarized in Table III.

Table II shows the duration, objectives and components of each
programme plus the target groups chosen and their coverage. An assessment
of the components of the 13 programmes, plus Chile and Cuba (Horwitz,
1987) reveals that 93% of them had nutrition/health education as one of their
activities (see Table III). The Supplementary Feeding Programmes formed
80% of the reported programme components. Health services including ORT,
immunization, deworming, treatment and control of gastrointestinal and infectious diseases were included in 73% of these cases (see Table III); and 67%
included growth monitoring.

It follows that the main types of activities included in intervention
programmes for nutritional improvement in infants and children would be
composed of one or more of the following:

Nutrition/Health education and counselling;

Supplementary feeding programmes;

Health services; and

Growth monitoring.

A brief description of what is involved in these activities is given next.

Nutrition Education

A high proportion of malnutrition results not only from food scarcity, but
also by incorrect nutritional practices, particularly in respect to the infant and
child feeding. Thus, it is possible to find, sometimes, malnourished children
in households with adequate food supplies, while -- as Haaga (1987) has
stated -- even very poor families have some resources which can be redirected
towards their children if it can be clearly and effectively demonstrated to them
that it will benefit their children's health and well-being.

Any communication system attempting to improve nutrition through enhancing knowledge and correcting related attitude and behavior is customarily termed nutrition education. These can include, - as summarized by Austin *et al.* (1978) -, mass media, non-formal face to face education or the combination of the two, formal education of adults, school children, health and other professionals and policy makers.

According to Hornik (1985), who has reviewed the results of the various evaluations of nutrition education programmes, more than the usual notions of nutrition education is currently incorporated in this field. Particularly effective, now recognized, is face-to-face nutrition education tailored to the individual needs and reinforced by right messages through various channels. Nutrition education is on most lists of potential policy options for malnutrition prevention and control. Table III shows, 93% of the 15 projects reviewed included nutrition education as one of the components necessary for achieving programme goals. Table II shows, nutrition education in most cases accompanies other approaches to nutrition intervention programmes (notably Growth Monitoring (GM)). However, it has been shown to have the potential of forming an effective intervention on its own (Ashworth and Feachem, 1985; Manoff, 1985; Devadas, 1987). Nevertheless, nutrition education as an independent intervention should only be implemented where inadequate knowledge is the primary cause of improper behavior with respect to the infant and child care practices, aiming to change the behavior, and not only nutritional attitudes and knowledge.

Supplementary Feeding Programmes (SFP)

These can be regarded as one of the most direct and the most common (in terms of the total number of beneficiaries reached) nutrition intervention programmes aiming at increasing food intake and improving nutritional status through non-commercial free or subsidized food distribution. Beneficiaries range from famine victims, households during economic/food crisis (economic recession, drought, seasonal food shortage) to nutritionally deficient individuals or communities. Target groups are usually nutritionally vulnerable groups mainly infants and preschool children, pregnant and nursing women, and malnourished, or individuals at risk of malnutrition *e.g.* during famine/drought. In school feeding programmes, school age children in poor areas, or communities form the target groups. There are different methods for food distribution, namely on-site, or take-home feeding programmes, and nutrition rehabilitation centers for severely malnourished subjects. The strengths and limitations of various ways of food supplementation and distribution have been investigated (Anderson *et al.*, 1981; Beaton and Ghassemi, 1982; Kennedy and Alderman, 1987; and others).

A variety of foods, both imported and/or locally produced have been distributed in such programmes. The ration is usually based on cereals and legume blends, but dried skim milk (DSM), sugar and oil are some other items reported to have been used (Beaton and Ghassemi, 1982). Either specific amounts of dry ingredients are collected by the beneficiaries at a regular intervals (weekly, bimonthly, monthly) on a take-home basis, or the supplement ration is prepared in the form of a meal/snack for daily (or 5 days/week) on-site consumption. The aim of a supplementary feeding programme is -theoretically- to compensate for the nutrient deficit of the current beneficiary's diet. Therefore, usually some kind of a dietary survey is first performed to determine current nutrient intakes in order to measure such deficits. In practice, however, many factors (mainly administrative) determine the actual amount of calories planned to be given and actually received by the intended beneficiaries (there is, for example, sharing, leakage,and substitution *etc.*). The calorie and protein contents of supplementary foods varies among different programmes. Beaton and Ghassemi (1982) have reported such variations ranged from 273 to almost 600 Kcal/day in some of the programmes they reviewed. According to Kennedy and Alderman (1987), the calories provided in different supplementary feeding programmes vary widely from 298 to 737, which would fill 67 to 88% of the estimated calorie gap respectively *if* totally consumed. The Integrated Child Development Services (ICDS) programme in India supplies moderately malnourished children with 300 Kcal and 8-10 grams of protein daily, for 300 days in a year. For pregnant and nursing women, the ration, in this programme, provides 500 Kcal plus 20-25 grams protein per day from the third trimester of pregnancy up to six months of lactation.

Another question is the optimum period of time necessary to give such assistance. Anderson *et al.* (1981) suggest at least one year is required for on-site and take-home programmes to show any effect. Similarly, Kennedy and Alderman (1987) recommend a length of one to two years of regular participation in both take-home and on-site feeding programmes for any significant effects resultant. A much shorter length of time, about 3-4 months, they suggest, is required for effective efforts taken in Nutrition Rehabilitation Centers, since here most of the nutrient needs of the child are provided and procedures can be closely supervised. The Tamil Nadu Programme in India (TNINP), however, provides supplementary foods for severely malnourished children under three years of age, for 90 days, extended to 120 days or more only in cases where response is slow. Growth monitoring is used in order to indicate when an individual child should be graduated from a feeding programme.

Apart from the actual food distribution, in other forms of supplementation it may be necessary to supply recipients with one or more micronutrients (Vitamin A, iodine, iron) in situations where either physiological needs have been raised (*e.g.* pregnancy, lactation) or related deficiency diseases are prevalent. These more specific types of supplementation are frequently performed in conjunction with health services.

Growth Monitoring (GM)

Frequent measurements and chart recordings of a young child's body weight (and less commonly so arm circumference, height *etc.*) have been used for early and timely detection of growth faltering in order to counsel, act and follow up results so that problems can be identified before they seriously affect health and nutritional status.

This strategy has gained much popularity in the last 2-3 decades and has been used in many countries as a means of detecting early and timely growth faltering of infants and young children. Such growth monitoring can be a diagnostic procedure, and also result in intervention leading to improved nutrition. More commonly, however, GM is used for screening purposes and in order to select beneficiaries for other nutrition intervention programmes, notably supplementary feedings. GM is also used as criteria for discharge from supplementary feeding programmes as well as admission into them. The procedure originated from clinic-based activities in Nigeria (Morley, 1973), yet it has caused controversy as regards its application, feasibility, cost and effectiveness (Gopalan and Chatterjee, 1985; Rohde, 1985 ; Yee and Zerfas 1987; Lotfi, 1988; Gerein, 1988; and others).

Although these controversies over GM have grown in recent years, the procedure has been shown to focus attention on at-risk children and to identify them before their health and nutritional status has seriously deteriorated.

Health Services

The close relationship between general health and nutrition means that interventions to improve both health and nutrition are compatible activities each reinforcing the effectiveness of the other. The health sector in reality has been one of the channels through which nutritional interventions have been implemented, like growth monitoring, micronutrient supplementation, promotion of breast-feeding and nutritional education and counselling. Here, the extent of health system coverage would be the main determinant as to whether substantial nutrition intervention efforts can reach those in need or not. In practice, health infrastructure in most developing countries suffers from serious inadequacies with respect to out-reach, coverage and both financial and manpower resources. In these cases other approaches need to be followed in order to cover the most out-reach and needy individuals as, for example, is done in the TNINP programme in India.

Increased nutritional requirements, anorexia, insufficient utilization and substantial losses of nutrients in diarrhoea are some of the nutritional effects of infectious and diarrhoeal diseases. Clearly, there are a range of health services to be included in heath-oriented programmes. The most useful of such programmes, with positive effects on nutrition, are immunization against communicable diseases, and control of diarrhoea and other infectious diseases. Thus, integrating health and nutrition programmes is believed to be the best approach for alleviating malnutrition problems in many situations.

Consideration of health services themselves, and their potential contribution to nutrition improvement, is beyond the scope of this chapter, but is well-covered in the literature (*e.g.* WHO, 1981). In summary, it should be understood that the nutrition programmes we discuss are frequently implemented through, or indeed are part of, health services. Perhaps growth monitoring, too, should equally be considered as a health or nutrition activity.

DESCRIPTION OF SOME LARGE-SCALE NUTRITION PROGRAMMES

In this section some details of six large-scale nutrition programmes are given, to illustrate the types of activities that are being carried out in different parts of the world. While we make no attempt here to assess their impact, the programmes have been evaluated - internally or externally - and reported to have achieved varying degrees of success (see also ACC/SCN 1989b).

Botswana Drought Relief Programme

In Botswana drought is a recurring phenomenon. For instance during the decades of 1970 - 1980, at least 4 and 6 years were drought years respectively (Moremi, 1988). However, Botswana suffers from inadequate food availability at the household level even when there is no drought. This situation has called for a permanent institutional organisation, recognition and establishment of which has been a major key factor in the Government's success to deal with problems that developed in earlier drought relief activities (Quinn *et al.*, 1988).

The Early Warning Technical Committee (EWTC) has had the responsibility to assess the incidence and severity of drought conditions and its consequences for the people all over the country. EWTC has also the task of formulating recommendations on types and amounts of drought recovery assistance required. The Inter-Ministerial Drought Committee (IMDC) coordinates activities of all the main Ministries and Departments in implementing relief programmes, based on EWTC reports and recommendations on current drought conditions. Distribution of food relief all over the country is the responsibility of a permanent food management and distribution office called the Food Resources Department. Three major activities of the drought relief programme (as described by Quinn *et al.*, 1988) are to deliver human, agricultural and human water relief. While all these components are equally important in the overall programme success, human relief programme activities are briefly described below being more relevant to the subject of this chapter.

The main components of human relief programmes are direct feeding, supplementary feeding and labor-based relief activities.

In remote areas, attempts have been made to re-habilitate severely malnourished children through direct on-site feeding (at health facilities) of several small daily meals providing daily nutritional requirements of these children. Only moderate success has so far been achieved with this approach as those in the greatest need of nutritional support are probably not reached effectively, as yet.

Food supplementary programmes provide food on a regular basis to specially vulnerable individuals under nutritional stress, for example, pregnant and nursing women, malnourished children under 5 years, primary school children, and tuberculosis patients. In drought years such programmes can be expanded to cover additional groups. Thus, during the drought period of 1981-1987, a programme covered all vulnerable groups in the rural areas with increased rations of supplementary foods. Moreover, the full adult daily energy and protein requirements of Remote Area Dwellers (RAD) were provided in the supplementary food rations. School and supplementary rations to the other groups, however, provided about one third of this amount. The Food Resources Department, responsible for distribution of the drought food relief throughout the country, has been successful in solving early logistical problems and also in reaching increasingly more vulnerable groups from 1982 to 1985.

The third component of the human relief programmes is labor-based relief which was complementary to food distribution programmes. This activity aims to supplement income by compensating the income lost due to drought and crop failure, and also to construct infrastructures necessary for increasing the income earning potential of the community. Cash for work is paid to those participating in work on projects selected by the Village Development Committee and approved by the relevant committee of the IMDC. This activity has been successful in creating almost equivalent number of work places lost as a result of the drought (Quinn *et al.* 1988), and by investment in socially useful and necessary infrastructures.

One important aspect of the Botswana drought relief programme is its coverage at a national level. For example, in the recent drought, 70% of the total population has received some type of food relief ration. The coverage of specific vulnerable groups was high, almost 100% for primary school children and over 80% of malnourished children under 5 years and around 48-64% of pregnant and nursing women. The majority of the rural Botswana people had indirectly benefited from labor-based relief programme and over 74,000 were paid during 1985-86 through this activity.

The extensive measures undertaken against drought in Botswana has two distinct benefits: First, it prevented widespread poverty and any sharp increase in malnutrition prevalence, and even, perhaps, decreasing it after some years of programme operation. Second, the effectiveness of these measures in combatting consequences of unfavorable economic and climatic conditions might have direct relevance to similar conditions in other countries.

Nutrition and Health Programmes in Costa Rica

Nutrition and health programmes have a long history in Costa Rica, and were substantially strengthened when a law of social development and family allowances was passed in 1974. This raised a 20% tax on most consumer transactions in the country, and allowed very substantial funding for nutrition and health programmes. There are two major programme types, which are considered distinctly (see Table II): these are the National Nutrition and Holistic Care Programme (NNHCP), and the Health and Social Development Programme (HSDP).

The NNHCP provides for a number of food programmes. The Ministry of Education provides for hot meals for school children, taking approximately half the NNHCP budget. Under the Ministry of Health, centers of education and nutrition also provide feeding and education, as do centers for integral child care, which cater particularly for working parents. Support for health centers, including milk distribution for pre-school children, provides the other component of this programme. In all, expenditure was nearly $9 million per year in 1982, increasing steadily to over $12 million in 1987. This amounts to over $20 per person per year, of which about half is used to purchase food. The coverage is wide, intended to be national, although outreach is incomplete in certain areas, but is estimated to reach some half a million children, that indicates rather complete coverage.

The HSDP has supported development of health services, particularly in rural areas. The coverage of the population in terms of primary health care is extensive, and substantial resources have been put into environmental health and sanitation. A network of hospitals and clinics in urban areas, and health centers and health posts in rural areas, has been developed by the Social Security Bureau and the Ministry of Health, and allows for effective referral. The cost of the HSDP is considered to be lower than that of the NNHCP, even allowing for the NNHCP food costs.

It is argued (Mata, 1989) that in Costa Rica priority should be given to health services, rather than to food distribution, on the grounds that inadequate food availability is no longer a major problem. This priority is used to support the argument that the health services are substantially more cost-effective than the nutrition programmes. It is conceded that the nutrition programmes have helped virtually to eliminate severe malnutrition, and indeed reduce moderate malnutrition to minor proportions. It is also suggested that the well-known significant and sustained improving trends in child health and survival in fact preceded the nutrition programmes. It may be that the experience of Costa Rica (see also Horwitz, 1987) provides lessons not only in the successful commitment to, and implementation of, health and nutrition programmes, but also to consider when during the process of development, it is most appropriate and effective to invest specifically in nutrition.

Tamil Nadu Integrated Nutrition Project (TNINP) in India

Although nutritional deficiencies are common almost across the board in Tamil Nadu, TNINP (with World Bank support) has adopted a strategy for identifying the most vulnerable and needy - that is severely underfed children (under three years) and pregnant and lactating women. This highly targeted programme (for a useful analysis, see Heaver, 1988) has set its main objective as reducing malnutrition and accompanied high mortality in under three year old children plus improving nutrition of pregnant and nursing mothers. Growth monitoring, health and nutrition education, short-term supplementary feeding and delivery of health care services and institutional building are the main components. To identify beneficiaries a double screening technique is used. Every three months, all households are surveyed and 6-36 months old children are registered for monthly growth monitoring. Those found to be malnourished (grade III and IV and recently also grade II) or not gaining adequate weight between successive weighings are registered as eligible for 90 days of supplementary feeding. Certain defined criteria are also used to select beneficiaries among pregnant and nursing women. To deliver nutritional services a Community Nutrition Center (CNC) is established in each village with an average population of 1500. The center is run by a Community Nutrition Worker (CNW). During growth monitoring sessions CNW administers Vitamin A prophylaxis and deworming drugs and checks on the health needs of the child (*e.g.* immunization, diarrhoeal management *etc.*).

In order simultaneously to upgrade the infrastructure and working skills of the existing health system, the following strategy has been adopted. A female Multipurpose Health Worker (MPHW) is assigned to every 4-5 villages (having about 5000 population). MPHW in the absence of a village-based health care worker, establishes a functional linkage between the nutrition and health care and social welfare systems through the CNW. The package of Maternal and Child Health services are likewise delivered by MPHW through the CNC.

The TNINP contains a very strong training component for both village workers and their supervisors. Nutrition services are delivered through an established infrastructure for selecting and training all those involved at various levels. Length of training time is, in contrast to many other projects, long enough and the components are reinforced further by on - job and in-field training and supervision. Employment of certain mechanisms enabled strong community participation in the programme. Some of these are criteria for CNW selection (to be a mother of a healthy child, village - resident with good communication ability), formation of Women's Working Groups and Children's Working Groups.

The regular collection, interpretation and analysis of data is supported through a management information system. A Project Co-ordination Office is responsible for the communication and monitoring activities. Data for compilation of the indicators flows from the village level to this office for review. Project monitoring and evaluation was intended to measure the degree of programme effectiveness in reaching its goals.

Tanzania Nutrition Programme (JNSP) in Iringa

Tanzania was one of the first countries to implement the WHO/UNICEF Joint Nutrition Support Programme (JNSP) in its Iringa region, with the aim of reducing infant and young child mortality and morbidity, through improving infants growth and development and maternal health and nutrition. The programme, locally known as the Iringa Nutrition Programme, was initiated in 1983 with funds from the Italian Government. A strong aspect of the programme was recognition of the fact that nutritional improvement should be achieved through increasing the society's capacity to assess and analyze these problems in order to establish appropriate actions to solve them. Thus, the conceptual framework to explain the causal relationship of various processes leading to malnutrition included what was known as a Triple-A-Cycle (Assessment, Analysis, Action). This was used to analyze the situation and to identify the most important causes for the problem and its solutions. Initial planning was based on this framework and all throughout the programme, processes of reassessment, reanalysis and modified actions continued at all levels from the village up to the central government.

The existing administrative structures were used to integrate programme management with Iringa Regional Development Director (RDD) as the overall manager. Initially a Management Team was established under the leadership of the Programme Co-ordinator with representatives from the Prime Minister's Office, the Ministries of Health, Agriculture, Education and the Tanzania Food and Nutrition Center. The decentralization of the programme was considered beneficial, therefore in 1986 the Management Team became known as the Regional Iringa Nutrition Support Team, providing required support to facilitate the transition of managerial responsibilities to the Districts. The Divisional and Ward secretaries, both Party and Government functionaries, played an important role in programme implementation at sub-district level. Every three months, the Village Health Workers reported data on growth monitoring and mortality - collected during community-based nutrition monitoring activities - to the Village Council and the Village Health Committees. Data gathered from this activity were first discussed at the village level, for problem/intervention identification, before being transferred to higher administrative levels. Village-based nutritional status and a death monitoring system served as a basis for decision making at higher administrative levels with respect to continuous monitoring of the effectiveness of the programme.

The components of the programme were: growth monitoring; nutrition education with emphasis on regular feeding; maternal and child health care including weaning food preparation; household food security through various activities including household food production, processing, storage, *etc*; income generation involving access to credit, *etc*; and environmental sanitation.

An extensive mid-term review in 1986, confirmed the effectiveness of the basic strategy and helped to make some modification of the programme structure. Outcome evaluation used information from the continuous assessment through a quarterly growth monitoring system, quarterly programme implementation/evaluation report, mid-term review and external evaluation and special studies on impact by National Institutions. The experience of the Iringa Nutrition programme in using a multisectoral approach to the malnutrition problem resulted in decreasing mortality - by establishing a community-based growth monitoring system, a village-based rehabilitation system for severely malnourished children, and increased immunization coverage *etc.* - This proved to be highly successful. Expansion of this experience to the other regions of the country has, thus, become a national decision in order to attack nutritional and health problems.

Supplementary Food Production Programme (SFPP) in Zimbabwe

Promotion of community awareness of nutritional problems, particularly in children of less than five years of age, and encouraging actions to address these problems through community mobilization and self-reliance were the main objectives for this programme. This programme emphasized supplementary feeding and weight monitoring of children under five. Appropriate technologies were used for food production using community participation and nutrition education aimed at providing nutritious foods with local available resources. External funds became available from Swedish International Development Agency (SIDA) through the Nutrition Unit in the Ministry of Health. The programme, started in 1981 on a pilot scale, has now extended to cover most districts having over 6000 ongoing projects nationwide. To meet nutritional goals, the programme adopted an intersectoral approach for organization and management. The project is implemented by the Intersectoral Committee under the chairmanship of the Ministry of Agriculture, with the Nutrition Unit of the Ministry of Health performing secretariat duties. Intersectoral Management Committees were set up at all levels to ensure effective programme implementation. Active participation of the major sectors like agriculture, community development, local government, education *etc.* strengthened the nutritional and health services offered to communities by extension workers. Initiation of activities for development of a Food and Nutrition Policy for the country has been one of the main duties of the National Intersectoral Committee. The programme has been successful in integrating nutrition into a broader development process.

Evaluation of the SFPP pilot project by a joint SIDA/Zimbabwe team in 1984 identified a number of needed improvements in planning and implementation. Lack of clear guidelines for programme implementation and a clearly defined mechanism for programme monitoring was noted. The programme was thus restructured particularly with respect to clarifying roles and responsibilities of the various sectors. A management Handbook was produced and a training strategy was adopted to overcome lack of clear objectives and guidelines. A process evaluation has been undertaken by the National Nutrition Unit early in 1989 to assess progress of the programme.

WHAT HAS BEEN ACHIEVED?

Nearly a decade has passed since Gwatkin and his colleagues (in the preface to their valuable monograph entitled "Can health and nutrition interventions make a difference?" published in 1980) raised the question: "Is our experience to date with health and nutrition intervention encouraging enough to justify augmented efforts to make primary nutrition and health care available to all?" Evaluating such programmes has been attempted by many trying to answer this same fundamental question on usefulness and effectiveness of direct intervention. This has proved no easy task. The diversity of nutrition/health projects regarding their approaches, magnitude, available resources, infrastructures, and the like, has made the evaluation of their impact on nutritional improvement difficult.

Gwatkin's answer - and others since, notably Beaton & Ghassemi (1982) - was a qualified "yes." Much of the information available at that time came from relatively small-scale programmes. Only quite recently have large-scale routine programmes been running for long enough that one can begin to consider the place of nutrition programmes as regular government activities.

In their extensive review of the literature on this subject, Beaton and Ghassemi (1982) have posed another question in relation to the first one: "What benefit should be expected in the individual or population," from an effective intervention, hence what should be measured? They argued that "the spectrum of potential effects of under-nutrition poses serious problems in the evaluation of the effectiveness of a food distribution programme," for example. Thus they concluded that presently available programme evaluations may in fact *underestimate* the real impact of the programme under review.

Results summarized by Austin *et al.* (1978), Habicht and Butz (1979), Drake *et al.* (1980), Gwatkin *et al.* (1980), Beaton and Ghassemi (1982), Berg (1987), Kennedy and Alderman (1987) and others provide the evidence that detectable changes do occur. Generally speaking, supplementary feeding programmes have often brought about at least some degree of success. In these cases they are likely to have contributed to increased growth rates reducing mortality and morbidity, and even to improved cognitive development in children (Gopaldas *et al.*, 1975; Freeman *et al.*, 1980; Kennedy and Pinstrup-Andersen, 1983; and others).

Gwatkin *et al.* (1980) analyzed 10 projects (generally pilot-scale) that they selected as being well-controlled and implemented. They concluded that, generally speaking, by effective implementation and careful design such programmes can decrease infant and child mortality and improve growth rates. Beaton and Ghassemi (1982) while not sharing this view directly, concluded that although food distribution programmes are rather expensive for the measured benefits "it would be deemed unwise to withdraw such food distribution programmes until there has been opportunity to assess their true effects and benefits." They focused their attention on reviewing over 200 reports on different types of supplementary feeding programmes for young children in developing countries. The objective of this exercise was mainly to learn from past experiences in order to improve planning and management of future programmes. Their general impression, gained from reviewing the literature, was that food distribution programmes directed towards young children, as being operated at the time of their study, have a rather disappointing overall impact. Particularly because a) only 10 to 25% of the estimated energy gap (instead of the 40 to 70% it was designed to meet) was closed for the target population as a whole, b) the programmes reviewed were not effective in reaching older infants and young children below the age of 2 years, and c) food distribution is inherently less efficient than feeding in targeting supplementary food to the intended beneficiaries.

Berg (1987) examined four large World Bank-assisted nutrition projects in depth. Survey was made on some 57 nutrition actions, that were components or sub-components of other Bank-assisted projects. Further, 75 items of nutrition related research supported by the Bank, and nutrition analyses in the Bank's economic and sector working were also surveyed. The four large projects were Tamil Nadu Integrated Nutrition Project (TNINP) in India; Nutrition Development Project (NIPP) in Indonesia; Integrated Nutrition Improvement Project in Colombia; and finally, Food Subsidy (PINS) and Pre-school Feeding and Education (PROAPE) in Brazil. He concluded that the delivery of nutrition services in Tamil Nadu, India; Nutrition Education in Indonesia; Pre-school Feeding and Stimulation (PROAPE) in Brazil; anemia control in Indonesia and the subsidy and marketing efficiency programmes (PINS, PROAPE) in Brazil, have worked most smoothly.

The JNSP nutrition programme in Iringa, Tanzania, is reported as a successful intervention. Data from the community-based monitoring system revealed that between 1984 and '88 severe malnutrition declined by as much as 70% and moderate malnutrition by 32%. But prevalence of both moderate and severe malnutrition in 442 villages in Iringa, outside the programme, had remained at the 1984 level. The percentage of severely underweight children decreased from 6.3% to 1.8 from 1984 to 1988. The infant mortality rate decreased similarly from 152 in 1984 to 107 in 1988, mainly as a result of decrease in number of deaths due to measles and diarrhoea. The programme also successfully increased full immunization rate from 50% to 96%. The programme is now planned to expand to other districts in the country.

Similarly, the Applied Nutrition Education Programme (ANEP) in the Dominican Republic was successful in reducing malnutrition prevalence by 31-43% in two to three years. Positive changes in mothers' behavior (*e.g.* increased breast-feeding, later introduction of supplements *etc.*) were observed. Significant differences were found between programme and non-programme participants.

The Tamil Nadu nutrition programme showed remarkable impact on physical growth, malnutrition prevalence and infant mortality rates. Further, as a result of programme operations, immunization rates increased from 44 to 88%. At the end of the project, ¼ instead of ⅓ of those weighed needed to be fed. This was an indication of positive programme impact on children's weight gain. The programme had a long-term effect as four and five year old children were still about 2 kg heavier than controls. (*i.e.* one to two years after graduation from the programme).

The Botswana Drought Relief programme has produced impressive results. At the beginning of the drought period (1982-88), and before intervention could have any effect, there was an observed increase in the prevalence of malnutrition, which appeared to fall in 1984 to just below the pre-drought levels of 25-30%. At the end of the drought in June 1988 national prevalence of underweight stood at 16% (Maribe, 1989) -- although it is not clear whether this figure is directly comparable with earlier data due to changes in the reporting system. Thus even under the unfavorable conditions of drought, the programme was able to control malnutrition.

In general -- and it is not the purpose here to review evaluation results -- there is a growing conviction that direct nutrition interventions *can* be effective under the right conditions. A key feature of success is appearing, well put by Heaver (1988) specifically in the context of nutrition programmes: "... the interests of the poor might best be served by a lowering of the policy makers' and program implementors' sights towards the daily realities of work in villages and slums, and the specific detail of designing doable jobs and providing adequate support for field workers and community volunteers."

FACTORS CONTRIBUTING TO THE PROGRAMMES' SUCCESS/FAILURE

The exact criteria for defining a successful programme are still unclear and the extent to which the various programmes have been considered to be effective, or otherwise, still differ. Nevertheless, certain specific measures, or features of programmes, have repeatedly been associated with useful outcomes. Such features are given in the literature (Gwatkin *et al.*, 1980; Beaton and Ghassemi, 1982; Kennedy and Alderman, 1987; and others). Highlighting the factors that appear to be responsible for the observed discrepancies in achieved outcomes, is necessary in order to improve on future efforts while learning from the past experiences. Certain factors that seem important are discussed below.

Objectives

One major determinant of programme success is the clarity of the programme objectives. Beaton and Ghassemi (1982) have stated that "a serious failing of many programmes now operating is that the real objectives have not been clearly identified and probably have not been sufficiently considered in programme design." Surely, all decisions, operational design and the selection of evaluation procedure should relate to the main programme objective, which should be explicit and agreed upon before programme implementation. For instance, in Zimbabwe, one of the key weaknesses of SFPP became apparent upon evaluation after three years of programme operation when the lack of clear objectives and guide-lines were found.

Too ambitious objectives should be avoided. Actions and efforts should be concentrated on a few critical problems. In practice, the less successful efforts are mainly those that do not concentrate on dealing with specific problems in specifically defined target populations.

Choice of what intervention to undertake should be based on careful analysis of the nature of the problem itself and of its related factors. There is evidence of failure due to having overlooked such very basic factors. As an example, when the primary cause of underweight is not food insufficiency, a supplementary feeding programme, no matter how well planned and performed, will have little or no impact on increasing body weights. In Costa Rica, NNHCP had little observable impact on malnutrition, because the cause of this problem was not food deprivation but presence of infection and disease.

Kennedy and Aldermen (1987) emphasize that if the programme objective is, for example, to increase or to maintain family calorie consumption in general, a well implemented food subsidy programme would be effective, but such programmes usually are much less effective for treating severely malnourished children. It follows that it might be inappropriate to evaluate successes of a food subsidy programme by measuring changes in the nutritional status of the severely malnourished.

Leadership and Management

Successfully conducted projects could not do without dedicated, strong and competent leaders who are capable of mobilizing communities, selecting the right individuals and being able to give them support and motivation.

Good administration is also needed for systematic mobilization and management of multiple resources to ensure effective implementation (Austin and Zeitlin, 1981). Effective programmes, as in India or Botswana, have also enjoyed strong political support. As Gwatkin *et al.* (1980) put it: "... a health and nutrition programme's overall effectiveness is likely to depend not just on what is done but also on how well it is done. The need is not just for an appropriate mix of programme components, but for an appropriate mix of effectively administered programme components."

Training and Supervision

Effective training of those involved in a programme operation is, obviously, an important feature of a successful programme. In fact, of the programmes listed in Table II, those having greater impact on the nutritional improvement of the recipients were those having also a strong training and supervision element in their initial planning (*e.g.* TNINP in India; Drought Relief Programme of Botswana; JSNP in Tanzania; ANEP in Dominican Republic). It is reported that the unusually strong training programme in the TNINP was the key to the success of that programme and its potential for long-term effects (Berg, 1987). Two aspects of training seem to be related to success in a more pronounced way. First, a long enough length of training performed in a systematic manner, and, second, relevant on-job and in-field training. Projects in Gambia and Thailand provided only a few days to one week of training, while ICDS programme in India tend to give such instructions to the field workers for as long as 3 months, and in TNINP (India) for two months. Another aspect is re-training of workers that has been given much attention in some projects (ANEP, TNINP *etc*).

Staff-to-client and supervision ratios need to be realistic. In the Indian programmes reviewed by Heaver (1988), worker-client ratios were around 1:200-300 families; supervision ratios were around 1:10.

Coverage

The effectiveness of a programme depends on how well it can reach those individuals or groups it intends to reach. For projects listed in Table II the more effective programmes managed to cover a great majority of their targeted population.

The ICDS Programme in India was able to cover 40% and 30% of malnourished pre-school children, and pregnant and nursing women respectively, all throughout the country. TNINP Programme covered over 90% of 6-36 months old children for GM in the state of Tamil Nadu, and succeeded in feeding 95% of them. The two programmes are not directly comparable since their scale of operation is widely different. In Botswana, the Drought Relief Programme could cover close to 100% of highly vulnerable individuals.

Targeting

The targeted programmes are most likely to demonstrate observable impacts (*e.g.* Food Subsidy scheme in the Philippines and in Colombia; TNINP, India). Most of the targeted programmes in Table II have used biological targeting procedures based on age and increased physiological needs (UPGK, Indonesia; WIC, USA; Drought Relief Programme and many others) as well as geographical targeting to high risk areas. Among these, those having a double targeting procedure by selecting malnourished individuals (usually from growth monitoring) have been considered more cost effective (TNINP, ANEP, Botswana Drought Relief Programme, *etc*).

Community Mobilization

No intervention can be implemented effectively in a community where the need for beneficial outcome is not felt by the population, and a demand for it is not created. Much of the success achieved in nutrition programmes such as those in Iringa (Tanzania), TNINP (India), Alternative School Nutrition Programme (ASNP) (The Philippines) *etc* was in fact related to active community participation. In the ASNP programme in The Philippines, families supported the intervention programme by producing foods and generating income to pay for the supplementary feeding of malnourished children, with improvements of school canteens and the like. Women's and children's Working Groups in TNINP, or making efficient use of community volunteers in Indonesia, are examples of effective ways in which the community can be mobilized.

Closely related to the above, is making use of local village workers - given adequate training, support or supervision - as a means of winning villagers' confidence in the programme goals. In India, great emphasis was put on selecting nutrition/health workers from local volunteers. Other successful projects in Jamaica, Guatemala, India, Iran, have all made good use of local trained workers (see Gwatkin *et al.*, 1980; Heaver, 1988).

Process Monitoring and Evaluation

Monitoring the process of programme operation in order to modify policy and adopted decisions should be responsible for - or can at least enhance - the programme effectiveness. For instance, Gwatkin *et al.* (1980) have reported that a process evaluation found that an initial emphasis on formal training led village health workers in the Kavar project in Iran to become primarily interested in curative services, paying little attention to preventive and public health activities. This was corrected before it could adversely affect the programme's effectiveness.

Among projects listed in Table II, in Zimbabwe, the process evaluation led to identification of both strengths and weaknesses of SFPP. This facilitated the restructuring of the programme in order to eliminate the observed limitations. In Costa Rica, on the other hand, a lack of process evaluation of NNHCP was said to have resulted in operation of a rather ineffective programme for many years. In Gambia, such evaluation was responsible to shifting recently the target group from under 5 year old children to pregnant and nursing women and under 2 year old infants in order to increase the programme effectiveness.

Integration of Health and Nutrition

A judicious mix of nutrition and health components have worked best in achieving programme's goals. Many of the projects reviewed have shown the beneficial linking of the two for a higher cost effectiveness and greater impact (Gwatkin *et al.*, 1980; Berg, 1987). The rationale behind this is the well-known interaction between nutrition and infection (Scrimshaw *et al.*, 1968; ACC/SCN, 1989c) and administrative considerations for the delivery of services.

COSTS AND EFFECTS

Certainly, no matter how effective these programmes might be, they should be affordable and within the means of governments in countries where implementation is intended. This is crucially important if these efforts are to be sustained after external assistance, if in place, has been withdrawn.

Cost assessment is perhaps one of the most difficult aspects of any programme evaluations. There are always hidden expenditures like cost to the beneficiary. For example, time spent for travelling and waiting in line, time and money spent to better look after children or family as a result of education received, cost of volunteers' time and energy, and the like. Theoretically, costs to the beneficiary using services, should be set against the costs the beneficiary has saved through participation in any effective intervention. Examples are having a better pregnancy and lactation outcome, having a healthier child, less episodes of diseases in the family, use of knowledge gained in the areas of nutrition and health for siblings not in the programme, or benefits for the family as a whole, and so forth.

The problem of cost comparing of different programmes is not only related to the variations in their objectives, components, or size but also to the differences in the whole context and environment in which these have been implemented. Cross-project comparisons are therefore complex.

Actually, costs or related data are seldom addressed in individual nutrition intervention programme reports. In cases where such data are available, cost components (food and non-food costs, management costs, *etc.*) have often not been distinguished clearly. Total costs, even when reported, have limited value by themselves. Frequently the cost of reaching an individual using the provided services (cost per beneficiary or recipient per year) is calculated (see Table IV), and this provides for some standardization for comparative purposes. But this measure has a number of limitations. Firstly, it does not reflect the quality of services provided, neither does it show whether the programme has any impact on the recipients. Moreover, the cost/beneficiary may change over time. In Tamil Nadu the cost/child in the programme fell by 19% between 1982 and 1985. Here, from the cost per beneficiary value alone it is not clear whether this has been due to a change in coverage, or as it has been in fact the case, fewer children required rehabilitation feeding as a result of the programme positive impact on the recipients. Secondly, from the cost per beneficiary value it is not known how many of the beneficiaries were in fact targeted. Methods for assessing effectiveness of targeting have been described by Mason *et al.* (1984). Third, there is a trade-off between close targeting to those who will respond (*e.g.* the most underweight in a feeding programme), the costs of this targeting, and the lowered effectiveness if many non-responders being included among the beneficiaries. For this reason in many supplementary feeding programmes the cost per individual enrolled in the programme has been several times lower than the cost calculated for those actually having been helped by the programme.

Previous reviews of nutrition programmes have tried to estimate costs-per-beneficiary, as well as per-caput, in project areas. We will focus on the former. Beaton and Ghassemi (1982) have calculated that, generally the cost of providing 300-400 Kcal/day would range from $15 to $25 per child (1976 US$ equivalent). They noted that the cost would be different for different types of food distribution. Anderson *et al.* (1981) reported a somewhat wider range: $10-30/year per child fed in take-home and on-site feeding program-

Country/ Project	Main Programme Components	Cost per Beneficiary	Notes and Sources
Table IV. Approximate annual costs of selected nutrition intervention programmes (US$)			
Philippines/ Subsidy	Consumer food subsidy	9	1984, quoted from Garcia and Pinstrup-Anderson (1987)
Botswana/ Drought Relief Programme	Direct feeding; cash for work, water, livestock, and agricultural relief	7	1985, Direct feeding programme
		38	1985, for all programmes
			Quoted from Quinn *et al.* (1988)
Tanzania/JNSP	GM	17	1987, calculated from 1983-1988 JNSP Evaluation Report (1988)
Dominican Republic/ANEP	GM, SFP, nutrition and health services	25	Quoted from Kennedy and Alderman (1987)
India TNINP	GM, SFP, health services	9	overall cost
		7	weighing-screening (Calculated from Balachander, 1989)
		12	weighing-feeding (from Berg, 1987)
ICDS	GM, SFP, health services	7.5	1989, not including food. Calculated from Chatterjee (1989). Based on central funds allocations to the states.
Costa Rica NNHCP	Feeding, nutrition education	21	1982, quoted from Mata (1989)
HSDP	Health service	2	1982, calculated from Mata (1989)
		3	1983
Colombia	Food Subsidy	35	1981, quoted from Berg (1987)
	SFP	42	1982, quoted from Kennedy and Alderman (1987)
Indonesia UPGK	GM, SFP	2	Weighing
		11	Weighing and feeding Quoted from Yee and Zerfas (1987)
NIPP	GM, SFP	13	Screening
		56	Screening and feeding. Quoted from Berg (1987)
Brazil PINS	Food subsidy	21	1980, quoted from Berg (1987)
PROAPE	Feeding and education	47	1980, quoted from Berg (1987)
Sri Lanka	Food stamp	9	1982, quoted from Garcia and Pinstrup-Anderson (1987)
Gambia	GM, food supplement, nutrition health education	55	Calculated from TAAL (1989)

mes. Kennedy and Alderman (1987) have estimated the costs of delivering a certain number of calories and found that this would change somewhat the overall picture. They have cited the examples from two programmes in the Philippines. The average cost of Mother and Child Health Programme at US$ 31.4/beneficiary is higher than the cost of the School Feeding Programme at US$12 per person, but in terms of the delivery of 1000 Kcal the former programme becomes cheaper than the latter (US$ 0.25 vs. 0.43). Seven out of the ten studies reviewed by Gwatkin et al. (1980) had reported cost values, although cost per person in the project area could not always be distinguished from cost per beneficiary (Wilcox, personal communication). In all the seven projects discussed, nutritional services were complemented by health measures with the exception of a project in Etimesgut, Turkey where services were predominantly medical support and family planning. The annual per capita costs of these projects ranged from $0.8 to $7.5. Among the World Bank assisted projects, the Indonesian Nutrition Education Programme cost only $4 per beneficiary per year initially, decreasing to $2 during expansion (Berg, 1987). These calculations are based without the cost of food provision, but when food cost is added the total cost would be around $11/beneficiary/year (Yee and Zerfas, 1987). The Indonesian weighing and feeding program (NIPP), at $56/beneficiary/year, was much more expensive. Ashworth and Feachem (1985) have cited annual costs of weaning education in 6 countries, most projects falling in the range of $2-10 per participating child per year. They point out that these costs are not directly comparable, due to differences in programme design and methods of cost calculations. They concluded, however, that weaning education may be an economically attractive diarrhoeal control measure in some countries.

The cost of controlling micronutrient deficiencies have been estimated as being very low when compared to dramatic benefits usually obtained, and the cost is mainly cost of delivery rather than supply. The cost of delivery, itself, depends on targeting strategies and availability of services. For vitamin A capsules, the costs have been estimated as 2 cents/beneficiary/year. This would be increased to 40 cents for capsule dose taken (ACC/SCN, 1987b). Salt iodization from the experience in S.E. Asia cost 5 cents/beneficiary/year, while intramuscular oil injection is reported to cost twice this figure in such programmes in Zaire and Nepal (ACC/SCN, 1988, p.15). Fortification of salt with iron costs 5-9 cents/beneficiary/year, and that of centrally processed grain products with vitamins and minerals would cost about 8 cents/person/year (Berg, 1987).

Annual cost per beneficiary estimates available for the programmes reviewed here are summarized in Table IV. An important factor explaining the differences between amounts is whether or not food (or feeding) costs are included. Generally the health and education programmes have the lowest cost/beneficiary/year, but then these are less directed toward undernutrition. Overall, the amounts are in line with -- if somewhat higher than -- those calculated from previous studies, that were generally smaller-scale projects. But they tend to confirm that the range of $10 - $30 per beneficiary per year is around that needed for programmes that are of sufficient scale to be likely to have a positive effect. One conclusion from this is that it has to be considered worth sustaining an expenditure of about this magnitude if direct nutrition programmes are to be undertaken.

The expected relationship between expenditure and effects is non-linear, a minimum level being needed to begin to affect nutrition (Habicht, Mason and Tabatabai, 1984). We can now start to calculate this relationship, considering that the range in which effect increases with expenditure may indeed be this estimate of $10 - $30.

IMPLICATIONS FOR FUTURE PROGRAMME POLICIES

Large-scale nutrition programmes are becoming routine in a number of countries. We have not tried here to bring together the experience of impact evaluation -- indeed this would be very useful -- but accepted that enough is known to support the view that such programmes are having beneficial effects on nutrition. Perhaps even more important, there is now a basis for more extensive and more effective programmes that will contribute to a significant reduction in malnutrition, particularly in some conditions in poorer countries. The situation has matured from the earlier Applied Nutrition Programmes through carefully designed and monitored pilot projects, together with a proliferation of small-scale projects, to the point where major efforts have been sustained for several years, and are continuing.

When are direct nutrition interventions appropriate? The experience outlined in this chapter suggests some answers. First, when food intake is a constraint, but not otherwise. That is, there are periods in the course of development when large numbers of families, and individuals notably women and children, just do not have enough of the right quality food to eat. Second, when there is a minimum level of organizational infrastructure on which to build programmes. This may, as in the Tanzania project, be the community itself -- but even in this case some substantial external input was needed to realize the potential. Perhaps it is sometimes the combination of *potential* organization and the willingness of others to support this. Third, when the resources needed are considered affordable, and in long-run terms. Too many programmes have been started and then not sustained.

Thus, at crucial times in the development of societies it may be particularly effective to tackle malnutrition in this direct way. It is argued, for example, that in Costa Rica direct food distribution may now be less of a priority than health targeted measures. On the other hand, in some of the poorest countries it may as yet be impossible to achieve the level of effort needed for direct programmes to be widely feasible, and then less direct methods, including production inputs, general food distribution, and indeed building up health infrastructure, may be pre-requisites to establishing large-scale direct nutrition intervention programmes.

Broad features of the design of nutrition intervention projects are becoming similar across programmes, and increasingly it is to the details of organization that attention is directed. Increased importance is being attached to factors such as staff-to-client and supervision ratios; criteria for entry to (and exit from) programmes; methods of communication; and other logistic matters. After a review of recent experiences, the following are considered major items when discussing design. First, the possible *objectives* of nutrition interventions are diverse. They can include not only nutrition improvement for supporting child growth, but also fostering optimum development through activity in the pre-school period, and during school; the nutrition of women, not only in relation to child-bearing and rearing, is gaining in priority; the income transfer effects of nutrition programmes is another possible objective. Clarifying such objectives and deciding their priority is essential.

Targeting methods evolve towards those that are simple to implement. Thus, almost all large-scale programmes now target by area, and then by age/sex -- usually pre-school children and their mothers. Selection as a final stage of targeting is common but not universal, and its place should depend on the objectives. Many programmes combine this with growth monitoring, so that children whose growth is faltering are selected for special treatment. This has clear advantages in terms of focussing resources. In some cases the targeting procedure changes as needs change, and this capability for flexible management is useful.

Third, the crucial interaction between nutrition and infection (see ACC/SCN, 1989c) is as important now as ever, and better understood. The key place of nutritional intervention in the prevention and management of many diseases means that nutrition activities have to become part of the means available for *health services* that aim at reducing morbidity and mortality.

Finally, it is striking that successful nutrition programmes not only need to be sustained into the future, but it is their long life itself that has allowed them to gradually adapt and become more effective. Long-term support, to allow programme management to solve problems and develop better methods for outreach and delivery -- without fundamentally altering their main approach -- has been crucial. Effective programmes do not just spring into existence. They depend on the long haul, and on the efforts of dedicated individuals, to whom, indeed, many women and children reached by these programmes owe their better health, and sometimes their lives.

REFERENCES

ACC/SCN. *Report on the Twelfth Session of the ACC Subcommittee on Nutrition and its Advisory Group on Nutrition*. ACC/1986/PG/10. Tokyo, 7-11 April, 1986. ACC/SCN, c/o FAO, Rome. (1986).

ACC/SCN. *First Report on the World Nutrition Situation*. ACC/SCN. United Nations Administrative Committee on Coordination/ Sub-Committee on Nutrition (ACC/SCN), November 1987. (1987a).

ACC/SCN. *Delivery of Oral Doses of Vitamin A to Prevent Vitamin A Deficiency and Nutritional Blindness. A State-of-the-Art Review*. By K. P. West and A. Sommer. United Nations Administrative Committee on Coordination/ Sub-Committee on Nutrition (ACC/SCN). ACC/SCN State of the Art Series. Nutrition Policy Discussion Paper No. 2, June, 1987. (1987b).

ACC/SCN. *Supplement on Methods and Statistics to the First Report on the World Nutrition Situation*. United Nations Administrative Committee on Coordination/Sub-Committee on Nutrition. December 1988. (1988).

ACC/SCN. *Update on the Nutrition Situation, Recent Trends in Nutrition in 33 Countries*. United Nations Administrative Committee on Coordination/ Sub-Committee on Nutrition. January/February 1989. (1989a).

ACC/SCN. ACC/SCN Workshop on Managing Successful Nutrition Programmes. In: *IUNS 14th International Nutrition Conference*. 20-25 August 1989. Seoul, Korea. (1989b). Proceedings Forthcoming ACC/SCN (1990).

ACC/SCN. *Malnutrition and Infection: A Review*. By A. Tomkin and F. Watson. United Nations Administrative Committee on Coordination/ Sub-Committee on Nutrition. The State-of-the-Art Review. Nutrition Policy Discussion Paper No. 5. (1989c).

Anderson, M. A.; Austin, J. E.; Wray, J. D., and Zeitlin, M. F. Supplementary Feeding. In: *Nutrition Intervention In Developing Countries. An Overview*. Austin, J. E. and Zeitlin, M. F. (eds.), Cambridge, MA, Oelgeschlager, Gunn and Hain. (1981).

Anderson, M. A. Targeting of Food Aid From a Field Perspective. In: *Nutritional Aspects of Project Food Aid*. M. Forman (Ed.). United Nations ACC/Sub-Committee on Nutrition. Rome, Italy. (1986).

Ashworth, A. and Feachman, R. G. Interventions for the control of diarrhoeal diseases among young children: weaning education. *Bull. World Health Organization* 63:6:1115-1127. (1985).

Austin, J. E., Anderson, M. A.,Goldman, R., Heimendinger, J. Overholt, C., Pyle, D., Rogers, B., Wray, J., and Zeitlin, M. *Nutritional Intervention Assessment and Guidelines. Harvard Institute for International Development*. United Nations ACC/ Sub-Committee on Nutrition. June, 1978. (1978).

Austin, J. E. and Zeitlin M. F. *Nutrition Intervention In Developing Countries. An Overview.* Cambridge, Mass., Oelgeschlager, Gunn and Hain. (1981).

Balachander, J. *Tamil Nadu Integrated Nutrition Project.* Paper presented at the ACC/SCN Workshop, Seoul, ACC/SCN (1989b), op. cit.

Beaton, G. H. and Ghassemi, H. Supplementary Feeding Programs for Young Children in Developing Countries. *American Journal of Clinical Nutrition.* 35: 864-916. (1982).

Berg, A. *Malnutrition: what can be done? Lessons from World Bank Experience.* World Bank Publication, Johns Hopkins University Press, Baltimore and London. (1987).

Corina, G. A., Jolly, R., and Stewart, F. (Eds.) *Adjustment with a Human Face, Volume I: Protecting the Vulnerable and Promoting Growth.* Clarendon Press, Oxford. (1987).

Cornia, G. A., Jolly, R., and Stewart, F. (Eds.). *Adjustment with a Human Face, Volume II, Ten country case studies.* Clarendon Press, Oxford. (1988).

Devadas, R. P. Currently Available Technologies in India to Combat Vitamin A Malnutrition. See ACC/SCN (1987b), op. cit., pp 97-104.

Drake, W. D. *et al. Final Report: Analysis of Community-Level Nutrition Programmes. Vol. 1.* Washington D. C. US Agency for International Development. (1980).

Fraser, D. R. *A Brief Report on Vitamin D-Deficiency Rickets.* Paper presented at annual meeting of Advisory Group on Nutrition, Sub-Committee on Nutrition. Geneva, 19-21 September, 1989. ACC/SCN. (1989).

Freeman, H. E., Klein, R. E., Townsend, J. W., and Lechtig, A. Nutrition and Cognitive Development Among Rural Guatemalan Children. *American J. of Public Health,* 70:1277-1285. December, 1980 (1980).

Garcia, M. and Pinstrup-Anderson, P. *The Pilot Food Price Subsidy Scheme in the Philippines: Its Impact on Income, Food Consumption and Nutritional Status.* Research Report 61, International Food Policy Research Institute, August 1987. (1987).

Gerein, N. Is Growth Monitoring Worthwhile? *Health Policy and Planning,* 3:181-194. Oxford University Press. (1988).

Gopaldas, T., Lansra, A. C., Srinivasan, N., Varadarajan, I., Shingwekar, A. G., Seth, R., Mathur, R. S., and Bhargava, V. *Project Poshak, Vol. 1.* New Delhi: CARE. (1975).

Gopalan, C. and Chatterjee, M. *Use of Growth Charts for Promoting Child Nutrition: A Review of Global Experience.* Special Publication Series 2, New Delhi:Nutrition Foundation of India. (1985).

Gwatkin, D. R., Wilox, J. R., and Wray, J. D. *Can Health and Nutrition Intervention Make a Difference?* Monograph 13, Overseas Development Council, Washington, D. C., Feb. 1980. (1980).

Haaga, J. *Priorities for Policy Research on Nutrition Intervention in Primary Health Care.* RAND Publication F-7378, RAND Corporation, Santa Monica, California, USA, , March. 1987. (1987).

Habicht, J-P. and Butz, W. P. Measurement of Health and Nutrition Effects in Large-scale Nutrition Intervention Projects. In: Kelin, R. E. *et al.,* eds. *Evaluating the Impact of Nutrition and Health Programs.* New York, Plenum Press. (1979).

Habicht, J-P., Mason, J. B., and Tabatabai, H. Basic Concepts for the Design of Evaluation during Programme Implementation. In: Sahn D. and Lockwood R. (Eds.) *Methods for the Evaluation of the Impact of Food and Nutrition Programmes.* pp 1-25. UNU, Tokyo. (1984).

Heaver, R. *Improving Family Planning, Health and Nutrition Outreach in India: Lessons From Some World Bank Assisted Projects.* Population, Human Resources, Urban and Water Operations Division. India Country Department, New Delhi Office. (1988).

Hornik, R. C. *Nutrition Education.* A State-of-the-Art Review, ACC/SCN State-of-the-Art Series, Nutrition Policy Discussion, Paper No. 1, ACC/SCN, January 1985. (1985)

Horwitz, A. Comparative Public Health: Costa Rica, Cuba and Chile. United Nations University. *Food and Nutrition Bulletin,* 3:19-29. (1987).

Kennedy, E. T. and Pinstrup-Andersen, P. *Nutrition-related Policies and Programmes: Past Performance and Research Needs.* Washington, D.C., IFPRI. (1983).

Kennedy, E. T. and Alderman, H. H. *Comparative Analyses of Nutritional Effectiveness of Food Subsidies and other Food-Related Interventions.* International Food Policy Research Institute, Joint WHO UNICEF Nutrition Support Programme, Washington, D. C., USA.

Kennedy, E. T. and Summer, L. (1989). *WIC - A U.S. Success Story.* Paper presented at the ACC/SCN Workshop. See ACC/SCN, 1989b.

Lotfi, M. Growth Monitoring: A Brief Literature Review of Current Knowledge. *Food and Nutrition Bulletin,* 4:3-10. The United Nations University. (1988).

Manoff, R. K. *Social Marketing.* New York: Paeger. (1985).

Maribe, T. *Botswana Drought Relief Programme (Human Relief).* Paper presented at the ACC/SCN Workshop, Seoul, ACC/SCN (1989b), op. cit.

Mason, J., Habicht, J-P., Tabatabai, H., and Valverde V. *Nutritional Surveillance.* Geneva, Switzerland: World Health Organization, Chapter V. "Nutritional Surveillance for Programme Management and Evaluation." (1984).

Mata, L. *National Nutrition and Holistic Care Programme (NNHCP) in Costa Rica.* Paper presented at the ACC/SCN Workshop. See ACC/SCN, 1989b. (1989).

Moremi, T. C. *Transition from Emergency to Development Assistance Botswana Experience.* Paper presented at the Conference on Nutrition in Times of Disaster. Geneva, 27-30 September, 1988. ACC/ACN. (1988).

Morley, D. *Paediatrics Priorities in the Developing World.* Postgraduate Paediatrics Series. London: Butterworths. (1973).

Quinn, V., Cohen, M., Mason, J. B., and Kgosidintsi. *See* Cornia *et al.* (1988). pp. 3-27. (1988).

Rohde, J. E. *Feeding, Feedback and Ssustenance of Primary Health Care.* Keynote address. In:Taylor, T. G., Jenkins, N. K., eds. Proceedings of the 13th International Congress of Nutrition, 18-23 August, 1985, Brighton, UK. London:John Libbey, 1985:19-25,(1985).

Scimshaw, N.S., Taylor, C. I. and, Gordon, J. E. *Interactions of Nutrition and Infection.* WHO Monograph Series No. 57. Geneva, Switzerland. (1968).

Taal, S. *Institutional Support for Health and Nutrition.* Paper presented at the ACC/SCN Workshop, Seoul, ACC/SCN (1989b), op. cit.

WHO. *The Role of the Health Sector in Food and Nutrition. Report of a WHO Expert Committee.* World Health Organization Technical Report Series No. 667. Geneva, Switzerland. (1981).

WHO/UNICEF (JNSP). *Joint Nutrition Support Programme in Iringa, Tanzania.* 1983-1988 JNSP Evaluation Report Dar es Salaam, October 1988. (1988)

Yee, V. and Zerfas, A. Issues in Growth Monitoring and Promotion (Summary). In: *Information Packet: GROWTH MONITORING.* Clearinghouse on Infant Feeding and Maternal Nutrition, American Public Health Association International Health programs, Washington, D. C., USA. (1987).

Index

A

adaptation mechanisms, 22
aflatoxin, 126, 139, 199, 211
albumin, 50
allergies, 74, 130, 221, 224
amenorrhea, 34, 52-54, 96, 98-99, 133-135, 138-140
anemia, 44-48, 55-58, 60, 211, 218, 222, 227, 229, 233, 243, 265, 284
anorexia nervosa, 38
anthropometric indicators, 24
appetite, 26, 37, 124, 132, 138, 156, 162, 164, 199, 207, 216, 226
arterial hypertension, 206
ascorbic acid, 60, 201, 210, 233

B

beikost, 193-195, 197-199, 203-204, 207, 210-211, 214, 224
birth weight, 24, 30, 33-34, 36-45, 48-49, 54-60, 64, 82, 94, 111, 126, 138, 145, 226-227
bonding, 127, 139, 255
Botswana, 276, 278, 285, 287-288, 297
boycott, 250, 252-253, 255
Brazil, 27, 82, 88, 92-93, 113, 116, 145, 173, 251, 257, 284
breast milk, 3, 7, 9, 12-13, 16, 33-38, 48-55, 58, 60, 62, 64-65, 68, 71-75, 79, 86, 98, 103, 111, 113, 118, 120, 122-126, 128-130, 132, 135-136, 138-140, 142, 145-147, 149, 151, 153-154, 156-157, 159, 161-162, 168, 173, 177, 181-182, 184, 187, 192, 194-200, 205-206, 212, 215, 220-221, 224, 226-228, 246-249, 253-255, 259, 262
breast milk substitute, 33, 136, 181-182, 187, 192, 246, 249, 253-254, 259, 262
breast-feeding, 1-7, 9, 11-18, 24, 36, 48-50, 53, 56, 60-66, 68-71, 73-76, 78-98, 100-101, 103, 106-116, 118-121, 125-140, 142-143, 145-146, 148-149, 151, 153-162, 168-190, 192-199, 201, 203, 205, 212, 214-216, 218-229, 234, 236-239, 241-243, 249-251, 254-256, 259, 261, 275, 285

C

Caribbean, 142-143, 148-149, 152, 154-155, 157-160, 166, 172-173, 179, 225
carnitine, 239-240, 243
cereals, 147, 149-154, 157-158, 160, 163-165, 199-200, 203-205, 207-211, 218-219, 223, 225, 242, 274
Colombia, 43, 88, 116, 180, 284, 288
colostrum, 73-74, 124-126, 137, 142-143, 145
composition of breast milk, 34, 36, 48, 51, 55, 57, 111, 120-122, 124, 125, 137-138
congenital deformities, 2
consumer demand, 3
corn syrup, 206, 208, 218, 223, 225
Costa Rica, 114, 233, 264, 278-279, 286, 289, 294, 296-297
cow's milk, 66, 68, 123, 125, 130, 135, 137-138, 146, 148, 150-151, 201-203, 205, 212, 214-215, 217, 219, 221-222, 224-225, 228-229, 242-244, 247-248
crèche, 4-5, 13, 16

D

developing countries, 29-30, 32-34, 36, 38-40, 44, 47-48, 54, 59-60, 81, 89, 100, 112-114, 116, 130, 134, 136, 141-142, 159, 168, 172, 178-179, 183, 190, 194-195, 198, 200, 209, 211, 220, 249-251, 253, 255, 258, 260-261, 264-265, 276, 284, 295-296
diarrhoea, 8-9, 18-19, 24, 26, 85, 95, 113, 129-130, 148, 151, 166, 171, 198, 206, 211, 213, 220-221, 229, 246, 248-250, 276, 280, 284, 292, 295
diet, 18, 23-24, 26-27, 29-30, 32-33, 35-39, 42-58, 60, 66, 73, 108-109, 111, 114, 122, 124-125, 131-132, 135, 137, 139, 142, 146-148, 151, 157, 161-165, 168, 171-173, 177, 183, 189, 192, 194-196, 199-203, 206-209, 211, 215-225, 227-229, 234-237, 239-244, 247, 255, 274
dietary fibre, 209, 218
dietary protein, 42, 44, 60, 234-236

E

education, 3, 13, 16, 27, 57, 92, 95, 106, 127-128, 130, 160, 165, 170, 173, 179, 182, 186-188, 198, 200, 219, 237, 272-273, 275, 278-279, 281-282, 284-285, 289, 292-293, 295-296

environment, 9, 23-25, 27, 33, 62, 68, 75-76, 85-86, 90-91, 94, 108-110, 112, 124, 126, 128-129, 131-132, 168, 171, 176, 185-186, 198, 216, 221, 246, 251, 256-257, 279, 281, 290

F

farinaceous foods, 9

feeding methods, 2-3, 62, 75, 145, 160, 237

feeding practices, 1-2, 8, 62, 76, 81, 85, 100, 107, 112-116, 137, 141, 145, 148, 151-152, 158, 168, 170-174, 176, 179-182, 188-190, 192, 199, 221, 224-228, 236-238, 242-243

feeding surveys, 8

fertility, 3, 18, 34, 37, 52-56, 60, 62-63, 85, 94, 96-98, 100-101, 103, 108, 110, 112, 114-115, 134, 137-140, 172, 179

fetal growth, 37-38, 41-45, 54-55, 58, 60

fluoride, 211-212, 222, 224, 229

folate, 45-47, 57, 125, 137, 221

food intake, 29, 33, 35, 43, 49, 56, 133, 161, 216, 273, 293

G

gestational age, 36, 39-40, 42-45, 59-60

goitrogen, 46

growth monitoring, 272-276, 279-281, 288, 294, 296-297

gruel, 146-153, 157, 161-166, 168, 170

gut mucosa, 74

H

health sector activities, 157-158

hunger, 59, 185, 196-198, 264

hygiene, 18, 130, 141, 165, 170, 172, 213, 221

I

India, 24, 27, 43, 45, 55, 57, 80, 113, 119, 129, 134, 140, 142-143, 145-146, 148, 153, 156, 160, 164, 166, 168-170, 172-174, 179, 194, 224, 274, 276, 279, 284, 287-288, 296

industrialisation, 1-3

industrialization, 33, 210

industry, 18, 107, 187, 233, 239, 245-254, 256-261

infections, 25-26, 33, 38, 44, 47, 64, 71, 73, 75, 77, 90, 93, 109, 111-112, 114, 118, 128-129, 131, 136, 145

intense exercise, 25

iron, 35, 38, 44-45, 48, 52, 54-55, 74, 123-125, 137-138, 198-199, 201-205, 209-211, 218-219, 221-229, 233-234, 238-239, 241-244, 264-265, 275, 292

iron deficiency, 44, 48, 55, 201, 204-205, 210-211, 218, 222, 228-229, 233-234, 243, 265

K

Kenya, 56, 142-143, 145-147, 150-151, 153, 156, 158, 160, 166, 168, 171, 173-174, 180, 200, 229

L

lactation, 32-34, 36, 38, 48-58, 60, 62-64, 94, 96-98, 111-113, 115, 117-119, 121-125, 127, 129, 131, 133-135, 137-140, 143, 145, 154, 156-161, 168, 170, 172, 174, 176, 186, 189, 192, 196, 198, 201, 205, 227-228, 274-275, 290

lactoferrin, 74, 123, 128, 197

lymphocytes, 74, 128

lysozyme, 74, 123, 128

M

Malaysia, 91, 93, 112, 142-143, 145-146, 149-150, 153, 156-160, 171-172, 174

malnutrition, 21-23, 25, 34-35, 38, 41, 50, 52-56, 59, 69-71, 75, 92, 112-116, 122, 147, 156, 171, 198, 209, 211, 218, 223, 227, 250, 256, 264-265, 272-273, 276, 278-279, 281, 284-286, 293-296

maternal beliefs, 182

maternal employment, 157-158, 180

Mexico, 53, 56, 112, 142, 145-146, 149, 154, 157, 171, 173

milk feeds, 123, 159

milk output, 36, 38, 48-52, 64-65, 120-122, 132, 161, 194-198, 200, 227

mineral deficiency, 34

morbidity, 3, 24, 46, 48, 62, 73, 75-76, 80-82, 89-90, 95, 108-109, 112-113, 115-116, 129-130, 171, 255, 294 mortality, 3-4, 7-9, 13, 18-20, 24, 29, 33, 46, 48, 58-59, 62, 69-71, 73, 75-83, 85-91, 93, 95-96, 101, 103, 106, 108-110, 112-116, 128, 130, 143, 171, 228, 248, 251, 255-256, 262, 265, 279-281, 283-285, 294

N

Nestle, 30, 225, 228, 250-255, 257
Nigeria, 27, 50, 56, 112, 119, 142-143, 147, 151, 153, 156-160, 162, 166, 169-174, 194, 257, 275
nipple stimulation, 98-99, 158
nutrient absorption, 32-33
nutrient content, 36, 51, 65, 161

O

obesity, 24-25, 59, 131, 139, 215-217, 224-226
oligosaccharides, 74, 124, 128
opiates, 4
orphans, 2
otitis media, 129, 140
ovulation, 35, 53, 97-99, 133-135

P

prolactin, 53, 57, 97, 115, 133-134, 140

R

rural communities, 154, 157, 172, 187

S

salt, 29, 46, 124, 146, 200, 203-204, 206-208, 211, 216, 221-224, 227, 234, 292
sanitation, 3, 17-18, 33, 85, 93, 112, 198, 250, 255, 279, 281
selenium, 240-241, 243
sevrage, 142, 154, 156-158
skinfold measurements, 41
social class, 8, 85-86, 106, 196, 198, 216
socioeconomic status, 50, 71, 108, 171
soya, 204, 206, 211, 214
stillbirth, 34
stress, 22, 25, 83, 96, 107, 133, 143, 156, 161, 264, 277
suckling, 2, 4, 7, 16, 53, 65, 96, 124, 127, 131, 133-135, 138, 184
sucrose, 204, 208
sudden infant death syndrome, 129

sugar, 122, 143, 146-147, 152, 204, 206, 208, 210-212, 216, 225, 248, 274
supplementary feeding programmes, 272-275, 283-284, 290
supplementation, 13, 17, 34-35, 43-48, 50-55, 57-60, 93, 107, 121-122, 125, 132, 134, 139, 142, 146-154, 159-160, 168, 174, 177, 179-183, 185, 203, 205, 212, 218, 220, 222, 227, 239, 273, 275
syphilis, 2

T

Tanzania, 164, 169-170, 280-281, 284, 287-288, 293, 297
taurine, 239-240, 242
traditional practices, 142, 146-147, 149

U

urban areas, 3, 6-8, 17, 97, 116, 150-152, 156, 160, 168, 173, 181, 279

V

vegetarians, 217-218, 221, 240, 243
viscosity, 161-165, 209
vitamin A, 45-47, 52, 57, 59, 218, 220, 228-229, 264, 275, 280, 292, 295-296
vitamin C, 45, 52, 198-199, 202, 218, 220, 249
vitamin D, 45, 47, 125, 139-140, 199, 211, 218-221, 233, 239, 265, 296
vitamin supplements, 46, 52, 226
vitamins, 22, 26, 35, 45, 47, 51-52, 58-59, 125, 142, 153, 164, 218-219, 228, 239, 292

W

wasting and stunting, 25
weaning, 13, 17, 72, 80, 87-88, 93, 95, 134, 136-137, 142, 163, 166, 168, 171-174, 178, 180, 182, 184-185, 191-203, 205, 207-209, 211-221, 223-229, 246-247, 251, 257, 259, 281, 292, 295
weight loss, 25-26, 49, 52, 58, 132, 139
wet nurse, 2, 8, 10-12, 247

Z

Zaire, 49-50, 53, 55, 119-120, 142, 147-148, 152, 156, 158, 160-161, 172, 292
Zimbabwe, 282, 286, 289

T - #0117 - 111024 - C320 - 229/152/15 - PB - 9780367450489 - Gloss Lamination